Palliative Care for Infants, Children, and Adolescents

T0198040

Palliative Care for Infants, Children, and Adolescents

A PRACTICAL HANDBOOK

Second Edition

Edited by

Brian S. Carter, M.D., F.A.A.P.

Marcia Levetown, M.D., F.A.A.P., F.A.A.H.P.M.

Sarah E. Friebert, M.D., F.A.A.P., F.A.A.H.P.M.

The Johns Hopkins University Press

BALTIMORE

© 2004, 2011 The Johns Hopkins University Press
All rights reserved. Published 2011
Printed in the United States of America on acid-free paper
9 8 7 6 5 4 3 2 1

The Johns Hopkins University Press
2715 North Charles Street
Baltimore, Maryland 21218-4363
www.press.jhu.edu

Library of Congress Cataloging-in-Publication Data

Palliative care for infants, children, and adolescents : a practical handbook / edited by Brian S. Carter, Marcia Levetown, and Sarah E. Friebert. — 2nd ed.
    p. ; cm.
Includes bibliographical references and index.
ISBN-13: 978-1-4214-0148-5 (hardcover : alk. paper)
ISBN-13: 978-1-4214-0149-2 (pbk. : alk. paper)
ISBN-10: 1-4214-0148-7 (hardcover : alk. paper)
ISBN-10: 1-4214-0149-5 (pbk. : alk. paper)
    1. Terminally ill children—Care—Handbooks, manuals, etc. I. Carter, Brian S., 1957– II. Levetown, Marcia, 1960– III. Friebert, Sarah E.
    [DNLM: 1. Palliative Care—methods. 2. Terminal Care—methods. 3. Adolescent. 4. Child. 5. Chronic Disease. 6. Infant. WS 200]
    RJ249.P356 2011
    618.92'0028—dc22   2010050249

A catalog record for this book is available from the British Library.

Special discounts are available for bulk purchases of this book. For more information, please contact Special Sales at 410-516-6936 or specialsales@press.jhu.edu.

The Johns Hopkins University Press uses environmentally friendly book materials, including recycled text paper that is composed of at least 30 percent post-consumer waste, whenever possible.

With thankful remembrance to Drs. William A. Silverman and Gerald B. Merenstein for encouragement and support.

BSC

In honor of my husband, Philip Blum, M.D., who encouraged me to follow my heart, regardless of the consequences; my children, Lila and Alex, who understood when I loved children in addition to my own; the Project on Death in America; my friends and colleagues over the years, for their support; and the patients and families who taught me about what is truly important by allowing me to "be with them" during the most intimate and sacred time of their lives.

ML

With gratitude and blessings to all of the children and families who have taught, led, inspired, indulged, and trusted me over the years.

SEF

CONTENTS

CONTRIBUTORS

M. Karen Ballard, M.C.M., B.C.C., Director, Chaplaincy Services
Department, Akron Children's Hospital, Akron, Ohio

Jennifer Brown, Parent and Consultant, Memphis, Tennessee

David Browning, M.S.W., B.C.D., Senior Scholar and Co-Director,
Patient Safety and Quality Initiatives, Institute for Professionalism
and Ethical Practice, Children's Hospital Boston and Harvard Medical
School, Waltham, Massachusetts

Lori Butterworth, Co-Founder, Children's Hospice and Palliative Care
Coalition; Founder, Jacob's Heart Children's Cancer Support Services,
Santa Cruz, California

Brian S. Carter, M.D., F.A.A.P., Professor of Pediatrics, Division of
Neonatology, Monroe Carell, Jr. Children's Hospital at Vanderbilt,
Nashville, Tennessee

Anita J. Catlin, D.N.Sc., F.N.P., F.A.A.N., Professor of Nursing, Sonoma
State University, Rohnert Park, California

Susan O. Cohen, M.A., A.D.T.R., C.C.L.S., Pediatric Advanced Illness
Care Coordinator, The David Center for Children's Pain and Palliative
Care, Hackensack Medical Center, Hackensack, New Jersey

Margaret Comeau, M.H.A., Director, Catalyst Center, Health and
Disability Working Group, Boston University School of Public Health,
Boston, Massachusetts

Devon Dabbs, Co-Founder and Executive Director, Children's Hospice
and Palliative Care Coalition, Watsonville, California

Deborah L. Dokken, M.P.A., Consultant and Parent Advocate, Chevy
Chase, Maryland

Elana E. Evan, Ph.D., Director, UCLA Children's Comfort Care Program; Assistant Professor of Pediatrics, Pediatric Pain Program, David Geffen School of Medicine at UCLA, Los Angeles, California

Betty Ferrell, Ph.D., R.N., F.A.A.N., Research Scientist, City of Hope National Medical Center, Duarte, California

Chris Feudtner, M.D., Ph.D., M.P.H., Director, Department of Medical Ethics; Director of Research and Attending Physician, Pediatric Advance Care Team and Integrated Care Service, Division of General Pediatrics, Children's Hospital of Philadelphia, Philadelphia, Pennsylvania

Kris Ford, parent

Sarah E. Friebert, M.D., F.A.A.P., F.A.A.H.P.M., Director, *A Palette of Care* Program, Haslinger Division of Pediatric Palliative Care, Akron Children's Hospital, Akron, Ohio; Associate Professor of Pediatrics, Northeast Ohio Universities Colleges of Medicine and Pharmacy, Rootstown, Ohio

Mary Jo Gilmer, Ph.D., M.B.A., R.N., Professor of Nursing, Vanderbilt University School of Nursing, Nashville, Tennessee

Robert J. Graham, M.D., Associate, Division of Critical Care, Department of Anesthesiology, Perioperative and Pain Medicine, Children's Hospital Boston, Boston, Massachusetts

Dianne Gray, B.S., President, Hospice and Healthcare Communications, Naples, Florida

Brian Greffe, M.D., Director, National Children's Hospital International, PACC; Professor of Pediatrics, Hematology, Oncology, and Bone Marrow Transplantation, Department of Pediatrics, University of Colorado, Denver, Colorado

Lee Ann Grimes, Faculty, Project DOCC—Delivery of Chronic Care; Parent, Houston, Texas

Richard Hain, M.D., LATCH Senior Lecturer in Paediatric Palliative Medicine, Department of Child Health, Cardiff University School of Medicine, University Hospital of Wales, Cardiff, United Kingdom

Melody Hellsten, M.S.N., P.N.P., Director of Community Programs, Center for Comprehensive Care of Children with Complex Chronic Conditions, Christus Santa Rosa Children's Hospital; Instructor, Department of Pediatrics, University of Texas Health Science Center at San Antonio, San Antonio, Texas

Kari R. Hexem, M.P.H., Center for Pediatric Clinical Effectiveness, Children's Hospital of Philadelphia, Philadelphia, Pennsylvania

Susan M. Huff, R.N., M.S.N., Director, Pediatrics at Home, Johns Hopkins Children's Center, Baltimore, Maryland

Nancy Hutton, M.D., Medical Director, Harriet Lane Compassionate Care Program; Director, Intensive Primary Care Clinic; Associate Professor, Pediatrics, Johns Hopkins School of Medicine, Baltimore, Maryland

Hollye Harrington Jacobs, M.S., R.N., M.S.W., former End-of-Life Nursing Education Consortium (ELNEC) Pediatric Coordinator, City of Hope National Medical Center, Duarte, California; Vice President of Programs, Dream Foundation; Author; Educator; Huffington Post Contributor, Santa Barbara, California

Barbara Jones, Ph.D., M.S.W., Associate Professor, School of Social Work, University of Texas at Austin, Austin, Texas

Patrick M. Jones, M.D., M.A., Assistant Professor of Pediatrics, Division of Neonatal-Perinatal Medicine, University of Texas Health Science Center Medical School, Houston, Texas

Jeffrey C. Klick, M.D., Director, Pediatric Palliative Care, Children's Healthcare of Atlanta, Clinical Assistant Professor of Pediatrics, Emory University School of Medicine, Atlanta, Georgia

Kendra D. Koch, Chair, Parent Advisory Council, Dell Children's Medical Center, Austin, Texas

Dexter Lanctot, M.Div., B.A.Ph., Chaplain, Pastoral Care Services, Children's Hospital of Philadelphia, Philadelphia, Pennsylvania

Steven R. Leuthner, M.D., M.A., Co-Director, Fetal Concerns Program; Professor of Pediatrics (Neonatology) and Bioethics, Medical College of Wisconsin, Milwaukee, Wisconsin

Marcia Levetown, M.D., F.A.A.P., F.A.A.H.P.M., Principal, HealthCare Communication Associates, Houston, Texas

Stephen Liben, M.D., Director, Pain and Palliative Care Services; Assistant Professor, Pediatric Critical Care, Montreal Children's Hospital, Montreal, Quebec, Canada

Maureen E. Lyon, Ph.D., A.B.P.P., Division of Adolescent and Young Adult Medicine Faculty, Children's National Medical Center; Associate Research Professor, Department of Pediatrics, George Washington University School of Medicine and Health Sciences, Washington, D.C.

Elaine C. Meyer, Ph.D., R.N., Director, Institute for Professionalism and Ethical Practice; Director, Program to Enhance Relational and Communication Skills; Staff Psychologist, Medical/Surgical Intensive Care Unit; Associate Professor of Psychology, Department of Psychiatry, Harvard Medical School, Boston, Massachusetts

Wynne Morrison, M.D., M.B.E., Director, Pediatric Critical Care Medicine Fellowship; Children's Hospital of Philadelphia; Assistant

Professor and Attending Physician, Department of Anesthesiology and Critical Care and the Pediatric Advanced Care Team, University of Pennsylvania, Philadelphia, Pennsylvania

Stacy F. Orloff, Ed.D., L.C.S.W., A.C.H.P.-S.W., Vice President of Palliative Care and Community Programs, Suncoast Hospice, Clearwater, Florida

Sara L. Perszyk, R.N., B.S.N., C.H.P.N., Stepping Stones (Child and Family Support Program), Suncoast Hospice, Clearwater, Florida

Cynda H. Rushton, Ph.D., R.N., F.A.A.N., Program Director, Harriet Lane Compassionate Care Program, Johns Hopkins Children's Center; Associate Professor of Nursing, Johns Hopkins School of Nursing, Baltimore, Maryland

John M. Saroyan, M.D., F.A.A.P., Assistant Professor of Pediatric Pain Management and Palliative Care in Anesthesiology and Assistant Professor of Pediatrics, College of Physicians and Surgeons, Columbia University, New York, New York; Medical Director, Pediatric Advanced Care Team, New York–Presbyterian Morgan Stanley Children's Hospital, New York, New York

Sally Sehring, M.D., Health Sciences Clinical Professor, Division of Neonatology, Department of Pediatrics, University of California, San Francisco, San Francisco, California

David M. Steinhorn, M.D., Medical Director, The Bridges Program— Pediatric Palliative and End-of-Life Care; Medical Director and Co-Founder, Judith Nan Joy Integrative Medicine Initiative; Professor of Pediatrics, Northwestern University's Feinberg School of Medicine, Children's Memorial Hospital, Chicago, Illinois

Carson Strong, Ph.D., Professor, Department of Medicine, College of Medicine, University of Tennessee Health Science Center, Memphis, Tennessee

Lizabeth Sumner, R.N., B.S.N., Director, Center for Compassionate Care, Elizabeth Hospice, Escondido, California

Suzanne S. Toce, M.D., Division of Neonatology, Departments of Pediatrics and Medical Humanities, Gundersen Lutheran Health Center, La Crosse, Wisconsin

Carol Tuttle, Parent, Madison, Ohio

Kathryn Weise, M.D., M.A., Program Director, Cleveland Fellowship in Advanced Bioethics; Pediatric Hospital Medicine, Cleveland Clinic Children's Hospital for Rehabilitation, Cleveland, Ohio

Cora K. Welsh, B.A., C.C.L.S., Senior Child Life Specialist, Johns Hopkins Children's Center, Baltimore, Maryland

Janice Wheeler, Ed.D., Founder and Executive Director, Project Joy and
 Hope for Texas; Bereaved Parent, Pasadena, Texas
Lonnie Zeltzer, M.D., Director of the Pediatric Pain Program and
 Professor of Pediatrics, Anesthesiology, Psychiatry and Biobehavioral
 Sciences, David Geffen School of Medicine at UCLA, UCLA Mattel
 Children's Hospital, Los Angeles, California

PREFACE

In the seven years since the publication of *Palliative Care for Infants, Children, and Adolescents*, the field of pediatric palliative care has undergone explosive growth in recognition, availability, and opportunity. It has been gratifying to have played a role in this transformation and to be witness to the success of a field that is a passion for all of us.

In 2008, the subspecialty of Palliative Medicine was granted official recognition by the American Board of Medical Specialties. This cemented the approval of a Section of Hospice and Palliative Medicine within the American Academy of Pediatrics (now boasting over 200 members) and led to the development of dedicated educational tracks and mentorship opportunities designed especially for pediatric caregivers within the Center to Advance Palliative Care and its Palliative Care Leadership Centers, as well as approval of subspecialty fellowship training programs in palliative medicine (some of which are pediatric) by the Accreditation Council for Graduate Medical Education. Simultaneously, additional pediatric-specific educational opportunities have emerged, including the End-of-Life Nursing Education Consortium (ELNEC) Pediatric Training Program, the National Hospice and Palliative Care Organization pediatric curriculum, developed within the Children's International Project on Palliative/Hospice Services (ChIPPS), and the Initiative for Pediatric Palliative Care. There is now an increasing frequency of publications addressing pediatric palliative care in the peer-reviewed medical and nursing literature, as well as other texts addressing palliative care for children, numerous pediatric-specific palliative care conferences and conference tracks, and pediatric interest groups within national palliative care organizations. Most importantly, there are a burgeoning number of clinical care experts and programs available to meet the palliative care needs of children living with life-threatening conditions and their families.

It has been a pleasure to work with our new editorial partner, Dr. Sarah Friebert, whose knowledge, skill, and work ethic have been well showcased in this endeavor. A broad array of professional and family authors, expanded since the first edition, has served as our mentors. What a privilege it has been for us to learn from, to appreciate, and to have the pleasure of creating this high-quality resource with them in the attempt to assist and to serve families and health care professionals.

It is our hope that this text will inspire caregivers new to pediatric and/ or palliative care, as well as those who have been practicing in the field, to reach new heights in their care of children and families living with life-threatening conditions. We also hope that families reading this text will be better prepared to advocate and care for their own children. We salute the bravery and caring of those involved in this field and are excited to have had the privilege to contribute to the ongoing growth of pediatric palliative care through the publication of this book.

PART I

SOCIETAL AND
INSTITUTIONAL ISSUES

Epidemiology and Health Services Research

Chris Feudtner, M.D., Ph.D., M.P.H., and Kari R. Hexem, M.P.H.

A team of pediatric health care providers—a social worker, a psychologist, a nurse, and a physician—convenes to design a new palliative and hospice care service for infants, children, and adolescents. Each member of the team has had extensive experience caring for youngsters who are living with life-threatening conditions. They realize, however, that their plans for this service would be best informed not by personal encounters, but by a systematic review of the medical literature appraising key issues:

- How can we define and identify the children we seek to serve?
- What are the demographic characteristics of children who live with and ultimately die from life-threatening conditions?
- What medical conditions do they have?
- What medical technology do they rely on?
- Where do they die?
- What kinds of health care services do they currently receive, and what might they and their families need that they do not currently receive?
- What disparities or difficulties in accessing care exist across groups of children or as the children age into adulthood?
- How are the answers to these questions changing over time, so we can plan for the future?

This chapter addresses the questions posed above, describing what we know about patterns of childhood suffering, death, and the use of medical care before death. We begin by considering how we define children who ought to be the focus of palliative care efforts. Examining problematic aspects of this case definition will then inform our interpretation of the epidemiologic and health services data presented in the rest of the chapter and suggest future opportunities.

The Problem of Case Definition

One of the first difficulties that the palliative care team encounters is that each of them has a different notion of which children to serve and under what circumstances. Discussions with other medical colleagues, with hospital administrators, and with third-party payers make the need for a clear target population urgent, yet still elusive.

Who needs palliative care? Any systematic attempt to study or improve the provision of pediatric palliative care must grapple with this question. The most common answer is: children who "will die" need palliative care. Even though this appears to be straightforward, in practice it is not, for four reasons.

The first reason arises from ambiguity in the term "will die." We all will die; what people usually mean when they say that someone "will die" is that, within a certain time frame, death is likely to occur. These aspects of the terms "will die" and "dying"—time frame and probability—are not specified. Is a person who has an 80 percent chance of death in the next 4 weeks "dying"? What if the probability of death for the same person were to climb over the ensuing 6 months to 97 percent, as could be the case if the patient had relapsed cancer? What if the patient had a 97 percent chance of death, but only over the next 10 years, as happens with neurodegenerative disorders: is this patient "dying"? Finally, if a patient has a persistently elevated risk of death because of a static injury or condition (e.g., severe cerebral palsy with seizures and swallowing dysfunction), is this patient "dying"? Each of these scenarios involves a distinct and common pattern of how the risk of death varies over time, based on the underlying disease or injury (fig. 1.1). Health care professionals would likely answer the question of whether the patient is "dying" for the scenarios differently, based on their experience and, more importantly, their individual personality, values, and beliefs. No consensus exists to clarify how high the probability of death needs to be, and over what time frame, for the term *dying* to be applied consistently.

The second reason stems from the term *need*. Ambiguity again besets us. Suppose we knew for sure that palliative care services would improve the quality of a child's remaining life by 20 percent; would that child "need" palliative care? Said differently, how much does a child have to benefit from a service before that service becomes a need? This question is further com-

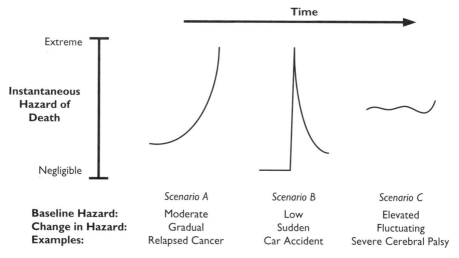

Figure 1.1. Hazard of death varies over time depending on underlying condition

plicated by potential trade-offs between the therapeutic goals of extending life and enhancing the quality of life: when does a patient benefit more from improvement in the quality of life, if securing this benefit potentially entails a shorter life span?

The third reason is the uncertainty that surrounds all attempts to predict the future, particularly medical prognosis. Even for expert clinicians, prognostication is hardly an exact science; instead, in most instances it is fraught with uncertainty and prone to optimistic biases (Christakis, 1999). The probability that any particular person will die during a given time frame, let alone how much this person would benefit from palliative care services, is impossible to estimate with certainty. This uncertainty in both realms hinders many physicians from raising end-of-life issues with their patients and making suitable, individualized plans.

The ambiguous aspects of the terms *dying* and *need*—the probability of death and the benefit from palliative care—along with the attendant uncertainty must be addressed in a rigorous manner to provide a systematized answer to the question, "Who needs palliative care?" These aspects can be thought of as key dimensions of any case definition, as they are important, definable, and potentially measurable (fig. 1.2).

The fourth reason that the statement "children who are dying need palliative care" can lead to problems in clinical practice emanates from the artificial boundaries separating palliative care from other forms of medical care, especially a mode of care called *curative* that contrasts with *palliative*

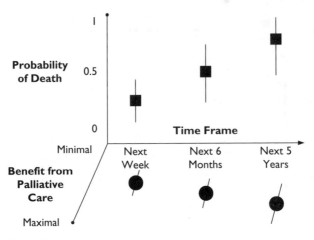

Figure 1.2. Case definition

(fig. 1.3). Over the past two decades, health care professionals attuned to the needs of patients who are living with life-threatening conditions have emphasized that curative (or life-prolonging) care and palliative care are not mutually exclusive; a gradual transition can be made to a greater proportion of care being in the palliative mode. In the community setting, this line of thinking has led to proposals for "open access" to hospice services, enabling all patients who could benefit from receiving hospice care but are not yet willing to relinquish access to "curative" treatments to receive both (Wright and Katz, 2007).

For many children who die, however, cure—meaning the eradication of the disease or normalization of the underlying condition—was never possible or became impossible. Instead, medical care for these children consists largely or exclusively of life-extending therapy and comfort- or quality-of-life-enhancing therapy. Often, trade-offs have to be struck between these types of treatments; however, some therapies that prolong life also promote comfort, as is the case of antibiotics used to treat people who have severe lung disease from cystic fibrosis. Grappling successfully with therapeutic trade-offs and "double effects" (a bioethical concept, whereby one action causes two things to happen, one desired and the other potentially not) is aided by a clearer sense of the goals of care, be they to eradicate disease, extend life, enhance comfort, promote quality of life in other realms, or support the family. Because these goals are not mutually exclusive, our understanding of the care we can provide is hindered if our model is based on mutually exclusive curative and palliative modes of care.

1. Incompatible Domains of Curative versus Palliative Care:

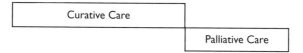

2. Competing Domains of Curative versus Palliative Care:

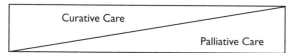

3. Complementary and Concurrent Components of Care:

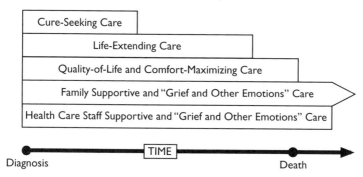

Figure 1.3. Domains of curative versus palliative care

These definitional difficulties impede efforts to prospectively identify children who will benefit from palliative care, whether these definitions be based on diagnoses with grave prognoses, extremely low quality of life (Huang et al., 2009), or medical frailty due to dependence on technology (Feudtner et al., 2005). Case definitions for retrospective studies have different but related challenges, which affect both generalizability and accuracy. Typically, retrospective studies have examined the experiences of children who died as a result of a specific cause, such as cancer, or in a particular place, such as a neonatal intensive care unit. Because of their focus on certain causes or places, these studies have been based on only a portion of the entire population of dying children and tend to overrepresent the final stages of living with a life-threatening illness (because children living with life-threatening conditions who did not die during the study period were not studied). Additionally, retrospective studies of the experiences of children before death—using either medical chart reviews or postdeath interviews—

are hampered by incomplete or recall-biased information, which makes accurate determination of palliative care needs and even accurate description of goals difficult.

One methodological approach to surmount the problems of generalizability is to study the broad population of children who die at the state or national level or within a varied assortment of children's hospitals. Much of the information presented in this chapter is based on this approach, using data from vital records and administrative hospital discharge records. "Complex chronic conditions" (CCCs) are defined as any medical condition that can be reasonably expected to last at least 12 months, unless death intervenes, and to involve either several different organ systems or one organ system severely enough to require specialty pediatric care, with a likelihood of some period of hospitalization in a tertiary care center. This generic definition led to the creation of a list of diagnoses used to identify children whose deaths might have been foreseeable. While this method is limited by the incomplete information contained in large data sets, it offers a reasonable assessment of the epidemiology and use of health services of children who die.

Deaths

> While acknowledging the lack of a precise case definition, the team forges ahead with greater clarity regarding various aspects of the concept of pediatric palliative care. To envision the kinds of children who might be enrolled in their service, they decide first to examine the characteristics of children who have died over the past several years.

In the United States in the year 2006, a total of 53,046 children and adolescents between birth and 19 years of age died (table 1.1). This count reflects a previously steady annual decline with a more recent plateau (due to the continued growth of the overall U.S. child population combined with no recent improvements in the rate of infant mortality), as there were 85,135 deaths in 1980, 69,429 deaths in 1990, and 53,728 deaths in 2000. Similar patterns are evident throughout the European Union (Lyons and Brophy, 2005). Several aspects of these mortality data have implications for pediatric palliative care.

AGE

The preponderance of deaths in 2006 (56.7%) occurred among infants, with the remainder among young children age 1–4 years (12.0%), school-age children 5–9 years old (8.5%), and preteen and adolescents 10–19 years old

Table 1.1 Causes of death

Age	Cause	No.	%	Rate per 100,000*
<1 year	Conditions originating in the perinatal period	14,321	50.2	346.7
	Congenital and chromosomal abnormalities	5,819	20.3	140.9
	Sudden infant death syndrome	3,462	12.1	83.8
	External causes of morbidity and mortality	1,598	6.0	38.7
	Diseases of the respiratory system	692	2.4	16.8
	Diseases of the digestive system	582	2.0	14.1
	Diseases of the circulatory system	543	1.9	13.1
	Certain infectious and parasitic diseases	479	1.7	11.6
	Diseases of the nervous system	373	1.3	9.0
	Endocrine, nutritional, and metabolic diseases	207	0.7	5.0
	Diseases of the genitourinary system	180	0.6	4.4
	Neoplasms	141	0.5	3.4
	Diseases of the blood and immune mechanism	102	0.4	2.5
	Total	28,527	100.0	690.7
1–4 years	External causes of morbidity and mortality	2,050	44.3	12.6
	Congenital and chromosomal abnormalities	515	11.1	3.2
	Neoplasms	437	9.4	2.7
	Diseases of the respiratory system	289	6.2	1.8
	Diseases of the nervous system	259	5.6	1.6
	Diseases of the circulatory system	221	4.8	1.4
	Total	4,631	100.0	28.4
5–9 years	External causes of morbidity and mortality	1,225	44.8	6.2
	Neoplasms	497	18.2	2.5
	Diseases of the nervous system	202	7.4	1.0
	Congenital and chromosomal abnormalities	182	6.7	0.9
	Diseases of the circulatory system	142	5.2	0.7

(continued)

Table 1.1 (*cont.*)

Age	Cause	No.	%	Rate per 100,000*
	Diseases of the respiratory system	136	5.0	0.7
	Total	2,735	100.0	13.9
10–14 years	External causes of morbidity and mortality	1,721	50.4	8.3
	Neoplasms	486	14.2	2.4
	Diseases of the nervous system	265	7.8	1.3
	Diseases of the circulatory system	226	6.6	1.1
	Congenital and chromosomal abnormalities	162	4.7	0.8
	Diseases of the respiratory system	133	3.9	0.6
	Total	3,414	100.0	16.6
15–19 years	External causes of morbidity and mortality	10,744	78.2	50.4
	Neoplasms	730	5.3	3.4
	Diseases of the circulatory system	478	3.5	2.2
	Diseases of the nervous system	447	3.3	2.1
	Congenital and chromosomal abnormalities	228	1.7	1.1
	Diseases of the respiratory system	200	1.5	0.9
	Total	13,739	100.0	64.4

Source: 2006 national data from Centers for Disease Control and Prevention, National Center for Health Statistics. CDC WONDER Online Database, compiled from Compressed Mortality File, 1999–2006. Series 20, no. 2L, 2009. http://wonder.cdc.gov/cmf-icd10.html.
* Infant rates are per 100,000 live births; beyond infancy, per 100,000 person-years.

(22.8%) (fig. 1.4). Among the infants, approximately 40 percent of the deaths occur within 24 hours of birth, 30 percent between the end of the first day and the end of the first month, and the final 30 percent of all infant deaths between a month and a year of age.

CONDITIONS

Child and adolescent deaths are caused by a wide variety of conditions. Cancer, which is perhaps the stereotypical condition associated with palliative care, in 2006 accounted for 141 (0.5% of 28,527 total) infant deaths and 2,150 (8.8% of 24,519) of deaths past infancy. As shown by these numbers, how-

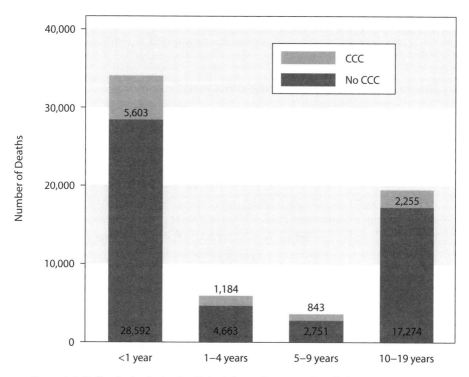

Figure 1.4. Pediatric deaths in the United States, by age and underlying cause, 2006

ever, cancer constitutes only a fraction of life-threatening conditions. Congenital and chromosomal abnormalities, for instance, caused 5,819 (20.3%) infant and 1,087 (4.4%) child deaths, while diseases of the nervous system caused 373 (1.3%) infant and 1,173 (4.8%) child deaths. Altogether, approximately one-fifth (18.6%) of all childhood deaths in 2006 were due to complex chronic conditions (fig. 1.4).

Meanwhile, beyond infancy, trauma of various types (such as motor vehicle crashes, suicide, homicide, or drowning) was the major cause of death. Although many traumatic deaths occur abruptly, not all do. Children who receive any medical care before dying from trauma are potential candidates for palliative care. Furthermore, all families whose children die from trauma warrant bereavement services, often requiring care of substantial intensity and duration.

Studies of patients enrolled in pediatric palliative care programs are starting to appear in the medical literature, providing a better portrait of the diversity of conditions in this patient population. For instance, in Canada, patients served by eight dedicated pediatric palliative care programs in 2002 had as their primary diagnosis either nervous system disorders (39.1%), cancer (22.1%), or perinatal-onset conditions or congenital anomalies (22.1%) (Widger et al., 2007).

MORTALITY RATES AND TRENDS OVER TIME

Improvements in child health and health care have, overall, decreased mortality rates associated with CCCs over the past few decades. Between 1979 and 1997, the annual rate of death due to noncancer and cancer-related CCCs declined to varying degrees for almost every age group (ranging from a 7.1% decline for infants with cancer to a 49.9% decline for 1- to 4-year-olds dying from noncancer CCCs). The notable exception regarded mortality attributed to noncancer CCCs among 20–24 year olds, for whom the rate of death was estimated to have increased by 11.6 percent over this 18-year interval (Feudtner et al., 2001). This observation fits the pattern of smaller declines in mortality over time seen in older age groups. One hypothesis to explain this finding is that advances in life-extending medical therapy postpone what proves ultimately to be unavoidable early death. If this hypothesis is borne out, then pediatric palliative care may be applicable to children for longer periods of time or at older ages. Indeed, palliative care services will need to assure that children living with life-threatening conditions who survive to adulthood do not "fall between the cracks" of the pediatric and adult worlds of medical care. For this reason, studies of "pediatric" deaths and palliative care should include experiences of young adults, into their twenties or thirties, who die from conditions with congenital or childhood onset.

ESTIMATED PREVALENCE AND TRENDS OVER TIME

For the United States, there are as yet no reliable data regarding the prevalence of children living with life-threatening conditions. The number of deaths due to these conditions does, however, provide a surrogate measure. Focusing on deaths due to CCCs, we can estimate the number of potential palliative care service days for children living with life-threatening conditions in the United States by retrospectively calculating the number of children who were alive on a particular day who subsequently died in the ensuing 6-month period (fig. 1.5). Between 1979 and 1997, these numbers have trended downward, especially for deaths due to cancer among the 10–24 year age group. By contrast, the 10–24 year age group deaths due to noncancer CCCs has remained fairly constant (Feudtner et al., 2001).

Another useful prevalence measure focuses on the deaths that occur within children's hospitals, as this allows one to determine how many children in a

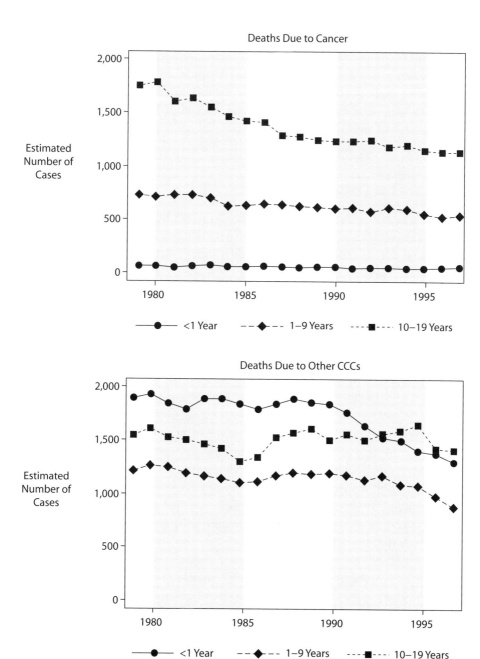

Figure 1.5. Estimated prevalence of children living within 6 months of death (national U.S. data, 1979–97)

hospital would potentially benefit from skillful palliative care. A study of 60 children's hospitals for the years 1991, 1994, and 1997 found that hospitals reporting 50–99 deaths per year had, on a typical day, 3.5 patients (median value) in the hospital who would die during that admission; hospitals reporting 100–149 deaths per year had 5.0 terminally ill patients on a typical day; and hospitals with 150 or more deaths per year had 7.0 patients on a typical day who did not survive to discharge (Feudtner et al., 2002).

Location of Death

The team considers whether their services should be designed to be mostly inpatient (following the model of many hospital-based adult palliative care services) or outpatient (following the model of hospice services) or both. They also wonder whether most of the suitable hospitalized patients would be located in the intensive care units or elsewhere in the hospital. To assess these questions, they examine where children were located when they died.

Across the United States, between 1989 and 2003, most deaths due to CCCs occurred in the hospital, overwhelmingly so for infants (fig. 1.6). Whereas the proportion of home deaths among infants rose only slightly (4.9% to 7.3%), among older children who died of CCCs, the proportion who died at home rose during this period from 17.9 to 30.7 percent for children between 1 and 9 years of age, and from 18.4 to 32.2 percent for adolescents 10–19 years of age. The rate of this rise, and the overall proportion, varied substantially depending on the underlying cause of death, with the greatest rise observed for children with respiratory CCCs (fig. 1.6). Furthermore, infants and children with CCCs who were classified on death certificates as white were more likely than either Hispanic or black children to have died at home (fig. 1.7) (Feudtner et al., 2007).

Several case series reveal that location of children's deaths within hospitals varies by hospital. A university teaching hospital in Chicago had 82 percent of the deaths occur in the pediatric intensive care unit (PICU), 13 percent in operating rooms, and 5 percent on the general wards (deaths occurring in the emergency department [ED] were not examined) (Lantos, Berger, and Zucker, 1993). More recently, a children's hospital in Tennessee documented that 87 percent of patient deaths occurred in ICU settings, with two-thirds in the PICU and one-third in the neonatal ICU (NICU; Carter et al., 2004). An Australian hospital reported that only 24 percent of its inpatient deaths occurred in the ICU, while 36 percent occurred in the ED (Ashby et al., 1991). A hospital in the Netherlands, by contrast, had 71 percent die in the

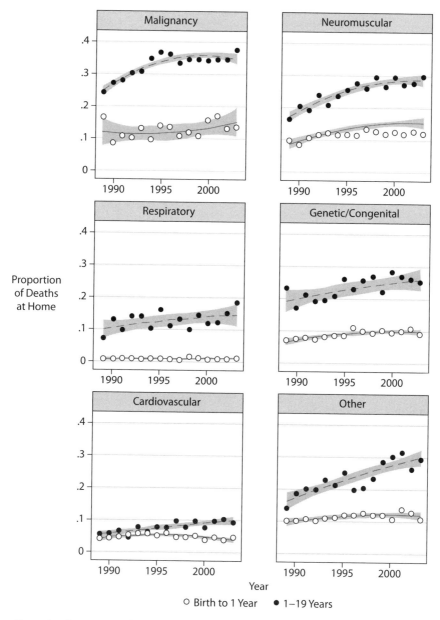

Figure 1.6. Proportion of home deaths due to complex chronic conditions (national U.S. data, 1989–2003)

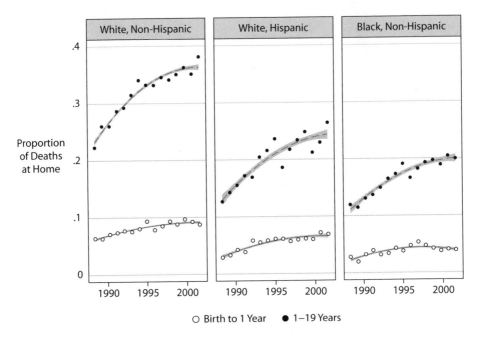

Figure I.7. Ethnicity differences in the proportion of home deaths due to complex chronic conditions (national U.S. data, 1989–2003)

PICU and 7 percent in the operating room (patients dying in the ED were excluded) (van der Wal et al., 1999). Eighty-three percent of children who died in a Canadian hospital died in the ICU (McCallum, Byrne, and Bruera, 2000). A report from a pediatric hospital in London noted a rising proportion of deaths in their ICU over time, from 80.1 percent in 1997 to 90.6 percent in 2004 (Ramnarayan et al., 2007).

Overall, then, most children died in hospitals, and more often than not in the ICU setting. Similar patterns, as noted above, are observed in non-English-speaking settings; for instance, among pediatric patients who died in the metropolitan areas of Mexico, most (85%) did so in hospitals (Cardenas-Turanzas et al., 2008). Importantly, in a multinational comparative study of pediatric deaths where patients and families had access to care in home, inpatient hospice, and hospital facilities, a third of the deaths occurred in each of the three locations (Siden et al., 2008).

In the U.S. setting, with time and alterations in payments and service structures, these patterns may continue to change. Furthermore, the location of death per se should ideally be a choice filled with meaning, which should be studied as such (Lowton, 2009). An investigation of how parents of children who had died from cancer considered their preparatory planning about the location of death showed that parents who planned the location were more likely to have had the child die at home, more likely to be comfortable with that choice, and less likely to have wished for a different location (Dussel et al., 2009).

Symptoms and Suffering

The relief of bothersome symptoms and suffering for children who are living with life-threatening conditions and their families was the team's primary mandate. To prepare for this clinical mission, they wondered, what kinds of symptoms and which forms of suffering would their patients likely have?

Several retrospective studies have sought to describe the epidemiology of symptoms and suffering among children who die. Parents of 103 children who died from cancer after treatment in Boston, interviewed on average 3 years after the death, recalled that the vast majority of children (89%) suffered substantially from one or more symptoms during the last month of life. Pain, fatigue, dyspnea, and poor appetite were the most prevalent, followed by nausea, vomiting, constipation, and diarrhea, each affecting 40 percent or more of these patients. Attempts to ameliorate symptoms, as judged retrospectively by the parents, were dramatically unsuccessful (Wolfe et al., 2000). A similar interview study of bereaved parents of 44 children, 0.5–2.5 years after their child's death, following treatment at a California pediatric tertiary care center for various conditions, also emphasized the importance—and suboptimal achievement—of pain management (Contro et al., 2002). A hospice in England reviewed the records of 30 children who had died in the inpatient hospice setting. Although the overwhelming majority of these children died of neurologic conditions, during the last month of life most of the children still experienced pain, and a substantial minority had dyspnea, cough, difficulty swallowing, excessive oral secretions, seizures, muscle spasms, anorexia, nausea or vomiting, and constipation (Hunt, 1990).

Family members—parents and siblings—have been observed to suffer from a broad array of psychological and physical forms of distress: parents report depression, feelings of grief, guilt, and anxiety as well as problems such as insomnia, headache, and musculoskeletal pain. Siblings struggle with fears, sensations of isolation, school and social difficulties, and resulting behavior problems (Mulhern, Lauer, and Hoffmann, 1983; Sirkia, Saarinen-Pihkala, and Hovi, 2000). Although data are limited, bereaved parents do not seem to divorce more often than the general population (Lansky et al., 1978).

Whether the impact of a child's death on parents and siblings differs between families who had a child die in the hospital and families in which death occurred at home in the context of special supportive care services is still unclear. No randomized studies have been performed, so at best conclusions are tentative. One set of follow-up studies suggested that parents who provided home care for their dying child fared better, with subsequent healthier patterns of adjustment (Lauer et al., 1983, 1989; Mulhern, Lauer, and Hoffmann, 1983), while other investigators have found no substantial difference between these families and those whose child died in the hospital (Sirkia, Saarinen-Pihkala, and Hovi, 2000).

Receipt of Health Care

With a clearer understanding of the demographic characteristics of dying children and their symptomatology (along with the problems confronted by the family), the team then turned to examining the kinds of health care that these children received before death. They believed that systematic review of what care was typically provided would enhance the likelihood of the delivery of optimal palliative care services, as well as inform them of what services might be necessary.

Population-based studies of health care services received by children before death are scant. Data from Washington State for the period 1990–96 reveal that 36 percent of infants who died were mechanically ventilated before death, while 11 percent of children and adolescents who died between 1 and 24 years of age had been mechanically ventilated. For infants and for children and adolescents who died with underlying CCCs, these proportions were, respectively, 50 percent and 19 percent. Chronically ill children and adolescents spent a median of 18 days hospitalized during the year preceding death, with a quarter of these cases having spent nearly 2 months (52 days or more) in the hospital (Feudtner, DiGiuseppe, and Neff, 2003).

In children's hospitals during the 1990s, the mean length of stay for children who died in the hospital was 16.4 days. Looking more closely, one sees that 25 percent of the stays lasted 1 day or less, 50 percent lasted 4 days or less, 75 percent lasted 16 days or less, and 90 percent lasted 42 days or less. Among children who died without CCCs, the mean length of stay was 8.7 days, whereas children with CCCs had a mean length of stay of 21.4 days. Using 2005 data, one can see that the duration of terminal hospitalizations also varied across age groups (fig. 1.8), with a substantial increase for children who had CCCs. Mechanical ventilation was provided at some point

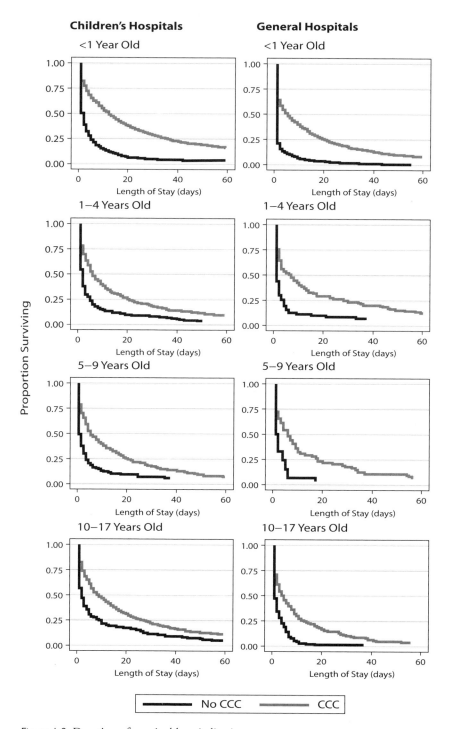

Figure 1.8. Duration of terminal hospitalizations

during the hospitalization for 66 percent of neonates, 40 percent of infants, 36 percent of children, and 36 percent of adolescents. Patients with CCCs were more likely than those without CCCs to have been mechanically ventilated (across all age groups, 52% vs. 46%) (Feudtner et al., 2002).

Empirical health services studies may help us to refine our ideas regarding modes of medical care for children who have specific diseases. For example, a retrospective study of patients who died from cystic fibrosis underscored "the combination of preventive, therapeutic, and palliative care given at the end of life," with three-fourths of the patients receiving intravenous antibiotics and oral vitamin or enzyme supplements on the day of their deaths (Robinson et al., 1997). Broadening the definition of the population in need to encompass children who have complex or special health care needs, one study demonstrated that a program located in an ED setting to provide telephone advice and care coordination enhanced parental satisfaction with emergency care (Sutton et al., 2008), while other studies have begun to underscore the problems of inadequate or lapsing health insurance status for this population of children (Satchell and Pati, 2005), especially as they transition into adulthood (Lotstein et al., 2008).

Several studies have examined the proportion of children who have medical interventions either withheld or discontinued before dying in hospital settings, with approximately a quarter having do-not-resuscitate orders that limited therapy and a third having treatments discontinued (Lantos, Berger, and Zucker, 1993; Vernon et al., 1993; Martinot et al., 1998; McCallum, Byrne, and Bruera, 2000). These studies all focused on children who were imminently dying or already deceased, so the true proportion of children who have interventions limited is not known (because not all patients who have limitations of medical interventions die). A prospective survey of nurses and physicians in a PICU found that, for the 503 patients admitted over a 6-month period, at least one of the health care providers thought that interventions (especially cardiopulmonary resuscitation and hemodialysis) should be limited for 63 (13%) of the patients. Of these 63 patients, 26 actually had DNR orders written, and 11 died during this PICU admission (Keenan et al., 2000).

Increasingly, investigators are examining how satisfied parents are with not only medical care per se but also their involvement in medical decision making. An Australian study of parents of children who died from cancer between 1996 and 2004 found high overall ratings of the quality of care for their child who had died, and parents who reported open and honest communication were the most satisfied (Heath et al., 2009). The emphasis on forthright communication, including supportive and clear discussions about end-of-life choices and care, is borne out in other pediatric and adult studies (Wright et al., 2008). Parents more completely informed about the severity of their child's prognosis have been reported to experience greater levels of hope emanating from their conversations with their child's doctors (Mack et al., 2007).

Bereavement Care

Published evaluations of bereavement counseling programs for surviving parents and siblings are few and of limited methodological rigor. A survey of parents of infants who died after discontinuation of interventions in NICUs in Scotland found that follow-up meetings between attending physicians and parents occurred within 2 months of the death in only 46 percent of one case series (McHaffie, Laing, and Lloyd, 2001). A postdeath interview of parents whose children had died traumatically assessed the overall benefit of a dinner meeting with staff of a regional trauma center and 15 "supporters" of the family: 77 percent believed that this meeting was of ongoing benefit (Oliver et al., 2001). While these types of interviews have been demonstrated to be of value, they seem to occur infrequently (Meert et al., 2007).

Future Work

> With their systematic review of the medical literature complete, the team continues to design their palliative and end-of-life care services with a firmer sense of the characteristics of dying children and the health services they receive, but also a keen awareness of how little is known in this realm.

A wise statistician once remarked that it is better to have an approximate answer to the right question than an exact answer to the wrong question (Salsburg, 2001). This maxim (credited to John Tukey) could be the motto for this chapter, which has prioritized formulating the key questions first and then seeking the best available evidence, even though this evidence often provides only approximate answers at best.

Clearly, pediatric palliative and end-of-life care warrants more research. All of the questions posed above could be answered much better. As we seek information to guide our care of individual patients (using the concepts of clinical epidemiology) or to devise better systems of care at local and national levels (using population-based epidemiology or health services research), we should consider seven principles that, if adhered to, would in the years to come improve our answers to the right questions.

1. *Study Valued Outcomes.* Ultimately, we strive to improve the quality of life for children living with life-threatening conditions and their families. Focusing on measures of the target population or of care processes (such as how many children died of specific conditions or were exposed to various types of medical treatments) are of value only insofar as we use this information to—in one way or another—improve outcomes that we value, such as the reduction of pain or the prevention of debilitating bereavement. Keeping this end in mind will enhance the impact of future epidemiologic and health services research.

2. *Assess Costs Thoroughly.* The costs involved in the evaluation of health care programs are often divided into direct costs (that is, the money spent by the program) and indirect costs (the money spent outside of the program budget by the patient and other participants, including the monetary equivalent for time). In the evaluation of palliative care programs, the meticulous accounting of both direct and indirect costs will be crucial, as will an understanding of how different programs affect families' finances.

3. *Evaluate Rigorously.* As new techniques of individual patient-level pediatric palliative care are developed, assessment must proceed in the most rigorous manner possible, which usually is a randomized controlled trial. The same standards should apply to new systems for providing palliative and bereavement care, be they in the hospital, home, or community settings.

4. *Consider Ethical Implications.* Too often advocates for services assert that randomized controlled trials are unethical, because the controls are not provided with the intervention that is being studied. The admirable passion of this view notwithstanding, rigorous evaluations are the best means to determine what interventions or changes are beneficial for children and their families and will be essential in convincing health care providers and third-party payers to adopt new practices.

5. *Keep the Entire Target Population in View.* For the purposes of planning services, be it at the level of a hospital or community-based palliative care program or a national consortium examining workforce or reimbursement issues, the entire population of children living with life-threatening conditions ought to be considered, with all members deserving equal attention.

6. *Use Available Data Thoughtfully.* Although privacy must be safeguarded scrupulously, vital statistics records and administrative health care records offer useful data with which to define target populations, discern patterns of use of health care, and identify changes in any of these parameters on an annual basis. Work in this area will also help guide the development of new and more perceptive data collection systems.

7. *Reassess Continuously.* The experience of children living with life-

threatening conditions and their families is influenced by a broad array of interacting factors, from medical interventions to reimbursement arrangements. Because this encompassing system of "people care" is always changing, our assessment of what is occurring to whom and with what impact needs to be ongoing.

Authors rarely hope for their work to become quickly obsolete, but this does not apply in the present case: it is to be hoped that, with each passing year, a cadre of investigators in pediatric palliative and end-of-life care, guided by these seven research principles, will have provided far superior answers to the questions posed above, to the betterment of the quality of life for children living with life-threatening conditions and their families.

Conclusion

Pediatric palliative and end-of-life care remains open to the conduct of more research. Such research must exceed empirical studies of childhood suffering, death, and the use of medical care before death. But the epidemiologic data necessary to monitor trends, mark progress, and understand the availability and use of resources for children living with life-limiting conditions, their families, and their communities must continue to be assessed. All of the stakeholders in pediatric palliative care have contributions to make toward the understanding of effective patient and family care, clinical management, communication, decision making, and caregiver competencies. They also have a stake in public policy decisions, which often rest on epidemiologic information and research emanating from populations such as those described in this chapter.

References

Ashby, M.A., Kosky, R.J., Laver, H.T., et al. 1991. An enquiry into death and dying at the Adelaide Children's Hospital: A useful model? *Med J Aust* 154:165–70.

Cardenas-Turanzas, M., Tovalin-Ahumada, H., Carrillo, M.T., et al. 2008. The place of death of children with cancer in the metropolitan areas of Mexico. *J Palliat Med* 11(7):973–79.

Carter, B.S., Howenstein, M., Gilmer, M.J., et al. 2004. Circumstances surrounding the deaths of hospitalized children: Opportunities for pediatric palliative care. *Pediatrics* 114(3):e361–66.

Christakis, N.A. 1999. *Death Foretold: Prophecy and Prognosis in Medical Care.* Chicago: University of Chicago Press.

Contro, N., Larson, J., Scofield, S., et al. 2002. Family perspectives on the quality of pediatric palliative care. *Arch Pediatr Adolesc Med* 156(1):14–19.

Dussel, V., Kreicbergs, U., Hilden, J.M., et al. 2009. Looking beyond where children die: Determinants and effects of planning a child's location of death. *J Pain Symptom Manage* 37(1):33–43.

Feudtner, C., Christakis, D.A., Zimmerman, F.J., et al. 2002. Characteristics of deaths occurring in children's hospitals: Implications for supportive care services. *Pediatrics* 109(5):887–93.

Feudtner, C., DiGiuseppe, D.L., and Neff, J.M. 2003. Hospital care for children and young adults in the last year of life: A population-based study. *BMC Med* 1(1):3.

Feudtner, C., Feinstein, J.A., Satchell, M., et al. 2007. Shifting place of death among children with complex chronic conditions in the United States, 1989–2003. *JAMA* 297(24):2725–32.

Feudtner, C., Hays, R.M., Haynes, G., et al. 2001. Deaths attributed to pediatric complex chronic conditions: National trends and implications for supportive care services. *Pediatrics* 107(6):E99.

Feudtner, C., Villareale, N.L., Morray, B., et al. 2005. Technology-dependency among patients discharged from a children's hospital: A retrospective cohort study. *BMC Pediatr* 5(1):8.

Heath, J.A., Clarke, N.E., McCarthy, M., et al. 2009. Quality of care at the end of life in children with cancer. *J Paediatr Child Health* 45(11):656–59.

Huang, I.C., Thompson, L.A., Chi, Y.Y., et al. 2009. The linkage between pediatric quality of life and health conditions: Establishing clinically meaningful cutoff scores for the PedsQL. *Value Health*, January 9.

Hunt, A.M. 1990. A survey of signs, symptoms and symptom control in 30 terminally ill children. *Dev Med Child Neurol* 32:341–46.

Keenan, H.T., Diekema, D.S., O'Rourke, P.P., et al. 2000. Attitudes toward limitation of support in a pediatric intensive care unit. *Crit Care Med* 28(5):1590–94.

Lansky, S.B., Cairns, N.U., Hassanein, R., et al. 1978. Childhood cancer: Parental discord and divorce. *Pediatrics* 62(2):184–88.

Lantos, J.D., Berger, A.C., and Zucker, A.R. 1993. Do-not-resuscitate orders in a children's hospital. *Crit Care Med* 21(1):52–55.

Lauer, M.E., Mulhern, R.K., Schell, M.J., et al. 1989. Long-term follow-up of parental adjustment following a child's death at home or hospital. *Cancer* 63:988–94.

Lauer, M.E., Mulhern, R.K., Wallskog, J.M., et al. 1983. A comparison study of parental adaptation following a child's death at home or in the hospital. *Pediatrics* 71(1):107–12.

Lotstein, D.S., Inkelas, M., Hays, R.D., et al. 2008. Access to care for youth with special health care needs in the transition to adulthood. *J Adolesc Health* 43(1):23–29.

Lowton, K. 2009. "A bed in the middle of nowhere": Parents' meanings of place of death for adults with cystic fibrosis. *Soc Sci Med* 69(7):1056–62.

Lyons, R.A., and Brophy, S. 2005. The epidemiology of childhood mortality in the European Union. *Current Paediatrics* 15:151–62.

Mack, J.W., Wolfe, J., Cook, E.F., et al. 2007. Hope and prognostic disclosure. *J Clin Oncol* 25(35):5636–42.

Martinot, A., Grandbastien, B., Leteurtre, S., et al. 1998. No resuscitation orders and withdrawal of therapy in French paediatric intensive care units. Groupe Francophone de Reanimation et d'Urgences Pediatriques. *Acta Paediatr* 87(7):769–73.

McCallum, D.E., Byrne, P., and Bruera, E. 2000. How children die in hospital. *J Pain Symptom Manage* 20(6):417–23.

McHaffie, H.E., Laing, I.A., and Lloyd, D.J. 2001. Follow up care of bereaved parents after treatment withdrawal from newborns. *Arch Dis Child Fetal Neonatal Ed* 84(2):F125–28.

Meert, K.L., Eggly, S., Pollack, M., et al. 2007. Parents' perspectives regarding a physician-parent conference after their child's death in the pediatric intensive care unit. *J Pediatr* 151(1):50–55, 55.e1–2.

Mulhern, R.K., Lauer, M.E., and Hoffmann, R.G. 1983. Death of a child at home or in the hospital: Subsequent psychological adjustment of the family. *Pediatrics* 71(5):743–47.

Oliver, R.C., Sturtevant, J.P., Scheetz, J.P., et al. 2001. Beneficial effects of a hospital bereavement intervention program after traumatic childhood death. *J Trauma* 50(3): 440–46; discussion 447–48.

Ramnarayan, P., Craig, F., Petros, A., et al. 2007. Characteristics of deaths occurring in hospitalised children: Changing trends. *J Med Ethics* 33(5):255–60.

Robinson, W.M., Ravilly, S., Berde, C., et al. 1997. End-of-life care in cystic fibrosis [see comments]. *Pediatrics* 100:205–9.

Salsburg, D. 2001. *The Lady Tasting Tea: How Statistics Revolutionized Science in the Twentieth Century.* New York: W.H. Freeman.

Satchell, M., and Pati, S. 2005. Insurance gaps among vulnerable children in the United States, 1999–2001. *Pediatrics* 116(5):1155–61.

Siden, H., Miller, M., Straatman, L., et al. 2008. A report on location of death in paediatric palliative care between home, hospice and hospital. *Palliat Med* 22(7): 831–34.

Sirkia, K., Saarinen-Pihkala, U.M., and Hovi, L. 2000. Coping of parents and siblings with the death of a child with cancer: Death after terminal care compared with death during active anticancer therapy. *Acta Paediatr* 89(6):717–21.

Sutton, D., Stanley, P., Babl, F.E., et al. 2008. Preventing or accelerating emergency care for children with complex healthcare needs. *Arch Dis Child* 93(1):17–22.

van der Wal, M.E., Renfurm, L.N., van Vught, A.J., et al. 1999. Circumstances of dying in hospitalized children. *Eur J Pediatr* 158(7):560–65.

Vernon, D.D., Dean, J.M., Timmons, O.D., et al. 1993. Modes of death in the pediatric intensive care unit: Withdrawal and limitation of supportive care. *Crit Care Med* 21(11):1798–1802.

Widger, K., Davies, D., Drouin, D.J., et al. 2007. Pediatric patients receiving palliative care in Canada: Results of a multicenter review. *Arch Pediatr Adolesc Med* 161(6): 597–602.

Wolfe, J., Grier, H.E., Klar, N., et al. 2000. Symptoms and suffering at the end of life in children with cancer. *N Engl J Med* 342(5):326–33.

Wright, A.A., and Katz, I.T. 2007. Letting go of the rope: Aggressive treatment, hospice care, and open access. *N Engl J Med* 357(4):324–27.

Wright, A.A., Zhang, B., Ray, A., et al. 2008. Associations between end-of-life discussions, patient mental health, medical care near death, and caregiver bereavement adjustment. *JAMA* 300(14):1665–73.

2

Goals, Values, and Conflict Resolution

Carson Strong, Ph.D., Chris Feudtner, M.D., Ph.D., M.P.H.,
M. Karen Ballard, M.C.M., B.C.C., Brian S. Carter, M.D.,
and Deborah L. Dokken, M.P.A.

Few tasks in pediatrics are as challenging as caring for children with life-threatening or terminal conditions. This challenge, unfolding over the course of a particular child's care, requires health care professionals to weave knowledge, skills, and values into an effective effort to promote the patient's quality of life and support the patient's family (table 2.1).

While this entire handbook strives to help caregivers provide such care successfully, this chapter specifically aims to improve the way ethical questions related to palliative care are addressed in order to optimize the effectiveness of care provided to the child and family.

These questions include the following: When is it the "right time" to discuss a poor prognosis with the patient and family? How should one resolve conflicts between parents and health care professionals regarding goals of care? How should disagreements among health care professionals about treatment decisions be handled? What are the obstacles to improved access to palliative care?

The objectives for this chapter are to

- describe the nature of palliative care and its goals;
- identify main types of ethically problematic situations that arise in palliative care;
- discuss practical approaches to resolving these situations.

The Goals of Palliative Care

Pediatric palliative care is comprehensive care for infants and children who may not or will not "get better." Palliative care is child centered, yet attends

Table 2.1 Steps in the provision of effective palliative care: interplay of values, skills, and knowledge

	Understanding and appreciation of benefit of palliative care	Recognition of patient's need	Individual initiation of effort to provide palliative care	Collaborative effort to provide palliative care	Effective provision of palliative care
Values	• Respect for persons • Emphasis on quality of life • Beneficence • Nonmaleficence	• Patient-focused care • Beneficence	• Fidelity • Conviction • Fortitude	• Conviction • Respect for colleagues	• Commitment to relief of suffering • Beneficence • Autonomy
Skills	• Training in palliative care techniques	• Awareness of patient • Assessment of patient's needs and desires • Self-awareness	• Forthright communication	• Forthright communication • Group facilitation • Conflict resolution • Values analysis	• Assessment of impact of care • Advocacy • Negotiation
Knowledge	• Understanding of causes of suffering	• Signs and symptoms of suffering	• Family context	• Ethical principles • Colleagues' potential contribution	• Control of pain and symptoms

to the needs of the child's entire family, striving to enhance the dignity of the child's time on earth and support the family's experience with empathy and culturally sensitive respect. Perhaps initially combined with cure-oriented or life-span-extending care, palliative care can intensify when these goals of care are no longer helpful or appropriate. A proactive and planned intervention, palliative care uses a team approach to prevent or relieve any physical, psychological, social, emotional, and spiritual suffering while improving the quality of life for dying children and their families (World Health Organization, 1990, p. 11).

The provision of pediatric palliative care is necessarily interdisciplinary, since no single discipline in pediatric health care can provide all of the support that the child or her family will require. Holistic care encompasses more than pain and symptom management, addressing also the psychological and emotional needs of the child and her family, tailored to their developmental needs. While palliative care may be applied within an inpatient treatment environment, its principles transcend the institutional setting and are applicable in home-based or outpatient care. Inpatient palliative care may be characterized by around-the-clock nursing assessment, physician management, and interdisciplinary support to prevent and manage symptoms that could occur in the dying child, such as pain, difficulty breathing, or seizures. These and other symptoms may persist and require planning, education, and 24-hour backup for parents or other home caregivers. Regardless of site of care, the holistic goals of palliative care remain the same.

Palliative care also attempts to address the spiritual needs of the family and, when applicable, the dying child. Spiritual concerns might include the interpretation of illness, dying, and death and the assignment of meaning to all that is happening. Some families approach these questions within a religious context, while others seek answers outside of religion. Varied value systems, beliefs, traditions, and rituals will find their place in providing comfort for the dying child and her family. These spiritual dimensions also may ease the acceptance of death, and the transition from life to death, with its attendant grief and process of bereavement by the family. Hospital chaplains or clergy of the family's choosing can be important members of the interdisciplinary team in addressing such spiritual concerns.

In summary, the goal of pediatric palliative care is the best quality of life for the child and family through the provision of proactive, comprehensive, family-centered, and holistic care for infants and children living with life-threatening conditions. In pursuing this goal, palliative care services will support the child and family in all matters pertaining to the control of pain and other symptoms across care settings and provide necessary support in managing the psychosocial and spiritual concerns associated with living with and dying from a life-threatening condition. Ultimately, the provision of the best quality of life for the child and family is sought.

Ethical Values in Palliative Care

The goals of palliative care are based on core values that form the basis of the relationship between the health care professional and patient (Beauchamp and Childress, 2009):

- *Beneficence:* the idea that the well-being of persons should be promoted. Health care professionals have a beneficence-based duty to promote the well-being of patients and to provide emotional support to patients' families. This gives rise to the duty to provide palliative care that addresses the well-being of the patient and family in a comprehensive way.
- *Nonmaleficence:* the principle that we should avoid causing harm to others. This implies a duty to attempt to recognize when continued disease-directed interventions are likely to cause more harm than benefit to the patient.
- *Autonomy:* the idea that a person's self-rule be free from both the control of others and personal limitations that interfere with choice, such as lack of knowledge. The principle of autonomy implies that health care professionals have a duty to respect the autonomy of minor patients who have the capacity to make their own decisions, to respect the moral right of parents to participate in medical decisions for their children who do not have capacity, and, where appropriate, to respect the developing capacity of minor patients who are not autonomous by means such as seeking the child's assent to treatment. Palliative care should be provided in a manner that is consistent with these autonomy-based duties.
- *Fidelity:* the core commitment to take care of patients as they progress through their illness experience, no matter what. This fundamental compact with patients—namely, that they will not be abandoned by their health care professionals—is acknowledged in professional codes of ethics (Baker, 1999, p. 34). Fidelity is important in all areas of medical care, but it is especially paramount when the condition is life threatening and the possibility of death increases.
- *Respect for Life:* the principle that human life should be protected. This duty to preserve life, however, must sometimes be tempered by the

duty to avoid causing undue harm to the patient. When life-prolonging efforts are likely to be unsuccessful and to cause more harm than benefit, the duty to avoid causing harm takes priority over the duty to prolong life. In this context, health care professionals should recommend to the patient and family that caregiving be directed toward maximizing quality of life rather than measures that attempt to prolong life at all costs.

- *Respect for Persons:* an overarching principle that, to the extent possible, the ethical principles discussed above should be followed. Treating the patient as a person requires the health care professional to attempt to recognize when palliative care is appropriate.

The duty to provide palliative care is thus an extension of the obligations already present in the health care professional–patient relationship. A responsibility to provide palliative care when appropriate is inherent in the nature of the relationship.

The Nature of Ethical Problems in Palliative Care

A wide variety of situations encountered in modern health care are, in one way or another, ethically problematic. Some of these situations arise when different ethical values suggest conflicting courses of action and there is disagreement or uncertainty concerning which values should be given priority. Such cases include, for example, a situation in which the decision makers are uncertain about whether to resuscitate an infant with hypoxic brain injury who has a prognosis of severe cognitive deficit and is having episodes of dangerously low heart rates (bradycardia). One consideration is that continued life support might cause more suffering than benefit for the child, thereby violating the principle to "do no harm." But another concern is protection of life and the idea that one should err on the side of preserving life. Resolution of this type of ethical dilemma involves, in part, deciding which of the conflicting ethical values should have priority in the particular situation. Here the conflict is between two competing goods—in this example, the ethical values of nonmaleficence and respect for life.

Ethical issues do not always, however, involve a dilemma about how to prioritize values. Another type of problem arises when there is widespread agreement concerning what the appropriate norms of behavior are, but a person or institution is not acting in accordance with those norms. Examples include treatment provided without consent, in a situation in which informed consent should and could be obtained, or a nurse who observes a physician failing to carry out a professional duty to relieve pain, but who feels too vulnerable to challenge the behavior. Again the ethical values are relevant, now because they help to define the problem. For example, failure to obtain consent is a violation of the principle of autonomy, and failure to relieve pain is a violation of the principle of beneficence. But resolution of this second type of ethical problem often involves recognition and management of additional factors, such as unequal power and authority (Feudtner, Christakis, and Schwartz, 1996), as well as the ability to engage effectively in "difficult conversations" (Stone, Patton, and Heen, 1999).

Both of these types of ethical problems arise in palliative care. Keeping these two types of problems in mind can be helpful in identifying the factors that are present in various ethically problematic situations. When one is faced with an ethical problem, the ethical values discussed above should be part of the thought process in deciding how to handle the situation, as illustrated in the next section, where the resolution of specific types of ethical problems is considered.

Main Types of Ethically Problematic Situations

Through the following fictional clinical vignettes, various types of ethically problematic situations are considered that are often encountered while caring for children with life-threatening conditions. In each case, underlying values are clarified that may be in conflict and behaviors that are interfering with effective palliative care are identified (table 2.1).

AVOIDANCE OR POSTPONEMENT OF BAD NEWS

Jason, 17, was critically injured when a car struck him as he was riding his bicycle, requiring care in the surgical intensive care unit (SICU). For the past week, he has developed one complication after another. Because the physicians want to monitor his neurological status, they have been judicious in their use of opiates and other analgesic pain medications. Each day, the surgical team discusses Jason's worsening prognosis outside the room in hushed tones. When discussing Jason's condition with the family, the attending physician adopts a much more optimistic tone. He tells the team privately that "we can't take away hope from the parents" and that he will discuss withdrawal of life support "when the time is right."

When is "the right time" to discuss the poor prognosis with the family in this case?

When should one raise the issue of reconsidering the goals of care, moving from a life-prolonging to a palliative framework?

How should the team members respond to the attending physician's unwillingness to discuss prognosis?

Forthright communication given compassionately and communicating bad news skillfully are of paramount importance.

The attending physician is concerned about the well-being of the family. This is commendable because the physician and other health care professionals have a beneficence-based duty to provide emotional support to the family. However, the physician believes that giving bad news will "take away hope" and constitute a failure to provide emotional support, and this way of looking at the case overlooks several other important ethical values. One is the right of the parents to have accurate information about their child's medical condition; truthfulness is a requirement of respect for persons. Moreover, if the parents are truly to participate in decisions about care, they need to understand the facts about the child's condition. Another value is the well-being of the patient; the delay in providing supportive care, particularly in providing adequate pain medication, may be causing unnecessary suffering to the patient.

The physician's approach to this case is creating a conflict between these ethical values. His attempt to protect the parents from inevitable emotional distress is preventing them from receiving information to which they have a right, and it may be causing harm to the patient. But this conflict need not occur. It can be argued that the attending physician's view about what needs to be done to provide emotional support is misguided. By keeping the family in the dark concerning the prognosis, the physician is setting them up for an even greater shock when the bad news is finally delivered. The family might be better able to cope if they are informed of the worsening prognosis as it develops (Mack and Wolfe, 2008; Mosenthal et al., 2008). This will also help prepare them for a conversation about changing the goals of care, a topic that should be raised relatively soon. Moreover, there is evidence that good communication with parents about prognosis does not necessarily diminish hope, and in some cases it can support hope (Mack et al., 2007). In addition, hope can be directed to matters other than survival, such as avoidance of pain and suffering.

All members of the health care team have duties to promote the well-being of the patient and the right of the parents to participate in decision making. If the team members fail to take issue with the attending physician's decision not to discuss prognosis, then they abrogate these duties. It would be reasonable to begin a discussion of this topic, perhaps on rounds, by asking, "When *is* it appropriate to discuss prognosis with the parents?" This would invite the voicing of alternative views, including the considerations in favor of prompt disclosure. Relationships of power and authority can make it difficult for nurses and residents to challenge the attending or discuss topics with parents that are disapproved by the attending physician. One tactic is to ask the family if they feel they have all the information they need and, if not, to arrange a family meeting with the attending to allow them to directly pose their queries. If resistance to change by the attending physician or others persists, an evidence-based educational forum on hope and disclosure might be feasible, at least at some institutions.

When prognosis is discussed, the social worker, chaplain, or psychologist could assist in several ways: they could help the health care team and family identify appropriate areas of focus for their hope, help the family contemplate the meaning they are assigning to this tragic situation, offer support to the team and family in giving bad news, and support the family as they attempt to deal with their situation.

GIVING BAD NEWS

This type of case is not unusual because many physicians have not been formally trained in giving bad news, and even when they have, some may feel uncomfortable doing so. Many interpret such conversations as an admission of failure. The ability to communicate well and with compassion in this type of difficult situation is extremely important to being a good physician; in fact, there is an ethical obligation to be competent in breaking bad news. There is a growing body of articles and books, written by clinicians, based on evidence from patients and families, giving advice about how best to give bad news (Buckman, 1992; Creagan, 1994; Browning, 2003; Strong, 2003; Feudtner, 2007; Levetown and the AAP Committee on Bioethics, 2008). Physicians can improve their skills by engaging in interactive training programs, such as the Initiative for Pediatric Palliative Care (www.ippcweb.org), and by consulting this literature as well as chapter 7 in this volume. Given the essential nature of possessing skill in breaking bad news and negotiating goals of care, it would seem that there is an ethical obligation for health care professions training programs to incorporate this topic into their curricula.

POOR COMMUNICATION

Polly's muscle biopsy results confirmed that the 8-month-old girl, who had been admitted to the hospital because she was growing weaker, had Leigh syndrome. A rare and uniformly fatal disease, Leigh syndrome causes brain cells to die, with almost all patients dying within a few months of diagnosis. The neurologist notified the hospital team and requested a care conference. Later that afternoon, the physician, a nurse, a social worker, and a physician-in-training sat together with the parents in a conference room. The neurologist started the conversation by stating, "Well, the test is back and your daughter, I am afraid to say, has Leigh syndrome," then launched into a 10-minute explanation of the cause of the condition, a defect of mitochondrial metabolism. At the end of his disquisition, the physician asked the parents whether they had any questions, and when they did not, he excused himself from the meeting, explaining that he would be happy to answer questions as they came up.

Clear, digestible, and forthright communication is a sine qua non of the ethical delivery of bad news.
Cognitive clarity is only half the issue; attention to emotional support is equally important.

This is an example of the second type of ethically problematic situation discussed above—a case of a health care provider not performing a vital task with the required level of skill. The skills in question center on the ability to provide information to the parents that will help them understand Polly's medical condition and to provide emotional support to them. Appropriate information includes the diagnosis and prognosis in terms the parents can understand, symptoms that might be expected, types of palliative care that might be appropriate, and a discussion of any other implications of the disease for the patient and family. How much to tell at one time varies because persons differ in the amount of information they can absorb. The physician should be prepared to have more than one session to present the relevant information in preparation for informed decision making. In addition to formal family meetings, brief interactions at the bedside are an essential element of building the parents' understanding (Mosenthal et al., 2008).

Although the provision of emotional support is an ongoing process, there are several things that can be done during a formal family meeting in which bad news is delivered (Girgis and Sanson-Fisher, 1995; Feudtner, 2007). Most importantly, the parents must be reassured that good care will continue without interruption and that the needs of the patient will be met. Also, because many people cope with crisis situations by seeking information, the physician should strive to help the parents understand the information that is being given to them, rather than devoting a great deal of time to medical details the parents do not understand. In addition, physicians should "show their feelings," allowing the family to see that they are concerned about the interests of the patient and family (Browning, 2003; Strong, 2003). It is important to respond to expressions of grief. Body language can be used to display warmth and sympathy; it may be acceptable to express concern by touching the parents, such as by gripping or holding hands. Cultural competence is required in knowing any cultural or faith-specific dictums about the appropriateness of touching. If the parents cry, expressions of sympathy followed by a period of silence might be appropriate, and facial tissue should be available.

At the end of the discussion, the physician should arrange a time in the near future to further review the situation with the parents. During the interim, the physician should either be personally available or identify someone else who will be available to address any questions or concerns. The physician should ask the parents whom they would like to tell about the situation and offer help in telling these people. For example, a family meeting might be arranged.

DENIAL OF POOR PROGNOSIS

Two days ago, Alex nearly drowned. Intubated and mechanically ventilated, the 2-year-old boy is still in a profound coma. The attending physician in the pediatric intensive care unit approaches the parents, who are seated alone at Alex's bedside. She tells them about their son's medical status, pointing out that he still is deeply comatose and explaining that this is a bad prognostic sign, as virtually all children who are still comatose 48 hours after a near-drowning injury either never awaken or suffer severe brain damage. The parents, who have heard this information before, nod their heads slightly in apparent understanding. The attending physician then goes on to suggest that at this juncture, given the high likelihood that Alex will be permanently impaired, they should consider withdrawing ventilatory support. Stunned, the parents manage to say that no, they couldn't possibly "give up"; they are sure that their son is going to "beat the odds."

Parents' difficulty in accepting a grave prognosis and responding to it cognitively and emotionally can be crucial aspects of ethically problematic cases.

Parents and professionals sometimes have a difficult time arriving at a common understanding of the meaning of a child's prognosis. Health care professionals' assessment of a child's future is primarily grounded in the facts—evidence of accurate diagnosis and reliable data to support their assessment of prognosis. They often convey these facts to parents and are confused and frustrated when parents do not assign the same significance to them. Hearing the facts is not the same as understanding them. Generally, parents understand their moral obligations as arising from their duty to be faithful to their child's life and to their role as a "good" parent, which characteristically includes both protecting their child from harm and preserving life, with an eye toward a hopeful future. Health care professionals can support parents in their efforts to understand the information and make sense of it by acknowledging the parents' advocacy for their child and by understanding their values and hopes concerning life, death, and disability.

THE MEANING OF HOPE

Expressions such as "not giving up" and hoping that their child will "beat the odds" reflect parental hope for a different outcome despite the fact that they have been told otherwise. Parental hope may appear disproportionate to the reality, yet hope is necessary for parents to endure an overwhelming situation. Hope is resilient. "Giving up hope" is not the same as accepting the reality of a child's death; hope may evolve as the situation unfolds. Ongoing counseling of the parents should continue to include information about prognosis, but it should also identify other things to hope for, such as freedom from suffering (Feudtner, 2005), acceptance, or peace.

Alex's parents have the task of adjusting to a new reality that has irretrievably changed the future for their child and family. Parents are vulnerable during such periods, and their need for time to arrive at acceptance must be honored. Often it is the health care professionals' need for closure that drives them to expect decisions to be made relatively soon. Shared decision making invites us to honor the parents' need for a process that allows them to live with the decisions they make for their child. This approach is based on the beneficence-based duty to support the well-being of the family.

The language of "giving up" implies that there are beneficial interventions that will be forgone. By being clear that the treatments thus far have not been and will not become successful, and by emphasizing non-abandonment, as well as palliative care goals and associated interventions, health care professionals have an important opportunity to make it clear that they are not giving up. The introduction of palliative care clinicians may prove helpful in clarifying this point and expounding on such options at this juncture. Options such as maintaining the current level of ICU intervention while attending to pain, symptoms, and family needs may give families time to accept their child's new reality. When appropriate, discussion about writing a do-not-attempt-resuscitation order may begin a process of defining other limitations of intervention. In these discussions, parental values and hopes should be explored and honored.

Health care professionals in these cases must be mindful of the power imbalance that exists between parents and professionals and openly work with parents to validate their feelings and concerns while continuing to address an appropriate balance of advocacy and interest on behalf of the patient. Clinicians should attempt to avoid adversarial situations leading to child protective services involvement or legal action; only rarely are such interventions necessary. Instead, health care professionals should ask themselves how they can best support this child and family during their difficult time and what measure of generosity and compassion will enable the family and professionals to preserve their integrity.

DISAGREEMENT OVER THE EFFECTIVENESS OF CARE

Three months later, Alex has continued to receive life-extending care. He remains deeply comatose; a recent MRI confirms the irreversibility of his condition, showing severe encephalomalacia (large cavities in the brain, representing loss of brain tissue) caused by the hypoxia that occurred during his accident. Alex continues to receive ventilatory support and medically administered hydration and nutrition. The nurses have been asking the physicians why they are continuing to keep Alex alive; they and the rest of the staff perceive that the treatment Alex is receiving is "futile." The attending physician in the intensive care unit has met regularly with Alex's parents to discuss his condition, and again she approaches them to discuss his prognosis and care plan. She explains that the MRI adds further evidence that Alex has suffered catastrophic brain injury, that there is no reasonable expectation that he will recover neurological function or any capacity for interaction with the world around him, and that he will most likely remain unconscious until such point as he dies, even with mechanical ventilation and other ICU care. After giving them a few minutes to absorb this information and ask questions, she states that she and Alex's other consulting physicians believe that the continued use of the ventilator has become futile and may be viewed as harmful, given the repeated episodes of ventilator-associated pneumonia that Alex has endured in the last 3 months. The attending physician recommends that the ventilator be discontinued. The parents react immediately, stating that they do not agree and want the respirator support to continue "for as long as it takes."

What does it mean to say that a treatment is "futile"?
A process of conflict resolution can be helpful in resolving disagreements over the futility of treatment.

For this type of case, it is helpful to understand several features of the concept of futility. To say that a treatment is "futile" implies a purpose for which it is futile. In some cases, the purpose is the achievement of a biological or physiological end point. For example, antibiotics are futile for the purpose of curing a viral infection. In this context, whether the purpose can be achieved is objective and measurable. In other cases, achievement of the purpose is not purely objective, but is a matter of evaluative judgment. For example, one might say, "Attempts to resuscitate a patient with metastatic cancer would be futile," and mean by this that it would be futile for the purpose of providing overall benefit to the patient. In this context, the futility claim involves a value judgment, along these lines: "The added duration of life that might be gained is not worth the burdens that would be imposed on the patient." When using the term *"futile,"* it is important to recognize whether one is using it to make an objective scientific claim or to make a value judgment. When a treatment is objectively futile—when it cannot achieve its biological end point, such as curing an infection or restoring a heartbeat—the physician has no duty to carry it out. This is what justifies a physician in halting an attempted cardiopulmonary resuscitation after sufficient effort has been unsuccessful. But when the claim that a treatment is futile is a value judgment, the values of the patient or surrogate decision maker should be considered, and the health care professionals should negotiate a resolution with the patient or surrogate. Because futility as a value judgment can be confused with futility as an objective fact, some prefer to avoid using the term *"futility"* in making a value judgment, in favor of an alternative term. The terms *"medically inappropriate"* or *"unduly burdensome"* are sometimes used, but it should be recognized that these could also be subject to the same confusion.

In Alex's case, the ventilator might accomplish an objective purpose such as maintaining his body, but when the physician says that ventilator treatment is "futile," she is claiming that it should not be continued because there is no reasonable expectation that it will resolve his neurologic injury and therefore, according to her values, there is no reasonable expectation that it will benefit Alex. People can disagree over what constitutes a benefit, and when disagreements over futility are evaluative in nature, a process of conflict resolution can be used. Here we discuss a version of this process that has been recommended by professional organizations (American Medical Association, 1999).

The process includes clarifying Alex's parents' values (prolonging life at all costs vs. hoping for resolution of his brain injury) and continuing to counsel them, addressing their grief and fear. Sometimes parents resist withdrawing "life-extending" treatment in part because they view agreeing to such a recommendation as being responsible for the child's death. Palliative care includes support for the family, suggesting a need to be alert as to whether parents are having such feelings of responsibility and associated guilt. Alex's parents might also be feeling guilt that they did not prevent his accident. Such guilt can complicate the parents' decision-making and grieving process. Because of these considerations, in discussing the options with the parents, it is best not to frame the decision making in such a way that the parents feel that they are the ones who are bearing the main burden of the decision. By coming forward with a recommendation, the physician in Alex's case was assuming part of the burden.

The process of conflict resolution includes offering to obtain a second medical opinion. If a second opinion is obtained that differs from that of the attending physician, then transfer of care within the institution can be explored. If no second opinion is desired by the parents, or if one is obtained that concurs with that of the attending physician, then an ethics consultation should be requested. Continued counseling and consultation can sometimes lead to an agreement to withdraw the interventions in question, while assuring the child's best comfort. If ethics consultants agree that the requested treatment is medically inappropriate, in the sense that there is no reasonable expectation that it will benefit the patient, and if the parents continue to request the treatment, then transfer of the patient to another institution should be explored. If no institution can be found that is willing to treat the patient on the parents' terms, then it is considered ethically permissible to withdraw the treatment with advance notice to the parents. The justification for withdrawal is that the resolution process has upheld the physician's judgment that the treatment is medically inappropriate and it has explored all other reasonable ways to resolve the conflict, such as counseling and transfer of care, to no avail.

At this point in the resolution process, many physicians will continue to provide the treatment because of concern about legal liability. To address these legal concerns in the United States, several states have enacted statutes permitting health care professionals to legally withhold medically inappropriate interventions if such a process is followed. Such statutes can reduce, although not necessarily eliminate, these particular concerns about liability. Even when legal concerns are a prominent factor, the process discussed can sometimes bring about agreement between the parties.

ENTRENCHED POSITIONS

Jane, although only 3 years old, is known to everyone at the nearby children's hospital. Perinatal intrauterine events, culminating in meconium aspiration at the time of birth, led to severe brain damage. This condition has left her unable to swallow anything safely, including her own saliva. Every month or two, she is readmitted to the hospital for yet another aspiration pneumonitis. On two prior occasions, she became ill enough to require intubation and mechanical ventilation. These episodes, together with the lung injury she sustained as a newborn and the ongoing damage of chronic microaspiration, have left her with horrible lung disease. Now she is quite ill again; the staff in the pediatric intensive care unit believe that the time has come to withhold intubation and mechanical ventilation. When this position is explained to Jane's parents, they insist that "everything" be done for their daughter, stating, "This isn't the first time we've been told by you doctors that she would die, and it won't be the last."

People's responses to new challenges presented by a child's evolving illness are shaped by their personal history of previous challenges, how they were handled, and what the outcomes were.
Fierce advocacy for the rights of children is one of the noblest behaviors parents can exhibit.

This case illustrates a failure of shared decision making and the limits of professional prognostication. Jane is one of a growing group of NICU graduates that spend many years on a roller coaster of exacerbation, improvement, and near-death episodes; often these spirals result in a chronic decline in function that occurs over a long period of time. Usually, parents and professionals begin their journey together by agreeing on goals of care focused on prolonging the baby's life. However, over time, especially with inadequate updates regarding the "big picture," parents and health care professionals can come to understand the child's prognosis for recovery and therefore the meaning of "giving a child a chance for life" differently. Health care professionals may regard the unfavorable balance of benefits and burdens that is likely for the patient, especially in the face of certain death in the near future, as grounds for curtailing further interventions. Alternatively, parents who have accompanied their child during these crises may see the current one as an opportunity to "beat the odds" again. When health care professionals declare that a child will certainly die during this hospitalization and the child does not, their credibility with the parent is undermined, and this may lead to adversarial situations.

This type of case illustrates the importance of developing a palliative care plan from the beginning. Although Jane may live for an extended period, it is essential to create a foundation for establishing goals, revising them based on her response to treatment, and altering the corresponding plan of care. Parents need to feel that they have advocated effectively for their child and may believe that health care professionals are no longer committed to their child's life when they constantly focus on limiting interventions and the negative aspects of the child's condition. Health care professionals often resort to this approach when they believe that parents do not understand the severity of the child's condition and must be forced to recognize the gravity of the situation.

The challenge is to give a realistic assessment of the child's condition and prognosis, simultaneously recognizing and respecting the parents' concerns, values, and advocacy. In cases where persons can reasonably disagree over what is best for the child, health care professionals have an autonomy-based duty to respect the parents' values. Health care professionals can share their concerns that a child might die without declaring that they *know* when a life will end. This difference in approach allows parents and professionals to remain committed to shared goals. Parents need guidance in interpreting how a current situation differs from past experiences and will need to have their previous experiences heard, understood, validated, and respected.

DISSENT AMONG HEALTH CARE PROVIDERS

Rachel was born prematurely, at the beginning of the 25th week of gestation, weighing only 600 grams. On the third day of her life, Rachel's condition suddenly deteriorates. A head ultrasound shows that she has had a severe hemorrhage (bleeding, stroke) in her brain. After discussing Rachel's prognosis and care options with the neonatologist, the parents decide to forgo further disease-directed care, and everyone agrees to embrace exclusively palliative goals of care. Plans are made to extubate Rachel later that day, after the family has had time to gather together and perform a meaningful ceremony. The attending physician writes the order for extubation, with a concomitant large dose of morphine to be given intravenously. The nurse, reading the order, informs the attending that she does not feel comfortable participating in euthanasia.

Does this disagreement over a medication relate more to poor communi-cation regarding the goals of care, unacceptable intentions, or inappro-priate dosing due to a lack of knowledge of proper dosing?

How should disagreements between health care providers be handled?

This case raises the importance of team communication and decision making. All members of the care team, particularly those who implement the decisions of others, must be engaged in a process that clarifies decisions, their justification, and the implementation plan. An essential part of this process is encouraging team members to attend family meetings and rounds and to freely express any concerns or perceived value conflicts in a respect-ful, nonpunitive environment. Based on the ethical principle of autonomy, health care professionals have a right to refuse to participate in activities to which they object on grounds of conscience.

Concerns regarding whether the plan of care constitutes euthanasia gen-erally arise when individuals question the propriety of the decision, when they perceive that they are being asked to participate in an act they find morally objectionable, or when communication about the goals of care has been insufficient. The first step is to clarify what euthanasia means to the nurse and to understand the nature of the nurse's objection and her concerns, including her perception of what euthanasia is. It may be that she is unaware of the decision-making process or the ethical justification for treating pain and suffering at the end of life. Alternatively, she may be concerned about her role in the timing and circumstance of Rachel's death. She may believe that using such a large dose of opioid gives the impression that the goal is to hasten death rather than to ease pain and suffering. This is a legitimate question that requires the team to examine its process for providing end-of-life care. The process should enable parents and professionals to be reassured about the goals of care being the relief of suffering rather than an intentional hastening of death.

If the primary goal is to relieve pain and suffering, it is ethically justifiable to accept the possibility that death might occur sooner. If Rachel has not had opioids or is receiving a much smaller dose without evidence of discom-fort, the nurse's concern may be justified. A process that incorporates an ongoing assessment of the infant's pain and suffering and uses titration of medications to achieve the desired effect would be a more appropriate and justifiable plan of care. Moreover, implementing end-of-life care requires that the community of caregivers and family support each other and bear witness to the process; embedded in the nurse's concern may be a fear of isolation and abandonment by other members of the team. While such concerns are not always articulated, good palliative care anticipates and attends to them.

It is possible that after clarifying the goals of care, the decision-making process, and the plan for implementing it, the nurse will continue to object on moral grounds. These objections must be taken seriously and handled in a respectful manner. Team members may benefit from calling an ethics consult to assist in achieving clear goals that are shared by all involved and then fashioning an associated plan of care (POC). Alternatively, if the POC is legal and ethical by majority standards, the nurse may choose not to participate based on her values. The Joint Commission on Accreditation of Healthcare Organizations (JCAHO) now requires that health care institutions have a process in place for responding to staff requests not to participate in actions they believe are morally objectionable.

GENUINE CONFUSION

Dan has mild mental retardation and a form of muscular dystrophy that always causes the breathing muscles to fail to adequately support gas exchange (causing "respiratory failure") sometime during early adulthood. Many people with this type of muscular dystrophy decide to have a tracheotomy and start mechanical ventilation, which can prolong life, but not indefinitely. This is what Dan's parents had envisioned happening. Now in his late adolescence, Dan is developing the predicted respiratory failure. When his doctors and parents talk to him about mechanical ventilation, however, he calmly yet firmly states that he does not want a "breathing tube" even though he knows that without mechanical ventilation he will die. His parents have always sought to respect Dan's autonomy, helping him to make meaningful decisions for himself. In this instance, however, they believe that his anxiety regarding the "breathing tube" would be transient and that he would subsequently enjoy an acceptable quality of life for several more years if "forced" to start mechanical ventilation.

Sometimes—despite forthright dialogue, mutual goodwill, and clear communication—deciding the "right thing to do" is genuinely confusing. In such instances, choosing among the therapeutic options under consideration often poses difficult trade-offs between ethical principles. Clarifying these trade-offs explicitly can be useful.

Creating new, possibly unusual, options may be pivotal.
Ethics committee consultation can be invaluable in these circumstances.

Dan's case illustrates poignantly how some circumstances create genuinely confusing ethical dilemmas. No one in this scenario is avoiding the implications of Dan's progressive illness, nor denying that he will die someday. Although each person who is involved has opinions regarding what should be done, no one is operating from an entrenched position, and "cooperative"— not "factious"—best describes the spirit of the conversation regarding what should be done. The problem encountered here, in other words, is not rooted in personal or interpersonal behavior, but rather in something else.

This "something else" is the standard bailiwick of bioethics, and this case represents a "classic" ethical dilemma of how to balance a respect for Dan's wishes regarding his care with a desire to protect what others consider to be his best interests (Johnston, 2009). In Dan's case, this dilemma is then compounded by one of the most difficult aspects of pediatric palliative care: how can we incorporate the preferences of our young or disabled patients into the decision-making process in a developmentally appropriate manner?

Like most genuinely confusing dilemmas, choosing among the therapeutic options being considered for Dan's care pits one set of legitimate concerns against another. If Dan's current wish is followed and no mechanical ventilation provided, then he may die a few years sooner than he otherwise would, losing time and life experiences that he and his family might have come to cherish. Conversely, if he is compelled by his parents and health care providers to undergo a tracheotomy and start a course of mechanical ventilation, not only will his fragile autonomy have been overridden, but he may experience complications or a diminishment in his quality of life not foreseen—and not of his choosing.

Spelling out the dilemma in clear terms—identifying not just what is at stake, but how much is at stake—can help clarify where the confusion lies (Hammond, Keeney, and Raiffa, 1999). For example, the debate here does not simply boil down to autonomy versus beneficence. Rather, the dilemma hinges on several questions: To what extent would Dan's preferences be violated in order to pursue what degree of benefit? How much of his autonomy would be sacrificed in order to secure how much longer, or better, life? These questions make clear that more work can be done to clarify all of Dan's preferences and priorities regarding his care, as well as to come up with the best estimate of how the use of mechanical ventilation would impact his and his family's life. It is also important to explore how fully Dan comprehends his likely quality of life on mechanical ventilation, the temporary pain from surgery, and his right to stop treatment at any time once it is started.

Conscious efforts to create new therapeutic options can also be pivotal. The confusing problem sometimes does not admit solution because a possible solution is not even being considered. These options may not be "standard operating procedure." For example, in Dan's case, suppose his health care team is unfamiliar with or simply has yet to use noninvasive mechanical ventilation, which does not require tracheotomy. Proposing a trial of noninvasive mechanical ventilation may be less threatening to Dan, so he might assent to this course of therapy. This treatment option would minimize any violation of his preferences; it would also enable him to examine his preferences under new circumstances and perhaps come to understand them better.

No guarantee exists, however, that clarification of trade-offs or attempts to create new options will lead to resolution of the dilemma. Under such circumstances, consultation with an ethics committee can be invaluable. While asking for help from an ethics consultative service is almost never a bad idea, here it can add value in two key ways. First, the members of the committee may help to discover a "breakthrough" with the trade-off clarification or option creation process. Second, if the consultation still results in deadlock, the committee can help absorb the psychological weight of making an incredibly difficult yet unavoidable decision, assisting all parties not simply to make the best possible decision, but to live with it in peace.

ARTICULATE DISAGREEMENT

Sara is a newborn with hypoplastic left heart syndrome. This condition, if left untreated, is always fatal. Alternatively, surgery can be done to create a partially functional heart from the existing malformed one, or a heart transplantation can be performed. Both of these surgical options entail extensive operations with prolonged and recurrent hospitalizations, significant morbidity, an unknown amount of suffering, and a significant probability that the patient will die despite these efforts. Sara's parents, after learning about this condition and the treatment options from both the neonatologist and the pediatric cardiologist, decide that they want to take their daughter home and keep her as comfortable as possible until she dies. Deeply religious, they believe that the most important thing they can do for Sara is to surround her with the love of family and friends, and then let God take her back, with them waiting until they can finally rejoin their daughter in the afterlife. The cardiologist, when informed of their decision, requests an ethics consultation, stating that to decline potentially lifesaving cardiac surgery is tantamount to medical neglect.

Should surgery be provided, and who should make the decision?

In this situation, all the parties want to do what is best for the patient, but there are differing views concerning what is best. Making a judgment about what is in the best interests of the infant involves a trade-off between improving the probability of long-term survival and avoiding reductions in quality of life. This case reflects the fact that reasonable people can disagree concerning how to weigh the duty to preserve life against the duty to avoid causing harm (Feudtner, 2008; Kon, 2008; Wernovsky, 2008; Ross and Frader, 2009).

The disagreement in this case gives rise to two distinct ethical issues—a substantive issue and a procedural one. Substantive issues have to do with the question of what is the right action, such as whether or not surgical treatment should be provided. Procedural issues pertain to the question of who should make the decision when there is disagreement. Added complexity arises because these two issues, although distinct, cannot be entirely separated; the question of who should make the decision sometimes depends on what the right decision is. Normally, parents should be allowed to make medical decisions for their children, for several reasons. First, the presumption that parents want what is best for their children is reasonable because experience shows that in most cases it is true. In a given case, we should presume that it is true unless the parents' behavior indicates otherwise. Second, parents should be permitted a domain of autonomy in making decisions about how to raise their children, a domain that encompasses the making of medical decisions for their children.

Despite this presumption, it is possible to have conflicts between parental autonomy and the well-being of the child; parents sometimes make medical decisions that are contrary to the child's interests. In such cases, it is considered ethical for the state to intervene in order to protect the child, and it is justifiable for health care providers to seek a court order authorizing treatment. But this raises the difficult question of distinguishing between cases in which intervention is justifiable and cases in which it is not.

FACTORS TO CONSIDER IN DECIDING
WHETHER TO OVERRULE THE PARENTS

Ethical analysis can help by identifying factors to consider that can vary from case to case. To identify these factors, it is useful to consider the ethical values that are central to the case: the well-being of the patient, the well-being of the family, and the autonomy of the parents. Several factors are relevant to the well-being of the patient. One such factor is the magnitude of the harm that the treatment would aim to prevent. Some cases involve life-threatening conditions, while other cases involve harms that are less severe. Another factor is the likelihood that the proposed treatment would be effective in preventing the harm in question. The more likely it is that the treatment would be effective, the stronger the argument for intervening. Other factors related to the patient's well-being are the likelihood that the treatment would have side effects and complications that would be harmful to the patient and the magnitude of such harm if it occurs. Factors related to the family's well-being include the likelihood that emotional and psychological harm would occur to the family if the parents' wishes are overridden and the expected magnitude of such harm. When there is prolonged treatment of seriously ill children, families usually need sustained emotional support from the health care providers. But forcing treatment undermines the ability of the health care team to provide such support. A factor related to parental autonomy is the degree of intrusion into family life that would be required in imposing treatment over the objections of the parents.

The argument for intervening is relatively strong when the treatment is lifesaving, highly likely to be effective, unlikely to have significant side effects, and can be accomplished quickly so that there is minimal intrusion into the daily life of the family. An example of a case in which these conditions for intervening clearly are satisfied involves parental refusal of lifesaving blood transfusions for an otherwise healthy child. By contrast, the strength of the argument diminishes when, as in the present case, there is substantial uncertainty whether the treatment would be effective, the treatment would likely involve complications that would significantly diminish the patient's quality of life, and the parents would be required to cooperate with treatment they disagree with over a sustained period of time. These considerations suggest that the argument for intervening is not strong enough in this case to justify overriding the parents' decision (Ackerman, 1980; Kon, 2008).

These are the sorts of considerations that should be taken into account by the ethics committee that is consulted. In this case, these considerations support the view that the parents should be the ones who decide. The committee should attempt to explain to the cardiologist that the current case differs in several important ways from the sorts of cases in which overriding the parents' wishes is justifiable. When persons can reasonably disagree over what is best for the child, we should defer to parental autonomy and respect the parents' wishes.

Bobby, a 7-year-old boy, has relapsed with leukemia 3 months after undergoing a bone marrow transplant. His parents and physicians, after considering Bobby's prognosis and the available treatment options, have agreed to focus on palliative goals of care to enable Bobby to enjoy life as much as possible, to maximize his comfort, and to keep him at home, far from the tertiary care center where he has received his cancer therapy. Unfortunately, when the health care team calls hospice and home nursing services in his rural home county, they all decline to accept him as a patient, citing the fact that "we don't know how to take proper care of children."

Access to palliative care is a policy issue as well as a clinical issue. What are the obstacles to improving access to palliative care? What can be done to overcome these obstacles?

Our health care system currently gives inadequate attention to palliative care. This problem is manifest in a number of ways. Many physicians have not recognized the value of palliative care and lack the technical skills required for its provision. Medical schools and residency programs are only recently beginning to provide any training in palliative care. Insurance often does not cover or inadequately covers the costs of providing palliative care, and community resources, such as hospice programs or home nursing services, are insufficient in many areas. The lack of pediatric palliative and hospice care, therefore, is the consequence of a multifaceted problem involving many aspects of our current health care system (Field and Behrman, 2003). To improve access to palliative care, all dimensions of this problem must be addressed through a variety of efforts, ranging from physician education to policy changes regarding reimbursement for services.

Persuading more physicians to join the bandwagon requires overcoming a number of obstacles. Many physicians still regard palliative care as an alternative to curative efforts, rather than something that can occur together with life-prolonging treatment. As a result, there often is reluctance to "switch" to palliative care because that means "giving up" on cure-oriented or disease-directed approaches. Some physicians regard stopping such efforts as an acknowledgment of failure. But palliative care or supportive care, to use another term, is often appropriate even as attempts to cure or prolong life are taking place (Sahler et al., 2000; Hubble et al., 2009). One key element in increasing access to palliative care is to educate physicians to embrace palliative care as an essential element of good care in the face of serious medical conditions. Unfortunately, many physicians are reluctant to use adequate pain medications for (sometimes legitimate) fear of being sanctioned by their state licensing boards. Their concern is that they might be accused of causing addiction or collaborating with addicts if they write large numbers of prescriptions for high doses of opiates, and that they might risk losing their medical licenses. In response, some states have passed legislation to reassure physicians that adequate treatment of pain will not result in the loss of one's license (Gilson, Maurer, and Jorenson, 2005).

There is a need for better insurance coverage for palliative care. In recent years many payers have not been especially responsive to consumer demands, and therefore legislation might be required to bring about improved coverage. Several studies have suggested that costs may indeed be reduced when palliative care is provided (Lonberger, Russell, and Burton, 1997; Morrison et al., 2008). Pragmatically speaking, further demonstrations of cost savings might be the most persuasive argument to motivate insurance companies to change their policies on reimbursement for services. Whether or not this pragmatic argument holds true in pediatric palliative care remains to be demonstrated. Ultimately, however, our medical system should not be governed merely by monetary considerations, as health care organizations are bound by ethical responsibilities similar to those that bind individual health care providers in a covenant with their patients (Reiser, 1994; Spencer et al., 2000). The provision of palliative care is a duty for health care providers, and facilitating the provision of palliative care services is a duty for health care organizations and the society that encompasses them.

CULTURAL DIFFERENCES

David, age 10, undergoes surgery for a malignant brain tumor. Tumor infiltration is extensive; tragically, he never regains consciousness following surgery. The physicians explain to David's parents that there is nothing else they can do for him that will eliminate the cancer. They encourage his parents to take David home or move him to a facility where he can receive palliative care. His parents refuse, saying that, as Orthodox Jews, they believe that every effort must be made to preserve their son's life. The hospital exhausts every possibility to find another facility to accept him, to no avail. Two months after the surgery, the physicians declare David dead, based on clinical criteria for brain death. They explain to his parents that his entire brain has stopped functioning, that this is irreversible and he is now legally dead, and that his body will be removed from the ventilator. The parents state that their religious beliefs do not recognize brain death, and that they consider him to be alive, reiterating that every effort must be made to keep him alive, and insisting that the ventilator not be turned off.

*Should the health care professionals act unilaterally and turn off the
  ventilator?*
How should cultural values enter into the resolution of the case?
*Can the conflict be resolved in a way that permits the health care team
  to continue providing emotional support to the parents?*

Cultural differences can lead patients and families to have different perceptions of clinical events, in comparison to health care professionals. Familiarity with the cultural beliefs and practices of their patients can help health care professionals provide culturally sensitive care. Orthodox Jews will often consult their rabbis to make sure their health care meets rabbinic standards, and some (but not all) Orthodox rabbinic authorities maintain that whole brain death does not constitute death of the person. When health care professionals and parents disagree over such matters, good communication is important to help all parties understand the perspectives of the others.

From the health care professionals' perspective, further use of the ventilator in David's case does not constitute treatment and is not correctly described as "life preserving" because the patient is already dead. Consideration of the health care professionals' various obligations, some of which conflict, can be helpful in deciding how to respond to the parents' request. From the health care professionals' perspective, it can be argued that there is an obligation *not* to continue ventilator support because doing so would use resources in a way that does not provide health-related benefit to the patient. But palliative care includes respecting the family's need for emotional and spiritual support, and this implies an obligation to respect their wishes if that is necessary in order to provide such support. The main question is which of these obligations should have priority.

There are medical considerations that are relevant to this type of situation. Attempts to maintain pregnant brain-dead patients for the sake of their fetuses have shown that it is extremely challenging to maintain circulatory function in such cadavers for an extended period of time (Field et al., 1988). With loss of all brainstem functions, the body's self-regulatory capacity ceases, and frequent and wide fluctuations in vital signs such as temperature and blood pressure result. Experience has shown that even aggressive efforts to maintain such bodies rarely succeed for long (Vives et al., 1996; Catanzarite et al., 1997). This contrasts with patients in a persistent vegetative state, whose continued brainstem functioning permits them, in many cases, to be maintained for extended periods.

With knowledge that aggressive efforts might not maintain cardiac activity for long, the health care team could acquiesce to the parents' request. This would avoid confrontation, show respect for the family's cultural values, and enable the team to maintain good rapport with the parents, thereby facilitating support for them.

Some health care professionals involved in David's care may be experiencing "moral distress" because of the disagreement about brain death, and perhaps because of earlier disagreements regarding the goals of care. For those professionals, a meeting with the ethics committee or a support group may provide a forum to share their own feelings about the case, to talk openly about the impact of differing cultural values and perspectives, and to discuss strategies for working with similar families in the future.

DISCONTINUING NON-ORAL NUTRITION AND HYDRATION

Abby was a previously healthy 4-year-old. She went to bed with a slight fever; however, her mother found her unresponsive in the morning. Admitted to the hospital with encephalopathy and seizures, she initially required intubation and mechanical ventilation because of her decreased mental status, but was able to breathe on her own after 4 weeks and was extubated. Despite the improvement in her brainstem function, enabling her to breathe on her own, her cortical function (thinking, remembering, interacting, motor control) deteriorated over the 6 weeks of her hospitalization, finally leading to a persistent vegetative state with severe brainstem dysfunction, resulting in frequent episodes of "autonomic storms." She could not eat or drink by mouth, and nutrition was supplied by gastrostomy tube. The episodes of storming were frequent and very distressing for caregivers and family members to witness. After weeks of struggling with how best to care for their daughter, thoroughly discussing the issues with their religious advisor, meeting extensively with their daughter's care team, and ultimately questioning the quality of her life, the parents requested that non-oral nutrition and hydration be withdrawn.

When is the withdrawal of non-oral nutrition and hydration appropriate?

Non-oral nutrition and hydration constitute medical treatments that may be withdrawn when the burden outweighs the benefit to the patient (Strong, 1981; Carter and Leuthner, 2003; Slomka, 2003; Diekema, Botkin, and the

Committee on Bioethics, 2009). Although such withdrawal can be ethically appropriate, clinical situations involving such removal are almost always emotionally charged. The act of feeding is one of the first bonding activities between parent and child. Eating and drinking are both so culturally and religiously significant that the idea of a dependent person *not* being fed is beyond what many people can tolerate as morally acceptable. It is critical that people be able to appreciate the many social and cultural values assigned to eating, such as joining the family at the table for a meal or participating in the rituals of bread and wine in religious practices, that are different from being medically nourished and hydrated through a tube. Even so, the challenge to accept this on an emotional level is rarely straightforward. A discussion of the goals of nutrition and hydration should be considered by all concerned. Parents have the legal and moral right to make medical and other decisions for their children. Although other parties may question parental decisions, there must be compelling evidence that the parents are not acting in the best interest of the child in order to justify overriding those decisions, as discussed above in Sara's case. If there are disagreements among the staff regarding withdrawing medical nutrition and hydration, a consultation from the ethics committee can be helpful.

When an intervention such as non-oral nutrition is withheld, other care measures need to be employed to reduce any associated pain and suffering—both for the child and also for the family and other caregivers. Such actions can include, depending on the situation, lip and mouth care, physical touching or holding, and judicious use of mild anxiolytic agents.

Conclusion

Ethically problematic situations occur across all stages of the delivery of pediatric palliative care, including the recognition of a patient's need for such care, the initiation of efforts to give such care, and the ongoing involvement of team members in providing it. Resolution of these ethical issues is aided by knowledge of the goals of palliative care and the values underlying these goals, as illustrated by the case discussions above. In analyzing these cases, we used the language of ethics, invoking terms such as "*autonomy,*" "*beneficence,*" and "*nonmaleficence.*" This language provides a useful means for thinking through ethical problems and discussing them with colleagues. In providing palliative care, knowledge of these concepts and the skill of ethical analysis must be combined with other knowledge and skills, as indicated in table 2.1. In the table, we attempt to identify various stages in the provision of palliative care. For each stage we give examples of knowledge and skills that are needed. The examples, of course, are not exhaustive, and some types of knowledge and skill are needed at more than one stage of the process, as suggested in the table.

References

Ackerman, T.F. 1980. The limits of beneficence: Jehovah's Witnesses and childhood cancer. *Hastings Cent Rep* 10:13–18.

American Academy of Pediatrics, Committee on Bioethics. 1994. Guidelines on forgoing life-sustaining medical treatment. *Pediatrics* 93:532–36.

American Medical Association. 1999. Medical futility in end-of-life care: Report of the Council on Ethical and Judicial Affairs. *JAMA* 281:937–41.

Baker, R.B. 1999. The American medical ethics revolution. In *The American Medical Ethics Revolution: How the AMA's Code of Ethics Has Transformed Physicians' Relationships to Patients, Professionals, and Society*, ed. R.B. Baker, A.L. Caplan, L.L. Emanuel, et al., pp. 17–51. Baltimore: Johns Hopkins University Press.

Beauchamp, T.L., and Childress, J.F. 2009. *Principles of Biomedical Ethics*, 6th ed. New York: Oxford University Press.

Browning, D.M. 2003. To show our humanness: Relational and communicative competence in pediatric palliative care. *Bioethics Forum* 18:23–28.

Buckman, R. 1992. *How to Break Bad News: A Guide for Health Care Professionals*. Baltimore: Johns Hopkins University Press.

Carter, B.S., and Leuthner, S.R. 2003. The ethics of withholding/withdrawing nutrition in the newborn. *Sem Perinatol* 27:480–87.

Catanzarite, V.A., Willms, D.C., Holdy, K.E., et al. 1997. Brain death during pregnancy: Tocolytic therapy and aggressive maternal support on behalf of the fetus. *Am J Perinatol* 14:431–34.

Creagan, E.T. 1994. How to break bad news—and not devastate the patient. *Mayo Clin Proc* 69:1015–17.

Diekema, D.S., Botkin, J.R., and the Committee on Bioethics. 2009. Forgoing medically provided nutrition and hydration in children. *Pediatrics* 124:813–22.

Feudtner, C. 2005. Hope and the prospects of healing at the end of life. *J Altern Complement Med* 11 (Suppl 1):S23–30.

———. 2007. Collaborative communication in pediatric palliative care: A foundation for problem-solving and decision-making. *Pediatr Clin North Am* 54:583–607.

———. 2008. Ethics in the midst of therapeutic evolution. *Arch Pediatr Adolesc Med* 162:854–57.

Feudtner, C., Christakis, D.A., and Schwartz, P. 1996. Ethics and the art of confrontation: Lessons from the John Conley Essays. *JAMA* 276:755–56.

Field, D.R., Gates, E.A., Creasy, R.K., et al. 1988. Maternal brain death during pregnancy. *JAMA* 260:816–22.

Field, M.J., and Behrman, R.E., eds. 2003. *When Children Die: Improving Palliative and End-of-Life Care for Children and Their Families*. Institute of Medicine Report. Washington, DC: National Academies Press.

Gilson, A.M., Maurer, M.A., and Jorenson, D.E. 2005. State policy affecting pain management: Recent improvements and the positive impact of regulatory health policies. *Health Policy* 74:192–204.

Girgis, A., and Sanson-Fisher, R.W. 1995. Breaking bad news: Consensus guidelines for medical practitioners. *J Clin Oncol* 13:2449–56.

Hammond, J.S., Keeney, R.L., and Raiffa, H. 1999. *Smart Choices: A Practical Guide to Making Better Decisions*. Boston: Harvard Business School Press.

Hubble, R.A., Ward-Smith, P., Christenson, K.P., et al. 2009. Implementation of a palliative care team in a pediatric hospital. *J Pediatr Health Care* 23:126–31.

Johnston, C. 2009. Overriding competent medical treatment refusal by adolescents: When "no" means "no." *Arch Dis Child* 94:487–91.

Kon, A. A. 2008. Healthcare providers must offer palliative treatment to parents of neonates with hypoplastic left heart syndrome. *Arch Pediatr Adolesc Med* 162: 844–48.

Levetown, M., and the American Academy of Pediatrics Committee on Bioethics. 2008. Communicating with children and families: From everyday interactions to skill in conveying distressing information. *Pediatrics* 121:e1441–60.

Lonberger, E.A., Russell, C.L., and Burton, S.M. 1997. The effects of palliative care on patient charges. *J Nurs Admin* 27:23–26.

Mack, J.W., and Wolfe, J. 2008. Early integration of pediatric palliative care: For some children, palliative care starts at diagnosis. *Curr Opin Pediatr* 18:10–14.

Mack, J.W., Wolfe, J., Cook, E.F., et al. 2007. Hope and prognostic disclosure. *J Clin Oncol* 25:5636–42.

Morrison, R.S., Penrod, J.D., Cassel, J.B., et al. 2008. Palliative care leadership centers' outcomes group: Cost savings associated with US hospital palliative care consultation programs. *Arch Intern Med* 168:1783–90.

Mosenthal, A.C., Murphy, P.A., Barker, L.K., et al. 2008. Changing the culture around end-of-life care in the trauma intensive care unit. *J Trauma* 64:1587–93.

Reiser, S.J. 1994. The ethical life of health care organizations. *Hastings Cent Rep* 24: 28–35.

Ross, L.F., and Frader, J. 2009. Hypoplastic left heart syndrome: A paradigm case for examining conscientious objection in pediatric practice. *J Pediatr* 155:12–15.

Sahler, O.J.Z., Frager, G., Levetown, M., et al. 2000. Medical education about end-of-life care in the pediatric setting: Principles, challenges, and opportunities. *Pediatrics* 105:575–84.

Slomka, J. 2003. Withholding nutrition at the end of life: Clinical and ethical issues. *Cleve Clin J Med* 70:548–52.

Spencer, E.M., Mills, A.E., Rorty, M.V., et al. 2000. *Organization Ethics in Health Care*. New York: Oxford University Press.

Stone, D.F., Patton, B., and Heen, S. 1999. *Difficult Conversations: How to Discuss What Matters Most*. New York: Penguin Books.

Strong, C. 1981. Can fluids and electrolytes be extraordinary treatment? *J Med Ethics* 7:83–85.

———. 2003. Fetal anomalies: Ethical and legal considerations in screening, detection, and management. *Clin Perinatol* 30:113–26.

Vives, A., Carmona, F., Zabala, E., et al. 1996. Maternal brain death during pregnancy. *Int J Gynaecol Obstet* 52:67–69.

Wernovsky, G. 2008. The paradigm shift toward surgical intervention for neonates with hypoplastic left heart syndrome. *Arch Pediatr Adolesc Med* 162:849–54.

World Health Organization. 1990. *Cancer Pain Relief and Palliative Care*. Technical Report Series 804. Geneva: World Health Organization.

3

Barriers to Integrating Palliative Care and Potential Solutions

Patrick M. Jones, M.D., M.A., Sally Sehring, M.D., Dianne Gray, B.S., and David M. Steinhorn, M.D.

Aaron, a 3-month-old boy who has Krabbe disease, is referred to the palliative care team. He has undergone a bone marrow transplantation, which unfortunately failed to reverse the symptoms of the underlying disease. The disease has progressed, and he now depends on a ventilator, is unresponsive, and is not expected to survive more than a few months. His mother, Alicia, a single parent, would like to spend time with him at home, where his 2-year-old sister, Abby, is waiting for him. Alicia would like Aaron to be able to die at home, but they live in a small, rural community, served only by an adult hospice in a nearby town. Alicia has begun to process the paperwork for a Medicaid waiver for medically fragile, ventilator-dependent children but has not yet received approval. The pediatrician practicing in the family's community is uncomfortable with technology-dependent and terminally ill children. Aaron seems destined to spend his remaining days in the acute care hospital because of the lack of suitable community resources, associated medical oversight, and systems to honor his family's wishes.

Recognition of the need for hospital- and community-based pediatric palliative care is growing. The public is increasingly aware of the presence of children who will not reach adulthood; however, relatively few children and their families are able to access high-quality, family-centered pediatric palliative and hospice care when needed. Wolfe and colleagues' documentation of unmitigated suffering experienced by children dying of cancer in one of the most forward-thinking medical settings in the United States is a call to action for individuals and organizations concerned about the well-being of children living with complex medical conditions. These data should serve as a potent stimulus to all health care providers, administrators, and public policy makers to evaluate why it is so difficult to meet the needs of children living with life-threatening conditions (Wolfe et al., 2000; Field and Behrman, 2003).

While advocating for the uniform and consistent integration of palliative care into health care for children, the reader needs to appreciate the difficulties that families face in obtaining optimal care for children living with life-threatening conditions. In the last decade, numerous authors have chronicled the obstacles (AAP COB, 2000; Meisel et al., 2000; Wolfe et al., 2000; Hilden et al., 2001; Himelstein, 2006; Löfmark, Nilstun, and Bolmsjö, 2007; Davies et al., 2008; Johnston et al., 2008; Steele, Bosma, and Johnston, 2008; Schickedanz et al., 2009). This chapter addresses the major barriers to pediatric palliative care as experienced throughout North America and in many other parts of the world:

- Lack of clarity regarding the nature of palliative care
- Poor communication
- Racial, social, and ethnic barriers
- Unrealistic expectations
- Reimbursement and financing
- Organizational obstacles

Lack of Clarity regarding the Nature of Palliative Care

An exciting opportunity for the emerging discipline of pediatric palliative care is to define the scope and modulate the public perception of the field. One of the fundamental obstacles to making palliative care services available is a lack of clarity among health care providers regarding what constitutes palliative care, including how palliative care differs from either skilled home nursing care or hospice care. Such misunderstandings arise in part from the fact that pediatric palliative care is a relatively new field and the majority of pediatric clinicians have no formal training in or exposure to systems for delivering effective pediatric palliative care. Pediatric palliative care programs ideally offer a broad set of services, integrating effectively to optimize the experience of illness for the patient and family, whether the goals of care are directed at the disease (including attempts to cure) or, at the other end of the spectrum, are focused on end-of-life care. As noted by the American

Academy of Pediatrics (AAP COB, 2000), palliative and curative therapies should not be mutually exclusive. It is generally accepted that

> the aim of palliative care is to improve the quality of life of patients and their families facing life-threatening illness, through the prevention, assessment and treatment of pain and other physical, psychosocial and spiritual problems. Palliative care provides relief from pain and other distressing symptoms; affirms life and regards dying as a normal process; intends neither to hasten nor to postpone death; integrates the psychological and spiritual aspects of patient care; offers a support system to help patients live as actively as possible until death; offers a support system to help the family cope during the patient's illness and in their own bereavement; and uses a team approach to address the needs of patients and their families. (Löfmark, Nilstun, and Bolmsjö, 2007, p. 685)

Pediatric palliative care providers are in the process of defining the optimal model of delivery across the spectrum of health care, developing strategies for reimbursement and sustainability, and even determining what constitutes core palliative care services for children. Thus, it is not surprising that clinicians, patients, and families are often not certain what services can or should be provided. While most medical specialties have come to define the boundaries of their fields, the range of services offered in a pediatric palliative care program is currently variable, depending on institutional support, availability of skilled individuals within each institution to provide such services, and the overall vision of how pediatric palliative care can close gaps in services provided by the institution. As clinical pediatric palliative care services and training programs develop further, it is likely that a consensus will emerge as to what constitutes basic and comprehensive pediatric palliative care. Improved reimbursement for services will also define pediatric palliative care, as the financial incentives supporting institutions drive availability, as discussed below. Finally, consumer demand for consistent, high-quality palliative care will further influence the final definition of needed services.

The transition from attempts to cure a condition to maximizing the quality of life as the primary goal is often subtle and cannot be precisely determined. Certain events, however, may herald a shift in goals. These include failure of a bone marrow transplant to restore health, recurrence of a cancer, repeated hospitalization for pneumonia for patients with severe neurodevelopmental disability, and inability to wean from mechanical ventilation. All too frequently, one hears the statement, "It is not time yet for palliative care," revealing the misconception that palliative care is of value only at the final phase of life, rather than functioning to enhance the quality of life throughout the trajectory of a potentially life-threatening condition. Improved access to pediatric palliative care will not occur until there is increased appreciation of the value of maximizing the quality of life throughout the course of illness. Pediatric palliative care (PPC) teams currently have to demonstrate their worth institution by institution, owing to a lack of universally accepted norms of care. Research is urgently needed to demonstrate the value of pediatric palliative care to clinicians, patients, families, and institutions. Further, a social marketing campaign directed at clinicians and families alike is needed to overcome existing misperceptions of the role and benefit of pediatric palliative care.

Sometimes clinicians are not ready to acknowledge the need for palliative care, and sometimes the family fears that accepting palliative care is tantamount to "giving up on their child" (Davies et al., 2008). While it may be impossible to identify the optimal time to begin a discussion of palliative care, many experts feel that early involvement of the PPC team is ideal (AAP COB, 2000). Early involvement of PPC teams enables improved communication, attention to symptom control, and continuity of care and sets the stage for greater involvement if the prospect for cure or satisfactory outcome diminishes or the uncertainty of goals mixed with grief becomes the dominant concern. Early involvement of the PPC team also prevents feelings of abandonment, as the end-of-life caregivers are then familiar with the family's journey—they have shared in the joys and sorrows—and are better prepared to accompany the family on the last leg as trusted caregivers, not new faces. Thus, it is vitally important for pediatric clinicians to understand that involvement of the PPC team does not imply that the patient is certain to die or that cure will not be achieved; rather, it acknowledges that the outcome is uncertain and that additional support focused on optimizing the experience of the child's life can be beneficial, even while struggling to achieve a cure or prolong life. The introduction of the PPC team to the family must be undertaken in the same manner as the offer of the assistance of chaplains and child-life therapists for support. The team becomes an added value, contributing to a more positive experience for the child and family.

The role played by the PPC team is typically supportive in the beginning, maintaining communication and facilitating discussions between the primary medical team and the family and assessing the patient's and family's overall response to treatment as the clinical course progresses. In some settings, the PPC team may also attend to the assessment and management of symptoms, the family's and child's experiences of grief and loss, and the interface between home and hospital. Their adjunctive role may change over time as the clinical realities change. For example, it is standard practice in some institutions to introduce the PPC team to patients and families before stem cell transplantation as one of the many available family support resources; frequent, brief visits with the patient and family allow this relationship to deepen and solidify. If all goes well, the PPC team can step back from direct involvement with the patient but is available if relapse or complications occur. If the transplant is unsuccessful or if life-threatening complications arise, the PPC team can provide an increased presence, helping the family to choose their best option. In the pediatric ICU and NICU settings, a similar role can be of benefit to patients and families if the initial prognosis is guarded. The PPC team may lead or participate in discussions regarding prognosis, goals of care, options to support those goals, probable response to resuscitation efforts, and the desire to limit no-longer-beneficial interventions. Importantly, the PPC team members may be the ones most attuned to the child's symptom distress, as well as the more general well-being of the family and child (Zhukovsky et al., 2009). In most settings, it is the primary team that writes the medical orders; therefore, the PPC team must be trusted by and integrate effectively with the primary team to see their recommendations implemented. This can be achieved in part by helping families manage tremendous uncertainties, constantly helping them assess the benefits versus burdens of therapeutic options. The interdisciplinary nature of the PPC team can benefit the family by eliciting an integrated, whole person and family-centered perspective on the situation. Unlike conventional multidisciplinary teams, in which each support service (e.g., social worker, chaplain, nurse, physician) operates within its own discipline and independent of the others, PPC team members frequently share the job of problem solving, counseling, and interpreting medical facts, functioning in an interdisciplinary or even transdisciplinary manner.

Confusion regarding the place and role of palliative care in some institutions has led to requests for PPC team consultation for many chronically ill children who have complex medical conditions but are not at risk of death in the next several years. Although it can be argued that many families and pediatric patients would benefit from the wide range of psychosocial and medical services provided by the PPC team, because of resource limitations, it is not practical to include the entire spectrum of children with medically complex conditions. Thus, clinicians must be selective regarding which children are offered palliative care to ensure care for those who will most benefit from it. In contrast to palliative care reimbursement, most states have well-established programs and waivers for the care of children who have various chronic and medically complex conditions. Thus, the PPC team must be aware of its own resource limitations and not become overextended by providing support to children whose lives are not genuinely threatened. The Center to Advance Palliative Care (CAPC) created a helpful list of conditions for which palliative care referral is most appropriate (available at www .capc.org/tools-for-palliative-care-programs/clinical-tools/consult-triggers/ pediatric-palliative-care-referral-criteria.doc).

Pediatric hospice and palliative medicine is an evolving specialty, differing from adult palliative care owing to the developmental variability of the patients and families served, their diverse medical conditions and responses to medical and pharmacological interventions, and the lack of societal acceptance of childhood illness and death. A general consensus exists among clinicians regarding the scope and purview of the specialty; however, there exist areas of significant overlap among palliative care and oncology, critical care services, the medical home, care of medically complex and chronically ill children, and each of the other specialties managing children living with life-threatening conditions (e.g., cardiology, neurology, genetics). While research in the field continues to reveal areas of unmet need for patients, families, and clinicians, we anticipate a gradual adoption of palliative care *principles* throughout medical practice, resulting in improved care for all patients. Perhaps one of the greatest contributions of the field of palliative care is improved awareness of the obligation to manage patients' illnesses in a holistic manner by attending to each patient's illness-related physical, emotional, social, and spiritual needs.

Impact of Ineffective Communication on the Provision of Pediatric Palliative Care

Difficulty in communication among physicians, nurses, and families is one of the most common obstacles to successfully integrating palliative care with other aspects of patient care. Problems may arise from language differences, cultural or values differences, and poor training of physicians regarding the use of appropriate language in discussing patients' conditions, likely outcomes, therapeutic choices, and family coping. It is also clear that uncoordinated clinician-family communication may lead to conflicting information and family confusion. Lack of confirmation of the family's comprehension of critical information is also common. Finally, lack of attention to the need to communicate with multiple family members may lead to one family member relaying confused information to other members, propagating misunderstanding and creating unnecessary conflict.

Language barriers constitute an enormous difficulty within our multicultural society. In any given community, it is impossible for clinicians to communicate with all of their patients' families with equal finesse and effectiveness. In palliative care, conversations have deep-seated emotional currents; nuanced wording and culturally expected pacing and other nonverbal cues are difficult to accommodate by a nonnative speaker or via a third-party conversation. Every clinician who has attempted a difficult family discussion using the services of a medical interpreter realizes that it is impossible to confer the same degree of understanding and empathy as can be accomplished with language-concordant families.

Additionally, cultural differences can lead to misunderstandings of critical clinical issues, such as what is meant by "limitation of life support" or "do not resuscitate." The lack of recognition by some cultures of certain Western medical concepts, such as "brain death" or the even more ethereal concept of "futility," makes it clear that effective communication requires an institutional commitment to reliable, effective, high-quality interpretation services. Each institution must address this issue based on available resources. Options include in-house medical interpreters for the most common languages, dial-in language interpreting by telephone service, or local interpretation services for large ethnic groups within the community. Family members are typically not the best resources for interpretation because of their lack of understanding of the medical terminology both in English and in their own native language, as well as the emotional blocking that can interfere with the transmission of information to the actual decision makers. One approach some hospitals are exploring is to offer orientation sessions to medical interpreters to enhance their understanding of palliative care principles and concepts. Such efforts will help these team members develop vocabularies and idiomatically correct jargon for discussing the subtle aspects of palliative care in the family's native language. It is beyond the scope of this chapter to suggest universal solutions for communication barriers; however, recognition of the linguistic challenges is an important initial step in achieving an effective exchange with families. Without superb linguistic support, discussion of family goals and values is difficult and can lead to misunderstandings that interfere with the development of trust between family and clinicians.

Several behaviors on the part of physicians in particular are recognized to impede effective end-of-life care and communication (Beckstrand and Kirchhoff, 2005). These behaviors include

- being evasive and avoiding frank conversations;
- offering uncoordinated or conflicting opinions from consultants;
- not involving bedside nurses in discussions of patients' care.

Heaston reported that good communication between physicians and nurses, as well as physicians' direct discussions with families, is critical in the end-of-life care setting, just as in other areas of medical care (Heaston et al., 2006; Löfmark, Nilstun, and Bolmsjö, 2007). Empathetic listening is the single most important requirement for effective communication (Penson et al., 2005). However, sufficient time must also be allocated for effective, supportive communications to occur (Davies et al., 2008). Families that feel forced into making decisions are frequently resentful and often resist making decisions, resulting in frustration and exasperation on the part of the medical team (Luce and White, 2007). Often the palliative care team member who has invested the time to develop a trusting longitudinal relationship with the patient and family is in the best position to understand their wishes. Thus, the PPC team can be an important communication liaison between the patient-family and the primary medical team.

In an earlier era of hospice as the only model of palliative care, the introduction of the "palliative care" team often signified that the patient was nearing death. In contemporary pediatric palliative care, the situation is very different, although confusion still exists (St-Laurent-Gagnon, Carnevale, and Duval, 2008; Thompson et al., 2009). Currently, the initial role of the PPC team is largely one of support, clarification of family values, and validation of the choices families make. The goal is to facilitate the articulation of realistic goals based on the patient's and family's values. Therefore, the team must be composed of clinicians who have exceptional listening and communication skills. Over time, the role of the PPC team changes, depending on the child's response to treatment, the child's and family's experiences of illness, and their evolving judgment of the burdens and benefits of the current care plan. Listening and communicating remain essential elements of care, although the PPC team may also take a more active role in assessing and managing symptoms, decision making, and discharge planning. Ideally, the PPC team proves itself essential to the child, family, and primary medical team as it shoulders the responsibility for challenging aspects of the care of children nearing the end of life.

There are many exciting opportunities for developing novel approaches to meet diverse families' needs. Close collaboration among experts in cultural sensitivity, interpretation, and palliative care will enable the discovery of new ways to most effectively communicate our collective concern, compassion, and caring for families in the most vulnerable circumstances.

Racial, Social, and Ethnic Barriers to the Provision of Pediatric Palliative Care

Disparities that various minority groups experience in the access to and quality of health care are the subject of a burgeoning body of health services research. Attempts are being made to understand both why such disparities exist and how to overcome them. Minorities and individuals of low socioeconomic and educational status experience obstacles to receiving palliative care for individuals of all ages, including children. One explanation is the lack of suitable services within local communities. However, a more formidable reason is often the tendency of some families to insist on more "life-prolonging" treatment in the face of overwhelming odds of suffering and death. In so doing, the burdens of disease-directed intervention often far outweigh the benefits (from the clinicians' viewpoint), rather than achieving the goal of maximizing the child's quality of life for the time remaining. Some of the greatest challenges to the acceptance of palliative care services are patients' and families' misconceptions of the likelihood of cure as well as their preconceived notions of the purpose and implications of palliative care. In such circumstances, the PPC team can play a vital role in assisting the primary care team to educate the family on the value of pediatric palliative care. While acknowledging the family's stress, love, and profound grief, the PPC team can nonjudgmentally assist the family to more clearly understand and reflect on the child's prognosis, associated family values, and the viable choices in the context of the child's best interests.

High-quality pediatric palliative care or hospice services are often available in medical centers and affluent, suburban areas. Such services for adults have evolved through consumer demand and the presence of patients with financial resources to support it. Children requiring palliative and hospice care, however, are still frequently unable to access care once they leave the medical center. There is great variability in the capacity of various community-based organizations to provide the services required by children at home. The availability of home-based pediatric palliative care services is often severely limited in inner-city and poor urban areas. The logistic difficulties of metropolitan areas can be enormous, such as encountering thick traffic while attempting to rapidly reach a patient in crisis, as well as ensuring personnel safety in some inner-city neighborhoods while transporting controlled substances or making emergency visits at night. While the high population density in large metropolitan regions favors the economic viability of adult palliative care and hospice services, most of these organizations cannot provide in-depth pediatric expertise or the full range of child-oriented services because of the far smaller number of children served by any given agency. While large metropolitan areas have a greater number of children requiring palliative care services, even these communities are unlikely to have a sufficient density of pediatric patients to support a single organization providing comprehensive pediatric palliative care. Logistic and financial challenges are compounded when the small population of patients in any region is cared for by multiple community-based palliative care organizations, diluting clinician experience and stretching the limited resources necessary to provide such care. A coordinated effort in each community could therefore better maintain standards and quality of care. A full discussion of the financial realities faced by community-based hospice organizations is beyond the scope of this chapter, although a brief review of reimbursement issues in pediatric palliative care follows.

Thankfully, many organizations focusing primarily on the palliative care of adult patients have committed to finding ways to create pediatric palliative care services. These often consist of pediatric home care nursing, part-time physician support, and part-time, volunteer, or ad hoc allied health care professional support to meet the psychosocial needs of the patient and family.

The specialized nature of pediatric palliative care and the very act of caring for ill children is often a difficult challenge for adult-oriented health care providers, sometimes weighing heavily on them both emotionally and financially. The provision of child-life and other expressive therapists' services tailored to the particular needs of young or developmentally disabled children, despite their clear benefit for patients and families, cannot be expected of agencies with small numbers of pediatric patients (AAP CLC/COHC, 2006). A possible solution to providing these services may be the development of regional coalitions of organizations that share the services of such specialized care providers, thus spreading out the costs while making services more broadly available.

Maintaining oversight for delivering high-quality service in a timely fashion can be a challenge when care is fragmented among multiple institutions and locations. The establishment of regional or national standards of pediatric palliative care, such as those recently promulgated by the National Hospice and Palliative Care Organization (www.nhpco.org), will make clear the expectations for each organization and allow families, referring physicians, and community organizations to assess the quality of care provided

(NHPCO, 2009). Additional standards may be defined in the future by national committees or by regional coalitions of community-based palliative care organizations, working cooperatively to determine community norms.

It has been difficult to obtain reliable data on the number of children who would be appropriate for palliative care services based on differing definitions of appropriate referrals. One estimate is that 100–200 children living within a 50-mile radius of a large metropolitan hub would benefit from palliative care; this estimate is based on the number of children referred annually from eight pediatric tertiary care centers, each in turn served by any of a half-dozen community hospice organizations in Chicago (based on average weekly census and referral rates). In addition, there are published data suggesting an average of 2 to 10 pediatric patients hospitalized for their terminal stay on any given day in each medical center (Feudtner et al., 2002). Clearly, the total number of pediatric candidates for palliative care is much smaller than the number of adult candidates (in the United States, there are 2.6 million annual adult deaths, compared to 50,000 annual pediatric deaths).

As can easily be imagined, pediatric hospice and palliative care services are frequently nonexistent in rural areas, although adult agencies will sometimes attempt to provide care for children within their communities. More often, these children and their families are given only the options of either receiving palliative care by staying at a tertiary care center far from home, family, and friends or having standard nonhospice home health care (at best) in their home environment. The most rapid way to resolve this access barrier, allowing more children to receive the benefits of high-quality palliative care services, is for agencies providing adult palliative and hospice services to partner with established pediatric palliative care programs. Other options might include applications of telemedicine to provide assistance with care management and even symptom control.

Finally, members of minority communities and socioeconomically disadvantaged individuals often have difficulty accessing high-quality health care because of lack of access to appropriate facilities, few resources within their communities, limited comprehension of medical conditions and associated recommendations, their own often chaotic social circumstances, and the medical problems associated with poverty (premature birth, chronic respiratory illness, etc.). The adult hospice literature makes it clear that disparities in access to end-of-life care (Crawley, 2005), adequate pain control (Cintron and Morrison, 2006), and even fulfilling eligibility requirements for hospice care for the most needy individuals (Fishman et al., 2009) continue to exist for patients of all ages. These challenges are particularly great for African

Americans (Washington, Bickel-Swenson, and Stephens, 2008), Latinos, and recent immigrants who have limited proficiency in English.

The Origin and Management of Families' Unrealistic Expectations

A major obstacle to providing suitable palliative care services for children derives from unrealistic expectations that the health care system will enable a miraculous recovery from a devastating injury or natural disease process. Unrealistic expectations lead some families to insist that every therapy with even the slightest chance of prolonging life or achieving the elusive cure be provided to their child, regardless of the child's associated suffering. While our society currently gives parents/guardians the right to insist on the continued application of nearly all interventions for their child, based on the notion that the parents have their child's best interests at heart, most hospital-based clinicians recognize that the most humane option may sometimes involve the heart-wrenching and difficult decision to limit no-longer-beneficial medical interventions, focusing instead on maximizing comfort and optimizing the quality of life during the time a child has left. This situation often leads to conflict between families and the clinicians caring for their child, who may feel that ongoing disease-directed intervention is unduly burdensome to the child, violating the clinician's sense of duty to his or her patient. In such situations, the communication skills of palliative care clinicians may be beneficial. However, parental distrust of any real or perceived limitation of treatment may prevent them from accepting palliative care, especially if it is offered as an alternative to the current plan of care. Often the choice of words used to explain that the goal of cure is no longer achievable is the true barrier. Sometimes the words chosen imply that the parents are *choosing* to give up on, or are medically abandoning, their child. Frequently, the words suggest disrespect for their relationship. For example, physicians may ask, "Do you *want* to stop *life support?*" This choice of words fails to recognize that no family *wants* to stop supporting their child. Other times, the family simply needs time to adapt to the new reality of the child's condition and prognosis. The flexible clinician can facilitate this acceptance using respect and empathy. When physicians become impatient at the thought of using resources for a patient who will not "benefit" from them, the family may perceive the physician's frustration as an attempt to force their decision. Such situations create an adversarial environment between families and clinicians, which is counterproductive to the maintenance of mutual trust.

Several strategies may prevent such disagreements. First and foremost is maintaining an open dialogue with the family regarding the *goals* of care, with frequent updates and frank discussions as the disease progresses. Consistently revisiting the goals of care in the light of these gradual changes can be helpful, avoiding the appearance of a sudden change of heart by the clinicians. A second strategy involves consulting the PPC team early, enabling the creation of a trusting relationship with the family while helping them explore care options based on their values. Last, for some minority families, but certainly not for all, having a clinician (physician, nurse, social worker, or chaplain) who is a member of their minority community can facilitate the establishment of trust. Generally, however, families will have far more comfort and trust based on the clinician's *attitude* of compassion, warmth, and openness (one human being to another) than on skin color or accent.

An additional resource when there is difficulty in achieving consensus between family and clinicians is the institutional ethics committee. Helping the family obtain a second opinion from an outside consultant can also be effective in reassuring them of the team's openness and desire to find the best possible path. It is important to shift the family's focus from the clinician delivering the message to the realities of their child's situation. An outside opinion from someone not previously involved in the case may help accomplish that shift.

Reimbursement and Financing of Pediatric Palliative Care

Integral to the debate regarding which services should be included in a pediatric palliative care program is the problem of how these services will be funded. A discussion of the financial and economic barriers to pediatric palliative care is complex, owing to the shifting nature of the U.S. health care system. As a result of the mix of private and public payers funding the care of individual patients, with significant variability between programs and health care providers, payment for services can be difficult to predict. Nevertheless, the reality is that these services are needed and should be equitably reimbursed. A fundamental change in health care structure and funding might be the key to opening the door for comprehensive and widespread pediatric palliative care services in the future.

WHO SHOULD FUND PEDIATRIC PALLIATIVE CARE SERVICES?

Families of children with special health care needs often incur significant out-of-pocket expenses. It is estimated that 33 percent of these families paid more than $500 in a 12-month period for their child's medical care; this proportion increased to ~45 percent if the family was either uninsured or covered only by a private insurance plan. As a result, 1 in 5 families reported that their child's health care costs caused them financial hardship (National Survey of Children with Special Health Care Needs, 2005/2006).

Who should be responsible for paying for pediatric palliative care and hospice services, lessening the burden on individual families? It seems reasonable that health care institutions should share some of this burden if they are to stay true to their goals of advancing the health of all children; much of this deliberation occurs once disease-directed treatments are over (successful or not) and the patient and family return to the community. Careful discharge planning, including close communication with community health care providers and support services, is critical for the care of children who have special health care needs. Also, medical centers should develop outreach services for pain and symptom management, hospice care, and bereavement counseling, which are often not available in the community. The goal of comprehensive child health promotion can best be met if medical centers give pediatric palliative care programs resources and funding support commensurate with other pediatric subspecialty programs. To go one step further, it is incumbent on all tertiary pediatric health care facilities caring for children who have advanced disease to provide pediatric palliative care services for those who do not respond to curative interventions. To not do so is tantamount to abandoning the patient and family at their time of greatest need for support.

Another potential source of funding for pediatric palliative care services is public health insurance. Programs such as Medicaid and the State Child Health Insurance Program (SCHIP) provide some funding for the health care of more than 35 percent of children who have special health care needs, and there are currently initiatives that work within these programs to provide pediatric palliative care. The remainder of this section will be devoted to a crash course in public funding for child health, as well as an example of a publicly funded pediatric palliative care program. This should not be seen as excusing health care institutions or private insurance carriers from their responsibility to support pediatric palliative care, but it is imperative to understand and learn from some successful attempts to overcome the financial barriers to providing palliative care for children.

A CRASH COURSE IN PUBLIC FUNDING OF PEDIATRIC HEALTH CARE

Governmental involvement in the health care of children can be traced to the 1912 creation of the Children's Bureau, a federal agency tasked with overseeing "all matters pertaining to the welfare of children and child life." The first federal grant program designed to assist state health agencies to establish services promoting the health of women and children arose from the Children's Bureau. The grant program led to several improvements, including a marked increase in the registration of births, the establishment of more than 1,500 maternal and child health centers, and an increase in the availability of public health nursing.

This experiment in federally subsidized health care ended in 1929 but was renewed and firmly established with the passage of the Social Security Act in 1935. Title V of this act created three grant programs focusing on different aspects of child health. The Services for Crippled Children program is most pertinent to this discussion because it provides funds for "the purpose of enabling each state to extend and improve . . . as far as practicable, under the conditions in each state, services for locating crippled children; providing medical, surgical, corrective and other services and care; and facilities for diagnosis, hospitalization, and aftercare for children who are crippled or who are suffering from conditions which lead to crippling."

With the exception of the outdated verbiage, the description of the functions of Title V should strike a chord with those interested in improving care for children who have special health care needs. The program's objectives were not only to improve acute treatment for chronically ill children but also to proactively identify and resolve problems that these children and their families experience (as demonstrated by the intention to *locate* such children, rather than passively wait for them to present to the health care system). Moreover, the authors of Title V realized the importance of community-based care following hospitalization (by emphasizing the need for "aftercare"). As proof of the federal government's commitment to this goal, states that submitted grant proposals without comprehensive health services were denied federal funding (Lesser, 1985).

The next major extension of child health care coverage came with President Lyndon Johnson's efforts to build a "Great Society." Originally, the focus of health care reform was on elderly Americans who had fallen into poverty as a result of their rising medical costs, but the legislation was amended to provide assistance for poor people of all ages as well. Thus, in 1965, Congress passed two amendments to the Social Security Act: Title XVIII established Medicare, the medical assistance program for individuals over 65, while Title XIX created Medicaid. While these two programs were passed together, they differed in many ways, including the public perception of Medicare versus Medicaid. Historian Rashi Fein notes that the names themselves show this difference: Medicare provides *care* to elderly people, while Medicaid provides *aid* to poor people (Palfrey, 2006). The administration of funds is also different: Medicare is a federal program, whereas Medicaid is administered by the states, with federal matching funds allocated based on that state's per capita income (ranging from 1:1 to 3:1 matching of state funds). This has led to significant state-by-state differences with respect to eligibility, reenrollment frequency, services provided, and reimbursement rates.

On paper, Medicaid provides a complete set of services that, as with Title V, includes many of the services championed by proponents of pediatric palliative care. However, as with Title V, Medicaid has been and continues to be chronically underfunded. States must fund a basic level of services to serve as a safety net for poor people. Unfortunately, the more impoverished states often have difficulties funding even their 25 percent contribution to the program, resulting in such low payment rates to health care providers that some refuse to participate in the program because they actually lose money by providing services. There is also the potential for the state Medicaid program to run out of funds before the end of the fiscal year, leading to a cessation of all provider payments and often of all patient services. Such imperfections in the administration of Medicaid funds have led not only to stresses for providers of direct care but also to severe cash flow shortages in medical centers dependent on these payments for services.

Despite the contributions of Title V programs and Medicaid, a significant portion of children in the United States remained without health insurance in the 1990s. SCHIP was proposed as a means to reduce this problem. Many families with uninsured children found themselves in a frustrating situation: their job (or jobs) did not provide health care benefits, yet the pay was enough to disqualify them from Medicaid. Although private coverage was available, many families, especially those who had children with chronic health care needs, found the coverage too expensive or simply not available because of the exclusion of coverage for expenses associated with the child's preexisting health conditions. SCHIP (1997) was the 21st amendment to the Social Security Act, providing states with funds to expand health care coverage to just such children. The states could use the funds to pay for the care of previously uninsured children, but not to replace existing public or private health care payments. As with Medicaid, funds were provided as a matching grant from the federal government, although substantial leeway was given to each state to design and implement its own programs to achieve these purposes (Lesser, 1985; Field and Behrman, 2003; Palfrey, 2006).

A SUCCESSFUL PUBLIC SECTOR MODEL:
FLORIDA'S PARTNERS IN CARE

An illustration of successful efforts to overcome financial barriers to the provision of pediatric palliative care can be seen in the work done by the state of Florida in conjunction with Children's Hospice International (CHI). Founded in 1983, CHI has worked to overcome funding barriers by working with the U.S. Congress. After the development of a pediatric palliative care demonstration model (Children's Hospice International Program for All-inclusive Care for Children and their families, or CHI PACC), CHI was able to obtain limited federal funding for supervision and technical support of pilot state demonstration projects. One of the recipient states was Florida, which in 2005 created Partners in Care: Together for Kids (PIC:TFK). Using the CHI PACC model to determine the scope of services, PIC:TFK worked with CHI to design and implement a program of pediatric palliative care to work with the existing Florida medical system. The Florida strategy was to reallocate funding from the Center for Medicare and Medicaid Services.

The waiver and amendments, in combination with the use or reallocation of existing resources, enabled the development of a more functional program to serve children who have special health care needs and their families, including children living with life-threatening conditions. For example, Florida's Children's Miracle Network (CMN, their Title V program) already provided care coordination for children who have special health care needs. Also, hospices that were previously funded only by Medicare and charitable contributions were eligible for these Medicaid funds and were therefore able to retool to provide needed pediatric services. These services were previously undeveloped owing to a lack of revenue (Medicaid hospice admission criteria are difficult to apply to the pediatric population because of a requirement to stop concurrent disease-directed interventions). The promise of funds from the state's Medicaid and SCHIP programs provided hospices greater potential to dedicate time and resources to developing pediatric programs. The Florida model demonstrates the importance of knowing how to work *within* the current system of care. While federal and private programs individually lacked the capacity to provide pediatric palliative care, by working together to change the allocation of existing resources, in part by educating public officials, these programs are now able to provide care for hundreds of children every year (Knapp et al., 2008).

POTENTIAL SOLUTIONS

As further data filter in from the CHI demonstration programs, work is already under way to ease the implementation of CHI PACC or similar pediatric palliative care programs. Introduced by a bipartisan group of U.S. representatives, the CHI PACC Act of 2009 proposed to amend Title XIX of the Social Security Act to allow states to implement pediatric palliative care programs without having to obtain a special Medicaid waiver. While appropriate federal and state funding may continue to be a problem, this act would remove a significant obstacle to the broader creation of statewide pediatric palliative care programs. If the demonstration program data confirm that pediatric palliative care is either cost neutral or cost saving, arguments for the implementation of these programs will be further strengthened. It is hoped that with the establishment and expansion of state-sponsored services and the associated demonstration of the benefit to those families as well as to the program budget, private insurance will also begin to routinely pay for PPC services, rather than each program having to advocate for payment on a case-by-case basis. An additional demonstration project organized in conjunction with CHI is currently in effect in Colorado, and CHI is working with states and health care providers in California, Illinois, Kentucky, New Jersey, New York, New England, North Dakota, and the U.S. Department of Defense to further expand the provision of pediatric palliative care by working to secure a reliable source of funding for health care providers (CHI, 2009).

Global economic challenges will continue to play a major role for each country in meeting the challenge of providing pediatric palliative care. On the positive side, the expense associated with providing palliative care to the small number of children requiring this service pales in comparison to the large amount of money required to provide quality end-of-life care for adults. On the other hand, one of the measures of a compassionate society is how well it is able to care for the most needy individuals, including those who have life-limiting conditions (HIV-AIDS, incurable cancers, intractable cardiopulmonary insufficiency, etc.), and the United States fares poorly with this metric. Following the lead of people who have chronic disabilities, health care providers and affected families can facilitate a global agenda for change in health care funding priorities by speaking up, helping the public and relevant regulators, officials, and lawmakers to recognize the importance of appropriate funding of palliative care. This will require data and being informed on issues of health care policy. Without such advocacy efforts, an important opportunity to change the experience of families and children facing life-limiting and life-threatening conditions may be lost.

Obstacles and Solutions Related to the Structure of Pediatric Medical Care and Education

In the United States, as in most developed countries, most children who die do so in tertiary hospitals that provide specialty care for children, which are often located far from the family's home, resulting in the loss of support by the family's community at the time that they need support the most. Until the availability of community-based pediatric palliative care is improved, the provision of holistic interdisciplinary palliative care falls on the often ill-prepared staff of the hospital and pediatric subspecialty clinics. As more infants, children, and adolescents survive with life-threatening and complex, chronic conditions, there is an increased need for the effective provision of upstream palliative care for these children and their families, long before the need for end-of-life care. The following discussion explores the barriers such institutions and their staff members encounter in trying to provide comprehensive pediatric palliative care, in contrast to end-of-life care, and how these obstacles might be overcome.

STAFF ALLOCATION, PALLIATIVE CARE TRAINING, EXPERIENCE, AND COMFORT

What are the staff's expectations, needs, and satisfactions in providing palliative or end-of-life care? Beckstrand and Kirchhoff (2005) surveyed adult critical care nurses regarding the frequency and intensity of barriers to providing end-of-life care. Tasks that remove the nurse from the bedside, behaviors that prolong patients' suffering or cause pain, and perceptions that the patient's family did not understand the implications of the use of "lifesaving measures" all created barriers to good end-of-life care. In this study, the three biggest obstacles to providing end-of-life care were (1) having multiple physicians whose opinions differed about the goals of a patient's care, (2) patients' family members and friends who continually called a nurse for an update on the patient's condition rather than calling the designated family contact person, and (3) physicians who were evasive and avoided frank conversations with patients' family members.

Similar concerns about unclear goals of care and lack of sufficient time for adequate patient care and support are described by Davies et al. (2008). In their survey of pediatric care providers based in an academic hospital, the most common factors interfering with optimal pediatric end-of-life care, according to both nurses and physicians, involve perceived uncertainty of the child's prognosis and discrepancies in treatment goals between staff and family members. Another common barrier was communication difficulties. Disagreements among health care providers about probable outcomes or possible treatment plans are both apparent and profoundly distressing to families; efforts to build consensus among consultants and health care providers from all disciplines are essential to preventing unnecessary family distress. In many hospitals, the PPC team facilitates the achievement of such a consensus. However, if palliative care is viewed as synonymous with end-of-life care or with cessation of all disease-directed interventions, then, in the presence of an uncertain prognosis, clinicians or parents may feel they are "giving up too soon" if they engage pediatric palliative services. Early introduction of palliative care can improve psychosocial support of the patient and family, enhance the control of symptoms throughout the illness, and trigger discussions of personal philosophy and values that might influence treatment choices if the child's clinical condition worsens. These anticipatory discussions allow the family to consider goals and treatment options in advance of a crisis, enabling more thoughtful decisions. This approach facilitates better family adaptation to a worsening prognosis or impending death. Thus, uncertainty should perhaps be viewed as a trigger to initiate palliative care, rather than a reason to avoid it (Davies et al., 2008).

Davies's group also found that nurses who work in non-ICU acute care units perceive differing barriers to pediatric palliative care than those who work in ICUs. Non-ICU staff reported time constraints and staff shortages as barriers to pediatric palliative care more frequently than did ICU staff, recognizing the intensive amount of staff time required to provide care and support to patients and families at the end of life. A solution to the problem of competing demands on the time and energy of bedside caregivers is the use of the PPC team to work with families and patients as the chance of recovery becomes less likely. Similar to ethics consultations, bedside caregivers should be empowered to access the PPC team to assist with caring for families and managing difficult conversations. By sharing the burden of care and painful discussions, bedside caregivers can alleviate much of their own distress and receive validation from the PPC team regarding the choices being made on behalf of the patient.

HOUSE-STAFF EDUCATION, CONCERNS, AND NEEDS

One of the most difficult and distressing events that pediatric residents (in the U.S. system, M.D. graduate learners in 1 of 3 years of pediatric specialty training) experience during training is the death of a patient. These physician trainees do not feel competent or comfortable providing palliative care to children (Michelson et al., 2009) and frequently lack suitable role models for how to conduct difficult discussions with families.

McCabe, Hunt, and Serwint (2008) surveyed their pediatric resident trainees about their experience of the death of a patient and their perception of the adequacy of their training to manage it. The resident curriculum included training in communication skills, symptom management, bereavement, communication with families after the death of a child, self-care after the death of a patient, accurate completion of death certificates, and obtaining consent for autopsy and organ donation. Despite the robustness of the didactic curriculum and complementary attempts to include residents in mentored teaching during clinical care, residents at all levels reported feeling unprepared. Neither the amount of time spent in palliative care activities nor the educational curriculum seemed to enhance the residents' feeling of competence in palliative care. Although many residents had taken care of patients who later died, they were present for few of the deaths and had limited participation in the events and tasks leading up to and following the death. As in most hospitals, the majority of deaths occurred in the NICU or PICU. Resident training time on these services is firmly restricted by the Accreditation Council for Graduate Medical Education Pediatric Residency Review Committee. Given the recent limitations on ICU time and duty hours, creative approaches must be explored to improve the opportunities to manage end-of-life care, including the acquisition of the practical and cognitive skills required. Equally important is gaining skill in understanding and addressing the emotional impact of the end of life of patients on their families, the caregiving team, and the trainee him- or herself. How this can best be done is not clear; McCabe, Hunt, and Serwint (2008) propose developing a longitudinal approach throughout the continuum of the medical education experience, beginning with basic education as students, then during residency expanding to the elements of palliative care necessary for the general pediatrician and honing skills during subspecialty training and continuing education. An important goal of training in end-of-life care is for the learner to develop insight about his or her own emotional response to the death of a patient and to learn how to survive with compassion intact.

As with many other aspects of end-of-life care, the PPC team can be of tremendous benefit to pediatric resident trainees by providing a compassionate "ear" for their concerns, affirming their actions when appropriate, educating and mentoring when mistakes are made, and offering a shoulder to cry or lean on when the emotions become overwhelming. The PPC team comprises familiar faculty and senior nursing staff members with whom the residents have interacted throughout their hospital-based learning experience. Where PPC teams exist, residents often view their members as trustworthy sources of information on symptom management and as sounding boards for residents' emotional concerns during difficult situations. As consultants, the PPC team members can maintain objectivity and can work with all members of the primary team to achieve the best outcome for all involved, including trainees.

INSTITUTIONAL OBSTACLES AND SOLUTIONS

Separate from the issues of training hospital-based care providers and adequate staff time to provide palliative care, barriers may arise from the "character" of the institution. Many hospitals mirror society, with its difficulty in speaking openly and supportively about the death of a child. Death may still be treated as a professional failure, something shameful and unmentionable. That this attitude is often unspoken makes it a no-less-powerful impediment to the development of good palliative care services. Hospital cultures that value the provision of excellent end-of-life care as the final phase of outstanding care for children facing inevitable death will find a way to provide it. Such institutions inculcate mores that the opportunity to care for children with complex diseases demands a willingness to care for those who will not be cured; providing such care is the privilege and responsibility of clinicians and institutions delivering care to children and their families. Excellent pediatric palliative care will be present in institutions whose leaders value and broadly acknowledge clinicians who provide good palliative care. Adherence to best practice principles and national standards will further support such efforts (see www.nhpco.org/i4a/pages/index.cfm?pageid=3409, www.ihi.org/IHI/Topics/PalliativeCare/, and www.capc.org).

Physical space and an environment conducive to quiet discussion, inclusion of the family at the child's bedside, and soothing end-of-life treatment not only facilitate excellent end-of-life care but also demonstrate institutional recognition of and commitment to its importance. Hospital policies outlining procedures for end-of-life care, resuscitation status, and withholding or discontinuing no-longer-beneficial interventions should specifically include sections appropriate for infants, children, adolescents, and young adults and should address the special assent and permission needs of minors. Education of hospital staff regarding the existence and content of these policies should be routine. Training including the policies, principles, and skills needed to provide good palliative care should be routinely offered to staff on pediatric units.

Each institution should attempt to estimate the required number of trained health care providers to address the longitudinal needs of children living with life-threatening conditions. Staffing ratios should accommodate the additional time required to provide individualized care during the last days of life and bereavement care thereafter. Feudtner et al. (2002) compiled national data reported to NACHRI (National Association of Children's Hospitals and Related Institutions) by children's hospitals. These data showed that on any given day the hospitals in this sample were caring for an average of 2.2 to 10.6 patients who would subsequently die there. Feudtner et al. note that "this method of estimating an average daily census could provide guidance as to the staffing required to meet the needs of just those patients who die in the hospital (and not necessarily the needs of patients who are discharged and die at home or who are never admitted)."

OBSTACLES AND SOLUTIONS TO THE PROVISION OF CONTINUITY AND COORDINATION OF CARE

Ideally, pediatric palliative care should be delivered seamlessly from the child's perspective, whether the child is in the hospital, at home, or in any other care location. Children and families benefit from consistency of health care providers. When feasible, it is helpful to have at least one home care provider visit the child and family in the hospital when admission cannot be avoided. One solution to providing continuity and consistency in care is to use the PPC team as a liaison between home and hospital services. The PPC team maintains contact by phone or via outpatient clinic visits with patients and their families following discharge, ensuring that the details of the child's course at home are known to the inpatient team. In so doing, continuity of care can be assured if the child requires future hospitalization.

Achieving the goal of seamless care requires a commitment to effective communication and concerted efforts on the part of the hospital-based and the home care teams. Conventional standards require biweekly interdisciplinary team meetings; this seems to be a reasonable interval as a minimum baseline for home care teams and hospital-based services to communicate regarding any changes in the child's medical condition, goals of care, medication regimen, or social circumstances. Organizations can routinely fax or e-mail the minutes of such team meetings to primary pediatricians and hospital-based teams for inclusion in the patient's office chart and hospital medical record. This information is often helpful when medications must be adjusted or to honor resuscitation status decisions that have already been made.

Continuity of services and support between care settings can also potentially be accomplished with regionally coordinated provision of palliative care services, assuming effective cooperation between service agencies and health care providers. The development of regional networks facilitates and formalizes the creation of continuity-of-care initiatives. In California, for example, three geographic regions have formed interdisciplinary collaborative work groups to focus the efforts of administrators based in hospitals, community hospices, and state governmental children's service agencies on improving coordination and quality of care for children living with life-threatening conditions (CHPCC, 2009). Such collaborative networks are models for the development of an infrastructure to care for these children more seamlessly in other parts of the country as well.

CARE IN THE EMERGENCY DEPARTMENT

A consistent problem nationwide is the emergency department (ED) approach to children with chronic, life-threatening conditions. On presentation, it is frequently difficult to know whether the child is already cared for by a palliative care team and whether advance care planning discussions have been initiated. While one would anticipate that parents could provide this information, in the heat of the moment they frequently do not, leading to confusion and sometimes the provision of unwanted medical intervention. Many organizations are developing electronic medical records and exploring ways to "flag" the patient's permanent record, indicating a previous inpatient or out-of-hospital do-not-resuscitate order or whether the palliative care team was involved during previous hospitalizations. The goal of such documentation is to provide the best overall quality of care, which may mean focusing on quality rather than duration of life, including when the patient presents to the ED for care.

A Parent's Perspective on Barriers to Pediatric Palliative Care

A parent's perspective can frame the issues raised in the preceding sections, emphasizing several important points to be addressed in planning and executing effective palliative care for children. Three major elements have significant impact on the likelihood of success in providing excellent palliative care to children and families:

1. Trust in the clinicians
2. Effective communication about difficult subjects
3. Early involvement of the palliative care team

Parents need to feel confidence and trust in the clinicians caring for their child. Trust is engendered by demonstration of the clinician's medical knowledge and acknowledgment that he or she does not have all the answers but will seek them for the family at each stage of the illness trajectory. Families recognize when physicians and nurses are being territorial and are engaged in power struggles over "who is right." Thus, disagreements between health care providers need to be resolved through frequent medical team discussions and with the goal of reaching consensus on the best course of action at each stage. Family confusion caused by clinician disagreement contributes to distress among all involved. Consensus of professional opinion and consistency in family guidance will ease an already difficult situation.

One situation that commonly begets loss of trust is an ineffective or delayed response to the child's symptoms. Poorly coordinated pain and symptom management makes parents feel they have to protect their child from the medical system, increasing their sense of abandonment owing to a perception that no one is listening to them and no one is concerned about their child's needs. While pain and symptom resolution can be difficult to achieve in patients with advanced disease, there must be open discussion and agreement about the day-to-day and hour-to-hour progress and ongoing plan for symptom management.

The clinician's comfort in discussing difficult issues sensitively and at a measured pace is critical to engendering and maintaining family trust. Clinicians who seem uncomfortable can create additional distress for families. In particular, those clinicians who see their own children in the faces of their patients or feel as if "they have failed the child" by not achieving a cure may create additional emotional burden for the family and patient, who sometimes end up feeling as if they need to care for the clinicians!

Early introduction of the palliative care team, a familiar and comfortable set of faces that know the entire clinical saga, ideally from the moment of diagnosis, prevents the distress associated with a new consultant brought in at the time of crisis. Families may resist the recommendations of clinicians whom they have known for only a short time in favor of more familiar individuals. While the primary pediatrician would be the ideal source of continuity of care, most will not feel comfortable in that role until palliative care education is better integrated into medical curricula. Effective palliative care can play an important role in normalizing the experience of families whose children have a limited life expectancy. Because the palliative care team has the greatest experience with children who will ultimately not survive, regardless of the underlying diagnosis, its members are in a unique position to help families understand that they are not alone in their suffering.

Institutions need to give clear priority to meeting the needs of parents of children who require palliative care. The provision of suitable rooms and furniture for parents and siblings to spend time with the patient, suitable facilities for showering and sleeping (both with and away from the patient when needed), and suitable facilities for family discussions with the medical team, both at the bedside and away when appropriate, are an important means of concretely demonstrating this priority (see the IPPC Institutional Self-Assessment Tool, www.ippcweb.org/quality.asp). Many hospitals have developed volunteer programs staffed by selected bereaved parents who can become allies with the ill child's parents as they negotiate the health care system and attempt to coordinate plans for discharge. Increased sensitivity to families undergoing social upheavals, such as marital or economic stresses due to the child's illness, is vitally important to help parents remain healthy and as supportive to the child as possible. Specialized social work and counseling staff may be needed to support such families as well.

Conclusion

Several issues impede the integration of pediatric palliative care into the spectrum of routine care for children. First and foremost is the lack of consensus regarding what constitutes high-quality pediatric palliative care, when it is best offered, and how it relates to the child's total care. Institutional reticence to embrace and support palliative care stems from society's discomfort with death in childhood as well as the costs of supporting a program that may lose revenue. The central role of communication in providing optimal palliative care has many ramifications, both for health professional education in effective and compassionate communication with families and for public discussion of the need to develop palliative care capacity in each community.

As in other areas of medical care, socially disadvantaged and minority communities may have unique and complex needs. Expertise in how best to help individuals of differing communities, cultures, and languages is needed to provide sensitive and effective care. In attempting to alleviate total suffering for patients and their families, palliative care must consider the patient in the greater social and family contexts. The focus must always be on optimizing the experience for both patients and their families. Some of the current problems in providing universal access to optimal, seamless, and high-quality pediatric palliative care seem daunting and insoluble. Nevertheless, the vision of widespread, accessible, and high-quality pediatric palliative care cannot be achieved without continued dedication to the ideal and ongoing efforts to accomplish these laudable goals.

As with all problems in health care, these challenges serve as a call to action. Health care providers, hospital administrators, and legislators must create new, effective, and economical solutions to meet the challenge of providing excellent care to children living with life-threatening conditions and their families. Integration of palliative care concepts in medical and nursing education will create a pool of future health care providers who have greater appreciation for caring for patients throughout life's continuum. Increased visibility of this population and new national standards for their care will encourage the greater allocation of resources for this critical clinical service. Lastly, parents' experiences of the palliative care journey teach us that early introduction of palliative care, trust, and effective communication are vitally important to the overall care of children living with life-threatening conditions and their families.

References

American Academy of Pediatrics, Child Life Council and Committee on Hospital Care (AAP CLC/COHC). 2006. Child life services. *Pediatrics* 118:1757–63.

American Academy of Pediatrics, Committee on Bioethics (AAP COB). 2000. Palliative care for children. *Pediatrics* 106:351–57.

Beckstrand, R., and Kirchhoff, K. 2005. Providing end-of-life care to patients: Critical care nurses' perceived obstacles and supportive behaviors. *J Crit Care* 14:395–403.

Children's Hospice and Palliative Care Coalition (CHPCC). 2009. Children's Hospice and Palliative Care Coalition. www.childrenshospice.org/benefit/collaborators/ (accessed February 10, 2010).

Children's Hospice International. 2009. Children's Hospice International Program for All-Inclusive Care for Children and Their Families. www.chionline.org/programs (accessed February 10, 2010).

Cintron, A., and Morrison, R. 2006. Pain and ethnicity in the United States: A systematic review. *J Palliat Med* 9:1454–73.

Crawley, L. 2005. Racial, cultural, and ethnic factors influencing end-of-life care. *J Palliat Med* 8:S58–69.

Davies, B., Sehring, S.A., Partridge, J.C., et al. 2008. Barriers to palliative care for children: Perceptions of pediatric health care providers. *Pediatrics* 121(2):282–88.

Feudtner, C., Christakis, D., Zimmerman, F.J., et al. 2002. Characteristics of deaths occurring in children's hospitals: Implications for supportive care services. *Pediatics* 109:887–93.

Field, M., and Behrman, R. 2003. *When Children Die: Improving Palliative and End-of-Life Care for Children and Their Families*. Washington, DC: National Academies Press.

Fishman, J., O'Dwyer, P., Lu, H.L., et al. 2009. Race, treatment preferences, and hospice enrollment: Eligibility criteria may exclude patients with the greatest needs for care. *Cancer* 115:689–97.

Heaston, S., Beckstrand, R.L., Bond, A.E., et al. 2006. Emergency nurses' perceptions of obstacles and supportive behaviors in end-of-life care. *J Emerg Nurs* 32:477–85.

Hilden, J.M., Emanuel, E.J., Fairclough, D.L., et al. 2001. Attitudes and practices among pediatric oncologists regarding end-of-life care: Results of the 1998 American Society of Clinical Oncology survey. *J Clin Oncol* 19(1):205–12.

Himelstein, B. 2006. Palliative care for infants, children, adolescents, and their families. *J Palliat Med* 9:163–81.

Johnston, D.L., Nagel, K., Friedman, D.L., et al. 2008. Availability and use of palliative care and end-of-life services for pediatric oncology patients. *J Clin Oncol* 26(28): 4646–50.

Knapp, C., Madden, V., Curtis, C.M., et al. 2008. Partners in Care: Together for Kids: Florida's model of pediatric palliative care. *J Palliat Med* 11:1212–20.

Lesser, A. 1985. Public programs for crippled children. In *Issues in the Care of Children with Chronic Illness*, ed. N. Hobbs and J. Perrin, pp. 733–57. San Francisco: Jossey-Bass.

Löfmark, R., Nilstun, T., and Bolmsjö, I.A. 2007. From cure to palliation: Concept, decision and acceptance. *J Med Ethics* 33:685–88.

Luce, M., and White, D. 2007. The pressure to withhold or withdraw life-sustaining therapy from critically ill patients in the United States. *Am J Resp Crit Care Med* 175:1104–8.

McCabe, M., Hunt, E.A., and Serwint, J.R. 2008. Pediatric residents' clinical and educational experiences with end-of-life care. *Pediatrics* 121:e731–37.

Meisel, A., Snyder, L., Quill, T., and American College of Physicians—American Society of Internal Medicine End-of-Life Care Consensus Panel. 2000. Seven legal barriers to end-of-life care: Myths, realities, and grains of truth. *JAMA* 284(19): 2495–501.

Michelson, K. N., Ryan, A.D., Jovanovic, B., et al. 2009. Pediatric residents' and fellows' perspectives on palliative care education. *J Palliat Med* 12(5):451–57.

National Hospice and Palliative Care Organization (NHPCO). 2009. Standards of Practice for Pediatric Palliative Care. Alexandria, VA.

National Survey of Children with Special Health Care Needs. 2005/2006. Guide to topics and questions asked. www.cshcndata.org/content/Guide2005.aspx (accessed February 10, 2010).

Palfrey, J. 2006. *Child Health in America: Making a Difference through Advocacy*. Baltimore: Johns Hopkins University Press.

Penson, R., Partridge, R.A., Shah, M.A., et al. 2005. Fear of death. *The Oncologist* 10: 160–69.

Schickedanz, A.D., Schillinger, D., Landefeld, C.S., et al. 2009. A clinical framework for improving the advance care planning process: Start with patients' self-identified barriers. *J Am Geriatr Soc* 57(1):31–39.

Steele, R., Bosma, H., and Johnston, M.F. 2008. Research priorities in pediatric palliative care: A Delphi study. *J Palliat Care* 24:229–39.

St-Laurent-Gagnon, T., Carnevale, F.A., and Duval, M. 2008. Pediatric palliative care: A qualitative study of physicians' perspectives in a tertiary care university hospital. *Palliat Care* 24:26–30.

Thompson, L.A., Knapp, C., Madden, V., et al. 2009. Pediatricians' perceptions of and preferred timing for pediatric palliative care. *Pediatrics* 123:e777–82.

Washington, K.T., Bickel-Swenson, D., and Stephens, N. 2008. Barriers to hospice use among African Americans: A systematic review. *Health Soc Work* 33:267–74.

Wolfe, J., Grier, H.E., Klar, N., et al. 2000. Symptoms and suffering at the end of life in children with cancer. *N Engl J Med* 342:326–33.

Zhukovsky, D.S., Herzog, C.E., Kaur, G., et al. 2009. The impact of palliative care consultation on symptom assessment, communication needs, and palliative interventions in pediatric patients with cancer. *J Palliat Med* 12(4):343–49.

4

Educational Initiatives

Betty Ferrell, Ph.D., R.N., Hollye Harrington Jacobs, M.S., R.N., M.S.W., Jeffrey C. Klick, M.D., John M. Saroyan, M.D., Elana E. Evan, Ph.D., Margaret Comeau, M.H.A., Sarah E. Friebert, M.D., and David Browning, M.S.W., B.C.D.

The provision of excellent pediatric palliative care is contingent on professionals who are prepared to deliver this complex care. Fortunately, in recent years there have been significant advances in the education of professionals both in formal training programs and through continuing education. This chapter summarizes several of these initiatives, including a model of nursing education, pediatric inpatient care, a model of interdisciplinary education, resident/fellowship medical education, and physician continuing medical education. Although there are differences across these programs intended for the unique needs of each population, there are also important "common threads," as each program has advanced both the core content needed in the field and innovative methods of teaching.

A Model of Nursing Education: The ELNEC Project

Nurses spend more time with patients and families facing life-limiting illness than any other health care professional. Despite the fact that nurses are intimately involved in all aspects of palliative and end-of-life care, research has demonstrated that major deficiencies exist in nursing education on these topics. To understand why deficiencies in care exist, researchers at the City of Hope National Medical Center implemented a project titled "Strengthening Nursing Education to Improve End-of-Life Care." This project occurred between 1997 and 2000 and was supported by the Robert Wood Johnson Foundation; it demonstrated that deficits in nursing textbooks, nursing school curricula, and continuing nursing education have all contributed to the lack of nursing readiness to provide palliative and end-of-life care for children and their families (Ferrell et al., 2000).

In 1997, the document "Peaceful Death: Recommended Competencies and Curricular Guidelines for End-of-Life Nursing Care" (AACN, 1997) was produced. It outlined key competencies and guidelines for nursing education and end-of-life care and has become recognized as a key statement describing the knowledge and skills required for nurses to provide quality care to children facing end-of-life issues. Results from comparable national studies also demonstrated that nurses were not prepared for or comfortable with providing optimum palliative and end-of-life care to children and their families (Ferrell et al., 2000; Field and Behrman, 2003).

In 1999, the American Association of Colleges of Nursing partnered with the City of Hope to propose a national effort to rectify these deficiencies and to create nursing education that would meet the recommendations of the "Peaceful Death" document. The national project, End-of-Life Nursing Education Consortium (ELNEC), was developed and launched in 2000. The original project assisted nurses in addressing the myriad of physical, psychological, social, and spiritual needs facing those in end-of-life settings (Sherman et al., 2005; Matzo and Hijjazi, 2008).

Even though the initial eight ELNEC courses, supported by the Robert Wood Johnson Foundation, were designed for patients across the life span, it became clear early in the project that a specific curriculum should be devoted to meeting the distinct and unique needs of children. A pediatric-specific ELNEC training course was conceptualized in 2001. A pediatric ELNEC course (ELNEC-PPC) was piloted in 2002, bringing together 20 pediatric palliative care expert advisors to adapt the ELNEC core curriculum to develop a pediatric-specific version. The curriculum was developed from this pilot course, and the first national ELNEC-PPC course was held in 2003.

Since its inception, more than 725 nurses from 50 states have completed ELNEC-PPC. To date, eight national courses have been offered. Support for the first course came from the Robert Wood Johnson Foundation, and the third and fourth courses were funded in part by the Aetna Foundation.

CURRICULUM

The ELNEC-PPC program is a 2-day "train the trainer" course implemented with the intention that the pediatric nurse participants will disseminate the information in clinical and/or university settings. The curriculum consists of 10 pediatric-specific modules: Nursing Care in Pediatric Palliative Care, Special Considerations in Pediatric Palliative Care, Communication, Ethical/Legal Issues, Cultural Considerations, Pain Management, Symptom Management, Care at the Time of Death, Loss/Grief/Bereavement, and Models of Excellence in Pediatric Palliative Care (table 4.1). During the

Table 4.1 ELNEC-PPC modules and overviews

Module	Overview
Introduction to Pediatric Palliative Nursing Care	Creates the foundation for the ELNEC-PPC curriculum. It is an overview of the need to improve care and the role of nurses as members of an interdisciplinary team in providing good-quality care.
Special Considerations in Pediatric Palliative Care	Focuses on the foundation of pediatric palliative care by highlighting the essential elements involved with caring for seriously ill children as well as addressing each child's multifaceted uniqueness.
Communication	Emphasizes the importance of good communication in pediatric palliative care. The complexities of communicating with children and families at this critical time are described along with suggestions for care.
Ethical/Legal Issues	Discusses some of the key ethical issues and legal concerns in palliative care for children and provides resources to address these in practice.
Cultural Considerations	Reviews dimensions of culture that influence pediatric palliative care. Assessment of culture is emphasized as essential to adequate communication and to providing culturally sensitive care.
Pain Management	Reviews basic principles of pain assessment and management in infants, children, and adolescents with a focus on pain in palliative care.
Symptom Management	Builds on module 6 (Pain Management) by addressing other symptoms common in children with life-threatening conditions.
Care at the Time of Death	Focuses on care at the actual time of a child's death, emphasizing the preparation necessary to ensure the best care at this critical event in the trajectory of illness.
Loss, Grief, and Bereavement	Addresses the challenging aspects of grief, loss, and bereavement of children and families as well as the loss experiences of health care professionals.

(continued)

Table 4.1 (*cont.*)

Module	Overview
Models of Excellence	Focuses on the role of nurses in achieving good-quality care for children living with life-threatening conditions and their families by reviewing limitations in existing systems and opportunities for change.

course, participants hear national pediatric palliative care experts use didactic lectures, case study discussions, role-play, and videos to teach the curriculum. Each participant receives the 1,000-page syllabus consisting of PowerPoint slides, talking points for each slide, case studies, teaching strategies, and key references for each of the 10 modules (www.aacn.nche.edu/ELNEC).

UNIQUE ISSUES IN PEDIATRIC PALLIATIVE CARE EDUCATION FOR NURSES

Nurses have a unique role in the collaborative, interdisciplinary palliative care team. Some of the key concerns of nurses are captured in eight major "common themes" incorporated throughout the ELNEC-PPC curriculum. The themes are as follows:

- It is important to recognize that the family is the unit of care.
- The important role of the nurse as an advocate is stressed.
- The importance that culture has in influencing palliative care choices is stressed.
- There is a critical need for attention to special populations such as ethnic minorities, the poor, and the uninsured.
- End-of-life issues for families, patients, and caregivers affect all systems of care across all settings.
- Many critical financial issues influence palliative care.
- Palliative care is not confined to cancer or AIDS, but rather it is essential across all life-threatening illnesses and in cases of sudden death.
- Interdisciplinary care is essential for quality care at the end of life.

MODELS OF SUCCESS

ELNEC-PPC trainers participate in the training program with the intention of educating other staff members and also ultimately improving the care of children and their families facing end-of-life issues. The ELNEC-PPC project has been an extremely effective educational endeavor to improve care for children on local, national, and international platforms.

For example, in 2001 in California, ELNEC trainers Lori Butterworth and Devon Dabbs founded the Children's Hospice and Palliative Care Coalition (CHPCC), an advocacy movement led by children's hospitals, hospices, and home health and grassroots agencies to improve care for children with life-threatening conditions and their families. As a result of their efforts, for the first time, Californian children diagnosed with a life-threatening condition have access to an innovative, comprehensive model of care that addresses their unique needs and those of their families. The benefit, approved in 2008 by the Centers for Medicare and Medicaid Services, includes a home- and community-based waiver that eliminates the requirement that children forgo potentially curative treatment to receive needed hospice and palliative care services (www.childrenshospice.org). Additionally, the CHPCC developed a resource guide for parents of children with life-threatening conditions (www.partnershipforparents.org).

In an effort to provide continuity of care for children navigating the complexities of the health care system, Jean Carroll, from the Children's Hospital in Philadelphia, Pennsylvania, developed "Partners in Pediatric Palliative Care." This program links hospital end-of-life care programs with community home hospice care organizations, including 32 agencies in the tristate area of Pennsylvania, New Jersey, and Delaware (Malloy et al., 2007).

In 2004, 10 associates from Children's Hospital of Orange County (CHOC) attended the ELNEC-PPC course. Intent on spreading their passion for pediatric palliative care and armed with an evidence-based curriculum, this group taught the first CHOC ELNEC-PPC course in 2004, which coincided with the opening of the Rainbow Room, the only hospital room of its kind in Orange County, designed with every amenity to make a child's last days as comfortable as possible.

Understanding the importance of children's grief, senior nursing students in the Baccalaureate Nursing Program at Nicholls State University experience hands-on service learning while providing follow-up bereavement care and compassion for children through guided group activities, under the supervision of ELNEC-trained nursing faculty. The students recognize the value of providing community, family, and peer psychosocial support by assisting children through this difficult time. The students translate their education into clinical experience at "Camp Brave Heart," a 1-day bereavement camp that provides a safe and wholesome environment of fun-filled activities for children from South Louisiana who have experienced the loss of a loved one, as well as the loss of property and other possessions such as from Hurricanes Katrina and Rita.

National collaboration is a natural progression from the networking at national ELNEC courses. Partnerships between the Children's Oncology Group (COG), an organization that develops research-based treatment protocols for childhood cancer, and the Association of Pediatric Hematology Oncology Nurses (APHON), the professional organization for nurses caring for children and adolescents who have cancer or blood disorders, have led to the development of educational resources for both associations (Malloy et al., 2007).

International ELNEC efforts also abound. In 2006 and 2007, the ELNEC staff hosted training sessions for representatives from 18 Eastern European countries at conferences in Salzburg, Austria, and an ELNEC course was held in Tanzania, Africa, in 2007. Using the expansive distribution system inherent in the Internet, Ayda Nambayan from St. Jude Children's Research Hospital, in Memphis, Tennessee, developed a Web-based version of ELNEC-PPC (www.Cure4Kids.org) and launched it in 2004. The ELNEC-PPC program has been accessed on the website more than 41,000 times by at least 1,060 unique users. The Spanish version was released on this site in 2008, and the Portuguese translation in 2009.

The ELNEC-PPC program is dedicated to supporting and connecting its ELNEC trainers through a variety of methods: a quarterly newsletter, *ELNEC Connections*; annual updates to the curriculum; project staff/investigator accessibility; and website networking, to name a few. Data have demonstrated that the ELNEC-PPC project has been a successful educational initiative (Malloy et al., 2007; Jacobs et al., 2009). Pediatric nurses are in a unique position to care for the most vulnerable population, children, at the end of life. Education is the key to ensuring that competent and confident nursing care is delivered to children and their families when they need it most.

Pediatric Inpatient Care

The World Health Organization's (2002) change in definition that palliative care can be provided alongside curative treatments, rather than only when curative treatments are *no longer* available, carried with it a dramatic shift in how individuals with life-threatening conditions could optimize their quality of life. Consequently, this conceptual shift has presented major educational challenges for how health care providers are relearning what palliative care is and how palliative care principles can be instilled in health care institutions. The American Academy of Pediatrics (2000) and Institute of Medicine (Field and Behrman, 2003) reports call for education, change in clinical practice, and research in pediatric palliative care, yet they explain that these changes also require behavioral change in the health care culture and clinical practice. From large tertiary care medical centers to smaller community hospitals, the challenges in bringing about behavioral changes often involve influencing systems that consist of practitioners with varying years of clinical experience and from multiple disciplines, all while working in pressured environments involving the care of children with life-threatening conditions and their families.

As pediatric palliative care programs across the country continue to develop, several behavioral strategies have been used and documented as contributing to the progress in educating health care providers in pediatric palliative inpatient care. Behavioral strategies such as role-modeling, group investment, and shaping can all be used in stimulating educational initiatives. Pediatric palliative care principles such as using an interdisciplinary (physicians, nursing, mental health clinicians, spiritual care, etc.) approach to inpatient care can be role-modeled, or demonstrated in its ideal form, by establishing an interdisciplinary team of administrative leaders (e.g., directors of various divisions and disciplines) as well as "unit-based" leaders or champions committed to pediatric palliative care (Browning and Solomon, 2005, 2006; Ellis et al., 2007). Having administrative leaders role-model or publicly endorse pediatric palliative care principles (such as establishing system-wide communication training seminars or symptom management order sets) can establish the expectation that these new principles are being reinforced on a larger "systems" level. Having unit-based champions designated on each shift can help role-model best practices, such as developmentally appropriate pain management strategies for children, and can answer questions, solve problems, and generally instill positive attitudes among staff. In the examination of unit-based education by Ellis et al. (2007), nursing champions were critical because they created a positive atmosphere for change and averted confusion or negative perceptions of the new protocol as difficult to use or burdensome. Role-modeling as a form of educating staff not only can occur during "teachable" moments at the patient's bedside but also can be taught through in vitro role-play sessions, modeling communication skills for delivering difficult prognostic information (Browning and Solomon, 2005, 2006).

Just as the practice of pediatric palliative care is patient centered and individualized to the quality-of-life needs of the patient, individualizing the palliative care educational objectives to the needs of the health care provider is pivotal in instilling motivation for positive change. Attempts to individualize the educational intervention to each group of pediatric clinicians or to the content specific to their area of involvement or expertise can promote a feeling of group investment in accomplishing change in inpatient practice (Ellis et al., 2007). Education can increase quality of and access to care, but it is only effective when clinicians perceive a "need to know" and a desire to learn. If they do not perceive a need and have little interest in expanding their knowledge or skills in this area, physicians can be particularly difficult to reach via education sessions or courses (Byock et al., 2006). Using this concept, Meier and Beresford (2006) used a challenging pretest as one method for motivating group investment in behavioral change with a sample of residents. The pretest assessed how much the residents knew about palliative care issues such as pain and symptom management, establishing goals of care, and eligibility criteria for hospice, as well as what they did not know. The examiner then gave them back their tests with the correct answers and annotated, referenced explanations. From this exercise it was observed that the resident physicians were especially motivated to gain knowledge and skills when their deficiencies were demonstrated, particularly when the content area was relevant to their day-to-day patient care responsibilities. Qualitative approaches, such as the one used by McIlfatrick (2006), that explore stakeholders' perception of palliative care needs are also helpful strategies for establishing group investment in educational objectives. McIlfatrick examined the perspectives of professional providers of care and key health care managerial professionals, along with those of primary caregivers and patients. The semistructured interviews and focus group formats enabled participants to talk freely about their experience, while maintaining a focus on the palliative care subject of interest.

Behavioral shaping (or reinforcing successive approximations toward the intended outcome) is another strategy that is especially relevant when introducing pediatric palliative care educational initiatives into a health care setting. Examples of shaping include "piggybacking" palliative care topics into existing grand round schedules, noon conferences, and other regularly scheduled activities and then positively reinforcing attendance with workplace incentives such as lunches, time for off-site conferences, and other motivators. After some time, the inclusion of palliative care principles in the ongoing staff and faculty education would be an expected standard of care wherein implementation of routine audits for quality pediatric palliative care would then be considered commonplace.

To make an impact with a particular pediatric palliative care educational intervention, one must investigate and assess the needs of the particular environment and then tailor the intervention according to the results of the needs assessment. The adult and pediatric palliative care literatures have described various assessment strategies used for documenting educational needs. Some of these methods involve using case-based tests to examine the knowledge of individual clinicians (e.g., Ray et al., 2006), while other strategies have included assessments of more global clinical knowledge and skills relative to other colleagues from the same discipline and what is entailed within their job description (Becker et al., 2007). A more open-ended needs assessment, such as semistructured interviews and focus groups, can be implemented with not only staff but also patients (when appropriate) and their caregivers (McIlfatrick, 2006).

The educational intervention employed will vary based on specific obstacles uncovered through the needs assessment phase. If it is determined, for example, that both the knowledge base and the communication style across multidisciplinary teams regarding symptom orders need improvement, the introduction of the computerized physician order entry (CPOE) system that incorporates evidence-based algorithms may be the appropriate educational intervention for optimizing the way in which clinicians make ordering decisions (Upperman et al., 2005). Other interventions may include using training modules from the Initiative for Pediatric Palliative Care (IPPC; Solomon et al., 2003), which is case based to enable discussion of individual barriers that prevent palliative care conversations. Ward-Smith et al. (2007) used teachable moments as educational opportunities while providing direct clinical service as a pediatric palliative care team. In other words, when the team encountered a challenging pediatric patient referral, education was most effective when it focused on the needs of a particular child and when implementation outcomes were readily identifiable and attainable.

CHILDREN AND FAMILY MEMBERS AS EDUCATORS

Pediatric patients and their families are powerful voices in bringing awareness to various educational objectives in pediatric palliative care and can be included in these interventions when appropriate. Factors such as the patient's and the family's physical fragility and mental status throughout emotionally challenging periods during the disease course and bereavement must be assessed when considering whether to include pediatric patients and families in any educational initiatives.

Currently, pediatric patients and/or family members have been included as educators through hospital and program parent advisory boards, multiple-learner forums, and research and other academic opportunities. Parent advisory boards have been established to steer policy change and education within the hospital (Zarubi, Reiley, and McCarter, 2008), act as a body of decision makers on residency selection committees (Conway et al., 2006), and create family-centered materials such as educational flyers and guides to be given to families on admission (Christopherson, 2008; Zarubi, Reiley, and McCarter, 2008).

Pediatric patients who have life-threatening illnesses along with their family members have also contributed as educators in multilearner (e.g., consisting of health care providers, hospital administrators, and health care policy stakeholders) forums. Examples of the multilearner model include the IPPC (Solomon et al., 2003), in which family members and multidisciplinary health care providers assemble for a 3-day experiential training workshop, and the Children's Hospital of Philadelphia (CHOP) model (Figueroa-Altmann et al., 2005) for health care providers, aimed at improving partnerships with children and families. Family leaders from CHOP co-present with nursing school faculty on various quality-improvement topics at national nursing leadership forums.

Including children with life-threatening conditions and/or their family in research and other types of academic activities not only empowers the patient and family but also offers tremendous insight for health care providers and researchers who are striving to better understand the phenomenological elements of experiencing a life-threatening condition. Patients and family members facilitate by teaching formal classes at the University of Pennsylvania School of Nursing, while families of chronically ill patients from the CHOP partner with faculty at the University of Pennsylvania School of Nursing, to expand the curriculum on family-centered perspectives in both the undergraduate and graduate programs.

At Harvard Medical School, patients living with a life-threatening condition are teachers of first-year medical students. In this course, students learn to elicit and value patients' perspectives and learn about the power of listening, about kinds of support that help patients and families manage illness, and about the experience of illness and treatment from the patient and the family (Block and Billings, 2005). While in some institutions including family members as part of the educational curriculum is a relatively new undertaking, in other programs, such as the University of Vermont College of

Medicine, partnering with patients and families has been part of physician education since 1985 as a requirement for all third-year medical students' pediatric clerkship; each session is co-taught by parent-to-parent staff (Kaufman, 2008). The teaching from real-life experience that patients and families contribute becomes essential to the advancement of pediatric palliative care within the health care system and also often acts as a legacy for patients who have life-limiting conditions and a way for families to honor the child who has died.

The Initiative for Pediatric Palliative Care

The IPPC, spearheaded by Education Development Center, Inc., was developed in collaboration with the National Association of Children's Hospitals and Related Institutions (NACHRI), the New York Academy of Medicine (NYAM), the Society of Pediatric Nurses, and the Association of Medical School Pediatric Department Chairpersons (AMSPDC). The project began with needs assessment research to uncover the views of bereaved parents (Heller and Solomon, 2005) and clinicians who care for critically ill children (Solomon et al., 2010). An expert panel developed a consensus-based description of quality domains for pediatric palliative care (Dokken et al., 2002) and two instruments that institutions could use to assess their own strengths and areas in need of improvement within those domains (Levetown et al., 2002; Solomon et al., 2003).

CURRICULUM AND EDUCATIONAL RETREATS

Through the process of establishing quality domains and learning parents' and clinicians' views, a core set of learning objectives were defined to guide the development of the curriculum. IPPC aims to enhance the capacity of children's hospitals and other health care organizations to

- maximize family involvement in decision making and care planning in the ways, and to the degree, that each individual family finds comfortable;
- inform and involve children with life-threatening conditions in decisions about their care and care planning as fully as possible, given their developmental abilities and desires;
- reduce pain and distressing symptoms for critically ill children;
- provide emotional and spiritual support to children and families as they cope with the multiple losses associated with life-threatening conditions;

- facilitate the resolution of families' practical needs, such as the need for respite, through coordination with the community;
- facilitate continuity of care across care settings, both within and outside the hospital;
- offer grief support to the child and the family before and after a child's death.

The curriculum (organized into five modules of three to seven lessons per module) was piloted in eight children's hospitals and peer-reviewed through two mechanisms: a review committee created by NACHRI and by two pediatric department chairs, identified by AMSPDC. Detailed facilitator guides, including learning objectives, procedures for running the interactive seminars, cases, and PowerPoint handouts, were developed. Curriculum materials can be downloaded from the IPPC website (www.ippcweb.org). In addition, a series of six films, which have won several national awards, was produced to provide triggers for discussion and learning. The five curriculum modules, designed to give equal weight to psychosocial and medical content, are organized around the following topics: engaging with children and families, relieving pain and other symptoms, analyzing ethical challenges in pediatric end-of-life decision making, responding to suffering and bereavement, and improving communication and strengthening relationships. There is particular attention given in the curriculum to the emotional challenges inherent for clinicians in working with this population of children and families, stressors that can contribute to emotional detachment and burnout.

In addition to the curriculum, which is a major resource in its own right, the IPPC team is conducting face-to-face retreats hosted by local health care organizations at venues across North America. Because there are approximately 100 learning objectives across the five IPPC modules, the retreats are *not* designed to include the entire range of content and skills addressed in the curriculum. Rather, the retreats are intended to expose participants to an overview of the curriculum's content and structure, so that they can further explore it and implement sessions when they return to their home institutions. Equally important, the purpose of the retreats is to inspire and equip clinicians to initiate change projects and to play leadership roles in the area of pediatric palliative care.

To date, IPPC faculty have trained more than 2,000 clinicians at 20 retreats conducted in regions throughout the United States and Canada. In a recently completed assessment of the effectiveness of the retreats in motivating institutional improvements, nearly three-quarters of respondents (74%) reported significant or moderate improvement in pediatric palliative care since the IPPC retreat, with another 25 percent reporting a little improvement; only 1 percent reported no improvement. Notably, 93 percent of respondents credited the IPPC retreat experience as being very or somewhat instrumental to the improvements, which ranged from new or enhanced forms of formal educational experiences to the establishment or strengthening of pediatric palliative care services, new methods for coordinating care, after-death support to families, new ways of communicating with children, more communication across disciplinary lines, and policies aimed at more fully involving parents and families in care and programs (Solomon et al., 2010).

PEDAGOGY

The underlying premise that forms the foundation for all IPPC educational activities is that pediatric palliative care occurs in the context of relationships, and that a pedagogy designed to convey the values, skills, and knowledge inherent in optimal care must be one that appreciates the social and contextualized nature of clinical practice and that focuses on what is happening in the relational space that exists among clinicians, patients, and families. The IPPC investigators originally described this approach to education as relational learning (Browning and Solomon, 2006) and more recently additionally conceptualized the approach as learning that occurs across existing boundaries (Solomon et al., 2010) in the health care world: boundaries between clinicians of different disciplines and between clinicians working in disparate care settings, and boundaries between clinicians and family members, including pediatric patients.

When pedagogy is viewed as a process of relational learning across boundaries, questions of who should be invited into the learning and whose voices need to be heard become critically important. The curriculum and retreats were designed to ensure that, as much as possible, all professional disciplines that most commonly are involved in working with critically ill children—physicians, nurses, social workers, chaplains, child-life specialists—are represented. In addition, professional participation should ideally represent the entire range of care settings—hospitals, rehabilitation facilities, home health, hospice, and community-based agencies—that serves this population of children and families. Because many clinicians lack more than superficial knowledge of the unique training and insight of professional disciplines other than their own, IPPC requests that organizations send interdisciplinary teams to the retreats. In addition to promoting interprofessional understanding and support, this also ensures that when participants return to their home institutions, their efforts to create change will be collective, rather than individual ones.

Because professional learning in health care settings routinely occurs in uniprofessional contexts (like individual silos), bringing together the wide range of professionals into a learning setting in which they will teach each other can be a powerful intervention. However, an even more profound context for learning can be created by including family members in substantive ways. With this value at the fore, IPPC retreats were designed to include family members as fully equal participants. In addition, selected family members with experience in small-group facilitation have been engaged as faculty members. When clinicians and family members are brought together for an intensive, 2½-day period of learning across boundaries in an atmosphere of trust and mutual respect, a remarkable process of transformational learning unfolds. This profound opportunity for meeting and the sharing of knowledge provides an incubator for the kind of robust and real partnerships necessary to improve the care of critically ill children.

Traditionally, the inclusion of family perspectives in medical education has most often taken the form of single, time-limited events in which patients or family members tell their stories to sensitize practitioners to "what it's like" to be in their shoes. Personal narratives presented in this format can be powerful in their own right. Part of their attraction rests, perhaps, in the familiarity of the format, involving a unidirectional transfer of knowledge from an expert (in this case, the family member) to an audience of learners. The reversal of the usual roles of the participants (with the patient or family member as teacher and clinicians as learners) can be innovative and instructive. However, single narratives may have limited utility when the goal is to create long-term, sustainable change in individual clinical and organizational practice and to establish health care environments in which compassionate, culturally competent, pediatric palliative care can thrive.

A comprehensive set of strategies for family participation—the use of short documentary films, the involvement of family members as curriculum developers and faculty, and most especially the inclusion of family members as equal learners in retreats—has had a meaningful impact on such goals as developing greater reciprocity between clinicians and family members, cultivating an understanding of the shared moral burden in difficult end-of-life decisions, and addressing power differentials that prevent optimal learning, clinical care, and the frank exchange of ideas. When a learning environment is established that is safe, nonjudgmental, and respectful of differing viewpoints, family members come to understand clinicians differently and clinicians see family members in a new light. Said one parent participant, "Before, I just saw my grief and my situation from my side of things. It wasn't until I was at the IPPC retreat and was put in a group with medical professionals that I heard their side of the story. I listened to them telling the stories about still remembering their first patient that died and how it still affected them, years later. I realized that health care professionals have a heart and do the best they can with what they have." A clinician commented, "The participation of family members at the retreat was huge in impact. It modeled that involving family members was not threatening but instead was helpful. Health care professionals witnessed and understood that the family perspective was unique and important. It's different hearing about family needs and perspectives directly versus having clinicians describe them."

Human beings who commit themselves to the love and care of critically ill children, whether health care professionals or family members, have a depth of knowledge and common bond that is insufficiently recognized in clinical contexts. This approach to the education of health care professionals—relational learning across boundaries—is proving to be a robust and effective method for cultivating the sharing of that knowledge, in the interest of providing better care to critically ill children and their families.

Graduate Medical Education

Graduate medical education (GME), clinically focused education directed toward medical students, residents, and fellows, forms the backbone of physician education and the foundation of clinical care. The general goal of GME is to help the learner develop competence in a specific area of medicine. More specifically, for hospice and palliative medicine, the goal is to build the foundation of knowledge, to develop the necessary skills, and to foster the attitudes and behaviors essential to provide care to and improve the lives of children with life-threatening conditions and their families.

The approach to GME can take two directions:

1. Learning experiences that address specific learning objectives in which prescribed approaches aim to address a specific competency or area of knowledge. This type of experience includes lectures and innovative learning experiences.
2. Formal curriculum that includes clinical experiences and didactic offerings over a set period of time. This type of experience is appropriate for electives, formal rotations, and fellowships.

In this section we will provide a framework and guide—the competencies in hospice and palliative medicine—for educational pursuits directed toward residents and fellows. We will discuss an abbreviated approach to curriculum development and briefly review some of the innovative educational tools for medical students, residents, and fellows in hospice and palliative medicine.

CORE COMPETENCIES

Each specialty of medicine defines the knowledge, skills, attitudes, and behaviors essential to clinical care. These then set the standards for education and attainment of competence. In hospice and palliative medicine, the *Companion Document: Core Competencies for Hospice and Palliative Medicine Fellowship Training* (Morrison, Scott, and Block, 2007; Education ACGME, 2008) established these competencies.

Hospice and palliative medicine is unique in that the essential competencies are not exclusive to that field. Skilled, open, and honest communication, excellent management of symptoms, and use of an interdisciplinary team are skills essential to all clinical practice. In the practice of hospice and palliative medicine, they are simply used in extreme circumstances. This fact is important to GME, as few clinicians will go on to specialize in hospice and palliative medicine. All clinicians, however, will go on to use the same competencies in the care of patients and will benefit from learning experiences focused on hospice and palliative medicine.

The core competencies and learning objectives can provide the framework and direction for all training programs and educational experiences in hospice and palliative medicine. While pediatric residents and non–hospice and palliative medicine fellows do not need to be expert in all of these competencies, they do need to be introduced to the knowledge, skills, attitudes, and behaviors described by them. For this reason, these competencies can provide a guide to what should be taught in any educational experience in hospice and palliative medicine. Each educational experience can provide a component of competency that, when taken as a whole, will help build competent clinicians and improve the care of children.

COMPETENCY VERSUS EXPERIENCE-BASED EDUCATION

Traditionally, GME has been focused on experience-based education. Competence is assumed if the learner is exposed to a certain number of similar clinical situations. The Accreditation Council for Graduate Medical Education, the governing body for accredited GME programs, recognizes that programs have a responsibility to ensure the competency of the learner to provide care. In other words, educational programs are responsible, and soon will be required, to ensure competence in clinical care. While this standard is in place only for accredited training programs, this vision should be in place for all GME opportunities, including didactic lectures, elective experiences, and core rotations.

DESIGNING A PROGRAM SPECIFIC TO THE LEARNER

The care of children with life-threatening illnesses and their families can be complex, requiring a mastery of using an interdisciplinary team and a process of life-long learning to become an expert in the field. Each learner has a different foundation of knowledge and understanding of patient care, making each learner's needs unique (Kolarik, Walker, and Arnold, 2006). Each experience should be directed at the level of competence of the learner but still accomplish progression toward increased competence in one or more of the competencies.

The beginning learner should get a start by participating in a didactic program of the basics of palliative care. Lectures, small-group discussions, and patient debriefings centered on introduction to palliative care, the scope and tasks of palliative care, defining an interdisciplinary team, and the basics of pain management are all appropriate.

As the learner becomes more advanced, clinical skills will improve only through practice in patient care. For this reason, learners with growing experience should be exposed to clinical experiences simply by integrating the learners as part of the clinical team and allowing them to directly observe and participate in patient care. Didactic offerings should expand to include journal clubs, debriefings after difficult patient interactions, and talks focusing on the psychosocial aspects of care and issues of self-care.

Advanced learners need to be exposed to a diverse set of experiences in an effort to apply their knowledge to other situations. This diversity should include other care settings, such as outpatient clinics, patients' homes, exposure to adult practitioners and patients, and hospital or hospice-based care. Partnerships with community groups and partnering agencies can help provide these experiences.

CURRICULUM DEVELOPMENT

Curriculum development can seem like a daunting task. The process, however, can be approached systematically over time, adding additional components to the curriculum as the program and faculty gain experience and the specific needs of the learners are more apparent. A curriculum can be defined as a combination of intended content and the set of learning experiences meant to teach that content and improve the competency of a group of learners. In general, these experiences should include clinical and didactic experiences that augment each other. Practically, the most efficient way to develop a curriculum is to design the experiences as part of normal patient care as follows:

Most excellent educational programs focus on patient care, providing direct exposure to a diverse range of pediatric care. Most adults learn best when placed in real situations that require them to apply the skills they are trying to learn, with direct and timely feedback and evaluation. For this reason, GME is most effective when a learner has practical experiences that are paired with didactic discussions that detail the subject. In addition, using the learner in direct patient care as part of normal patient and team flow can relieve some of the time burden spent on providing this education.

The didactic component of a curriculum is designed to augment the clinical experience by providing a framework of knowledge, as well as to cover topics not traditionally found in a clinical setting. In general, these experiences should be case based and refer to actual patient interactions as much as possible. Some programs and hospitals do not have the patient volume or diversity to support a meaningful clinical experience. In these situations, an excellent didactic program can still be achieved with offerings remaining case based and interactive.

Many pediatric palliative care teams include members with clear areas of expertise in symptom management, communication, psychosocial issues, or another competency. This expertise should be used through lectures and small-group, patient-based discussions. In general, the best and most efficient way to use these resources is by having the faculty teach to their strengths.

A STEPWISE APPROACH TO BUILDING A CURRICULUM OVER TIME

For beginning programs in the early phases of initiating educational programs, a proper curriculum simply includes a didactic program that aims to teach the basic knowledge essential for palliative care. These offerings should include lectures and small-group discussions on topics such as principles of pediatric hospice and palliative medicine, communication skills in delivering bad news and determining goals of care, and pain and symptom management. Skill development and improvement in clinical care, however, require practice and use of these skills in patient care (Allard et al., 2001; Ferris, von Gunten, and Emanuel, 2001). For this reason, the program should quickly evolve to include a clinical component.

Once the program gains exposure through its didactic offerings, it should then focus on adding a clinical experience by simply integrating learners as part of the clinical team. Allowing learners to directly participate in patient care and family meetings will facilitate a role-modeling experience and place them in situations where they can practice these skills. This system can be especially valuable for the professional just beginning to understand the scope and practice of hospice and palliative medicine. More specifically, the role-modeling can be an acceptable initial way to expose the learner to communication styles, working with an interdisciplinary team, and working with colleagues as part of self-care. While participation on the team is a great initial experience, the learner must have a direct, hands-on role in patient care. Role-modeling is valuable only if the learner is able to solidify the experience with direct patient care.

Didactic offerings can then expand to small-group, patient-based discussions; journal clubs with topics pertinent to patient care; and participation in debriefings after difficult patient interactions or the death of a child. Small-group discussions focused on the psychosocial aspects of care and issues of self-care are also valuable. Some programs also sponsor a morbidity and mortality conference in which the psychosocial aspects of care are discussed in addition to the pathophysiology and medical decision making.

Once a program has an established institutional-based clinical and didactic curriculum, the program should begin to diversify this experience by providing experiences in other care settings, such as outpatient clinics and the home environment, and even provide exposure to adult patients. To accomplish this, the program should establish relationships with community groups that can provide experiences that will augment the curriculum. Community hospices can take the learner into the homes of pediatric and adult patients. This experience has proven invaluable to helping the learner understand the challenges a family faces outside the vast resources of the hospital, as well as the challenges a hospice and palliative medicine team has in caring for a child at home. In addition, given their higher patient volume, regional adult-focused hospice and palliative care programs can provide diverse clinical and didactic offerings that may be outside the expertise of the pediatric program. While the pediatric program will then have to translate this knowledge to be applicable to children, many of the principles of communication, psychosocial issues, and even pain and symptom management are applicable.

Significant experience in GME can be accomplished in a short period of time. By building a program based on the competencies, including didactic and clinical experiences and building relationships with community hospices and adult-focused programs, the program will quickly evolve to be able to support non-pediatrics-trained physicians, such as adult-focused hospice and palliative medicine fellows, and even establish an accredited pediatric-focused fellowship training program.

One of the main barriers in developing a pediatric-focused training program is the development of a curriculum. Once the program has experience providing GME, the development of a fellowship curriculum is simply ensuring that all of the competencies can be addressed and the evaluation methods are in place.

SPECIFIC TEACHING STRATEGIES

The deficiency in educational offerings in hospice and palliative medicine has been well established, most notably by the Institute of Medicine reports *Approaching Death: Improving Care at the End of Life* and *When Children Die: Improving Palliative and End-of-Life Care for Children and Their Families.* With this deficiency in mind, a number of institutions have reported their programs in the literature. They include

- didactic focused offerings (Martin and Wylie, 1989; Grauel et al., 1996; Linder et al., 1999; Fins and Nilson, 2000; Lewin, Agneberg, and Alexander, 2000; Fischer et al., 2003; Schuh et al., 2007);
- clinical rotations (Von Roenn et al., 1988; Linder et al., 1999);
- small-group workshops and conferences (Knox and Thomson, 1989; Baile et al., 1997; Vaidya et al., 1999; Magnani, Minor, and Aldrich, 2002; Balmer et al., 2007);
- evaluation tools based on patient interaction (Han et al., 2005);
- simulated patients (Garg, Buckman, and Kason, 1997; Greenberg et al., 1999; Freer and Zinnerstrom, 2001; Roter et al., 2004).

All of these programs offer unique strategies for providing pediatric hospice and palliative medicine education. An innovative and comprehensive program would likely include strategies used in each of these programs.

As discussed in other parts of this chapter, online resources and modules such as the IPPC and the End of Life / Palliative Education Resource Center (EPERC) can further augment a curriculum. While some of these resources were developed for nonphysicians, certain modules are applicable to physician education.

There is some evidence that residents and fellows learn from role-modeling experiences (Balmer et al., 2007). While shadowing alone is not a sufficient learning experience, allowing a medical student or resident to witness and debrief about a family meeting focused on delivering bad news or establishing bad news can help impart templates for interpersonal communication. These competencies, however, will become solidified only if the learner is allowed to participate and practice.

Communication is an essential skill recognized as a core competency in all medical fields. Few proven standard methods for teaching communication exist. There are, however, some innovative techniques, including patient simulation (Greenberg et al., 1999), video feedback after interaction with standardized patients (Serwint, 2002; Roter et al., 2004), and role-play with timely direct feedback. The two most important common factors in all of these tools are direct interaction with a patient or patient substitute and timely, direct feedback to the learner. Importantly, skill development requires practice (Allard et al., 2001; Ferris, von Gunten, and Emanuel, 2001) and should be facilitated and supported in direct patient care.

Medical students, residents, and fellows rarely experience caring for patients in the home. In hospice and palliative medicine, visiting the home environment often enlightens the clinician to many insights into the patient's challenges and supports. If the clinical team is not able to do a home visit, many area hospice agencies and nurses will take the learner on their clinical rounds.

While it is clear that all areas of clinical medicine share many of the competencies essential to hospice and palliative medicine, few other fields, including pediatric residency programs, formally recognize many of these competencies. Using the *Companion Document: Core Competencies for Hospice and Palliative Medicine Fellowship Training* as a guide in initiating education offerings can provide a framework to building a curriculum. Building the curriculum using a stepwise approach over time can lead a program to establish an excellent GME experience. Finally, integrating the learner as part of the team can be a meaningful experience for both the program and the learner.

Continuing Medical Education

SELF-ASSESSMENT BY PEDIATRIC PRACTITIONERS

Self-assessment of pediatric practitioners' knowledge and skill in pediatric palliative care and pain management has been reported in subspecialist and general pediatrician samples. Of 110 attending physicians in a single-institution survey with approximately one-third general pediatricians and two-thirds pediatric subspecialists, 43 percent felt inexperienced with the management of symptoms of dying patients and 49 percent felt inexperienced with pain management (Contro et al., 2004). In the same study, the proportions of attending physicians who felt inexperienced with communicating with dying patients, communicating with patients' families, discussing transition to palliative care, and discussing do-not-resuscitate status were 40, 30, 50, and 35 percent, respectively. Of the general pediatricians and subspecialists (n = 223) surveyed from a single health care system, less than half were confident in their ability to describe palliative care concepts to children and families (44%), and approximately one-quarter were confident using opioids to manage pain (27%) and other end-of-life symptoms (23%) (Sheetz and Bowman, 2008). In contrast, the majority of practicing pediatric oncologists (n = 228) in the United States, Canada, and the United Kingdom reported competence in managing pain (91.1%), communicating with dying patients and their families (96.3%), and transitioning to palliative care (94.6%) (Hilden et al., 2001). Discordance between reports of parents and physicians regarding children's symptoms in the last month of life has been reported (Wolfe et al., 2000). Admittedly, self-assessment is not necessarily a measure of actual practice.

PEDIATRIC AND FAMILY MEDICINE BOARD CERTIFICATION REQUIREMENTS

The 2009–10 American Board of Pediatrics content outline for maintenance of certification for general pediatrics includes Palliative Care and Pain Management with the objective "to recognize and apply ethical principles involving palliative care and pain management." Pediatric subspecialty content specific to palliative care is lacking. Maintenance of certification for pediatric critical care medicine refers to the ethical issues around termination of care (Subboard of Pediatric Critical Care Medicine, 2008), pediatric hematology/oncology refers to arranging for terminal care for the patient and counseling for family in fatal illness (Subboard of Pediatric Hematology-Oncology, 2006), and neonatal medicine refers to aspects of grief counseling before, during, and after the death of a newborn infant (Subboard of Neonatal-Perinatal Medicine, 2008); the remaining subspecialty requirements do not contain any pediatric palliative care content. The Curriculum in Pediatric Palliative Medicine prepared by the education subgroups of the British Society for Pediatric Palliative Medicine and Association of Children's Hospice Doctors is a much more detailed account of the knowledge and skills needed for physicians specific to their level of training and area of expertise (Education subgroups of the British Society Pediatric Palliative Medicine and Association of Children's Hospice Doctors, 2007). The American Board of Family Medicine's recertification requirements include palliative care and end-of-life care under examination content (American Board of Family

Medicine, 2007). End-of-life issues and pain management are specifically included under geriatrics in the examination modules but are absent from child and adolescent care (American Board of Family Medicine, 2005).

STATE LICENSING REQUIREMENTS IN PALLIATIVE CARE

State medical licensing boards have required that continuing medical education include end-of-life, palliative care, pain management, or some combination thereof in California, Florida, Oregon, Rhode Island, West Virginia, and the District of Columbia (Advanced Studies in Medicine, 2008; American Academy of Dermatology, 2008). Specifics of how the requirement must be filled vary in these states. Other states are considering the addition of this requirement for licensure, and both allopathic and osteopathic physicians should check with the board in their state of practice. More specific requirements for what constitutes expertise in pediatric pain and palliative medicine will be required as state-specific waiver programs following the Children's Hospice International Program for All-inclusive Care for Children and their families (PACC) model provide reimbursement for pediatric pain and palliative physician expertise and services (Armstrong-Dailey and Koppelman, 2007).

TEXTBOOKS

Expertise in pediatric palliative care for the pediatrician or family medicine physician in practice is increasingly available. Textbooks dedicated to (Goldman, Hain, and Liben, 2006) or with chapters about (Liben, 2000; Ablin, 2003) pediatric palliative care have been published. The Compendium of Pediatric Palliative Care (Children's International Project on Palliative/ Hospice Services, 2000) contains multiple program-specific documents, as well as delineation of how the principles of pediatric palliative care may be applied in outpatient and inpatient settings. An updated and online version of the educational curricula published by the Children's Project on Hospice/ Palliative Services (ChiPPS; Papadatou et al., 2003) is planned.

NATIONAL MEETINGS AND ONLINE LEARNING

State and national meetings provide opportunities for physicians to attend oral and poster presentations, network, and participate in special interest groups. The yearly national meetings of the American Academy of Hospice and Palliative Medicine (AAHPM), the National Hospice and Palliative Care Organization (NHPCO), and the American Academy of Pediatrics frequently include neonatal, pediatric, and adolescent palliative care content.

NHPCO also offers a pediatric Listserv that is available through their website (www.nhpco.org). Online courses for "Pain and Symptom Management for Children Receiving Hospice and Palliative Care" and "Caring for Children Coping with Death: Providing Psychosocial and Spiritual Assistance" have been offered through Mount Ida College (www.mountida.edu/sp.cfm ?pageid=1730).

INTENSIVE TRAINING

Intensive training programs have also evolved from education models in adult palliative care. Most of these programs require participants to submit an application before enrollment. The Program in Palliative Care and Education Practice provided by the Harvard Medical School Department of Continuing Education began in 2000. In 2008, a 2-week-long pediatric track was offered for the first time based on feedback from pediatric care providers. Formats included didactic lecture presentation as well as more interactive formats that include role-playing.

The Children's Institute for Pain and Palliative Care (CIPPC) in Minneapolis first offered the "Ahlaya Seminars" for comprehensive training in pediatric palliative care in 2004. Sponsored by the NHPCO and Clinics of Minnesota, they were developed to train health care providers in pediatric palliative care and to create a resource and consultation network for those clinicians. The course continues to be offered one to two times per year. An annual Pediatric Palliative Care Master Class began in 2010. CIPPC also offers an annual week-long Pediatric Pain Master Class in response to pediatric palliative care providers' requests for more advanced training in pain management. Presentations are made by a multidisciplinary faculty of physicians, an advanced practice nurse, and a clinical social worker.

The Center to Advance Palliative Care (CAPC) has training and mentoring sessions specific to pediatric palliative care programs that meet for 2 days four times per year. In contrast to programs that prepare the clinician to work at the bedside, this curriculum addresses program development and growth. Trainings are designed for teams, providing intensive, hands-on operational training and year-long mentoring, to start and/or expand their palliative care programs. Akron Children's Hospital (Ohio) and Children's Hospitals and Clinics of Minnesota are the two PCLC pediatric training locations selected for 2009. Topics covered include systems assessment and mission statement, clinical models of staffing, financial case and sustainability, continuity of care, measurement, internal marketing, palliative care education, and program implementation.

Conclusion

There is a continued need to advance professional education in pediatric palliative care, as professional competence is the foundation of improved care. The programs described above serve as models with demonstrated effectiveness. Continued evolution of these programs and new innovations are needed, and methods for evaluation of outcomes of education will strengthen our efforts to improve the quality of care.

References

Ablin, A.R. 2003. Caring for children dying from chronic disease. In *Rudolph's Pediatrics*, 21st ed., ed. C. Rudolph, A.M. Rudolph, M.K. Hostetter, et al., pp. 563–72. New York: McGraw-Hill.

Advanced Studies in Medicine, Johns Hopkins University School of Medicine. 2008. Physician CME requirements. www.jhasim.com/template.cfm?TEMPLATE=phys_cme_req.cfm (accessed February 10, 2010).

Allard, P., Maunsell, E., Labbe, J., et al. 2001. Educational interventions to improve cancer pain control: A systematic review. *J Palliat Med* 4(2):191–203.

American Academy of Dermatology. 2008. Continuing medical education for licensure reregistration. State Medical Licensure Requirements and Statistics. www.aad.org (accessed February 10, 2010).

American Academy of Pediatrics, Committee on Bioethics and Committee on Hospital Care. 2000. Palliative care for children. *Pediatrics* 106:351–57.

American Association of Colleges of Nurses (AACN). 1997. *A Peaceful Death: Recommended Competencies and Curricular Guidelines for End of Life Care [Report from the Robert Wood Johnson End-of-Life Care roundtable].* Washington, DC: AACN. www.aacn.nche.edu/ELNEC/ (accessed February 10, 2010).

American Board of Family Medicine. 2005. Certification/recertification examination modules. www.theabfm.org/cert/DescriptionsModulesCert.pdf (accessed February 10, 2010).

———. 2007. Certification/recertification examination content. www.theabfm.org/cert/CertRecertExaminationOutline.pdf (accessed February 10, 2010).

Armstrong-Dailey, A., and Koppelman, J. 2007. Settings for pediatric palliative care in the United States. *Medical Principles and Practice* 16(Suppl 1):42–43.

Baile, W.F., Lenzi, R., Kudelka, A.P., et al. 1997. Improving physician-patient communication in cancer care: Outcome of a workshop for oncologists. *J Cancer Educ* 12(3):166–73.

Balmer, D., Serwint, J.R., Ruzek, S.B., et al. 2007. Learning behind the scenes: Perceptions and observations of role modeling in pediatric residents' continuity experience. *Ambul Pediatr* 7(2):176–81.

Becker, G., Momm, F., Gigl, A., et al. 2007. Competency and educational needs in palliative care. *Wiener Klinische Wochenschrift* 119:112–16.

Block, S.D., and Billings, J.A. 2005. Learning from the dying. *N Engl J Med* 323(13): 1313–15.

Browning, D.M., and Solomon, M.Z., for the Initiative for Pediatric Palliative Care, Investigator Team. 2005. The Initiative for Pediatric Palliative Care: An interdisciplinary educational approach for healthcare professionals. *J Pediatr Nurs* 20:326–34.

Browning, D.M., and Solomon, M.Z. 2006. Relational learning in pediatric palliative care: Transformative education and the culture of medicine. *Child and Adolescent Psychiatric Clinics of North America* 15:795–815.

Byock, I., Sheils Twohig, J., Merriman, M., et al. 2006. Promoting excellence in end-of-life care: A report on innovative models of palliative care. *J Palliat Med* 9:137–51.

Children's International Project on Palliative/Hospice Services. 2000. *Compendium of pediatric palliative care.* Alexandria: National Hospice and Palliative Care Organization.

Christopherson, T.M. 2008. Staff development story. *J Nurses Staff Develop* 24:252–55.

Contro, N.A., Larson, J., Scofield, S., et al. 2004. Hospital staff and family perspectives regarding quality of pediatric palliative care. *Pediatrics* 114(5):1248–52.

Conway, J., Johnson, B.H., Edgman-Levitan, S., et al. 2006. Partnering with patients and families to design a patient- and family-centered health care system: A roadmap for the future—a work in progress. www.familycenteredcare.org/pdf/Roadmap.pdf (accessed February 10, 2010).

Dokken, D.L., Heller, K.S., Levetown, M., et al., for the Initiative for Pediatric Palliative Care. 2002. Quality domains, goals and indicators of family-centered care of children living with life-threatening conditions. Newton, MA: Education Development Center. Available at www.ippcweb.org (accessed February 10, 2010).

Education ACGME. 2008. Companion document: Core competencies for hospice and palliative medicine fellowship training. www.acgme.org/acWebsite/downloads/RRC_progReq/540_hospice_and_palliative_medicine_companion_02122008.pdf (accessed February 10, 2010).

Education subgroups of the British Society for Paediatric Palliative Medicine and Association of Children's Hospice Doctors. 2007. Curriculum in paediatric palliative medicine. www.act.org.uk/page.asp?section=169&sectionTitle=Curriculum+in+Paediatric+Palliative+Medicine (accessed February 10, 2010).

Ellis, J.A., McCleary, L., Blouin, R., et al. 2007. Implementing best practice pain management in a pediatric hospital. *J Spec Pediatr Nurs* 12:264–77.

Ferrell, B., Virani, R., Grant, M., et al. 2000. Beyond the Supreme Court decision: Nursing perspectives on end-of-life care. *Oncology Nursing Forum* 27(3):445–55.

Ferris, F.D., von Gunten, C.F., and Emanuel, L.L. 2001. Knowledge: Insufficient for change. *J Palliat Med* 4(2):145–47.

Field, M., and Behrman, R. 2003. *When Children Die: Improving Palliative and End of Life Care for Children and Their Families.* Washington, DC: National Academies Press.

Figueroa-Altmann, A.R., Bedrossian, L., Steinmiller, E.A., et al. 2005. Improving partnerships with children and families: A model from the Children's Hospital of Philadelphia. *Am J Nursing* 105(6):72A–72C.

Fins, J.J., and Nilson, E.G. 2000. An approach to educating residents about palliative care and clinical ethics. *Acad Med* 75(6):662–65.

Fischer, S.M., Gozansky, W.S., Kutner, J.S., et al. 2003. Palliative care education: An intervention to improve medical residents' knowledge and attitudes. *J Palliat Med* 6(3):391–99.

Freer, J.P., and Zinnerstrom, K.L. 2001. The palliative medicine extended standardized patient scenario: A preliminary report. *J Palliat Med* 4(1):49–56.

Garg, A., Buckman, R., and Kason, Y. 1997. Teaching medical students how to break bad news. *CMAJ* 156(8):1159–64.

Goldman, A., Hain, R., and Liben, S., eds. 2006. *Oxford Textbook of Palliative Care for Children.* New York: Oxford University Press.

Grauel, R.R., Eger, R., Finley, R.C., et al. 1996. Educational program in palliative and hospice care at the University of Maryland School of Medicine. *J Cancer Educ* 11(3):144–47.

Greenberg, L.W., Ochsenschlager, D., O'Donnell, R., et al. 1999. Communicating bad news: A pediatric department's evaluation of a simulated intervention. *Pediatrics* 103:1210–17.

Han, P.K., Keranen, L.B., Lescisin, D.A., et al. 2005. The palliative care clinical evaluation exercise (CEX): An experience-based intervention for teaching end-of-life communication skills. *Acad Med* 80(7):669–76.

Heller, K.S., and Solomon, M.Z. 2005. Continuity of caring: What matters to parents of children with life-threatening conditions. *J Pediatr Nurs* 20(5):335–46.

Hilden, J.M., Emanuel, E.J., Fairclough, D.L., et al. 2001. Attitudes and practices among pediatric oncologists regarding end-of-life care: Results of the 1998 American Society of Clinical Oncology Survey. *J Clin Oncology* 19(1):205–12.

Jacobs, H.H., Ferrell, B., Virani, R., et al. 2009. Appraisal of the Pediatric End-of-Life Nursing Education Consortium (ELNEC) training program. *J Pediatr Nurs* 24(3): 216–21.

Kaufman, J. 2008. Patients as partners. *Nursing Management* 39:45–48.

Knox, J.D., and Thomson, G.M. 1989. Breaking bad news: Medical undergraduate communication skills teaching and learning. *Med Educ* 23(3):258–61.

Kolarik, R.C., Walker, G., and Arnold, R.M. 2006. Pediatric resident education in palliative care: A needs assessment. *Pediatrics* 117:1949–54.

Levetown, M., Dokken, D.L., Fleischman, A.R., et al., for the Initiative for Pediatric Palliative Care. 2002. A pediatric palliative care institutional self-assessment tool (ISAT). Newton, MA: Education Development Center. For information, contact: M.Z. Solomon, c/o EDC, 55 Chapel Street, Newton, MA 02458. Also available at www.ippcweb.org (accessed February 10, 2010).

Lewin, L.O., Agneberg, B., and Alexander, G.C. 2000. A course in end-of-life care for third-year medical students. *Acad Med* 75(5):519–20.

Liben, S. 2000. Pediatric palliative care: The care of children with life-limiting illness. In *Nelson Textbook of Pediatrics*, 16th ed., ed. R.E. Behrman, R.M. Kliegman, and H.B. Jenson, pp. 129–33. Philadelphia: W.B. Saunders Co.

Linder, J.F., Blais, J., Enders, S.R., et al. 1999. Palliative education: A didactic and experiential approach to teaching end-of-life care. *J Cancer Educ* 14(3):154–60.

Magnani, J.W., Minor, M.A., and Aldrich, J.M. 2002. Care at the end of life: A novel curriculum module implemented by medical students. *Acad Med* 77(4): 292–98.

Malloy, P., Sumner, E., Virani, R., et al. 2007. End-of-Life Nursing Education Consortium for Pediatric Palliative Care (ELNEC-PPC). *MCN: Am J Maternal/Child Nursing* 32(5):298–302.

Martin, R.W., III, and Wylie, N. 1989. Teaching third-year medical students how to care for terminally ill patients. *Acad Med* 64(7):413–14.

Matzo, M., and Hijjazi, K. 2008. There's no place like home: Oklahomans' preferences for site of death. *PCRT* 1:3–12.

McIlfatrick, S. 2006. Assessing palliative care needs: Views of patients, informal carers and healthcare professionals. *J Advanc Nursing* 57:77–86.

Meier, D.E., and Beresford, L. 2006. Palliative care has a role in the essential task of educating medical residents. *J Palliat Med* 9:842–46.

Morrison, L.J., Scott, J.O., and Block, S.D. 2007. Developing initial competency-based outcomes for the hospice and palliative medicine subspecialist: Phase I of the hospice and palliative medicine competencies project. *J Palliat Med* 10(2):313–30.

Papadatou, D., Corr, C., Frager, G., et al. 2003. *Education and Training Curriculum for Pediatric Palliative Care*. Alexandria: National Hospice and Palliative Care Organization.

Ray, D., Fuhrman, C., Stern, G., et al. 2006. Integrating palliative medicine and critical care in a community hospital. *Crit Care Med* 34:S394–98.

Roter, D.L., Larson, S., Shinitzky, H., et al. 2004. Use of an innovative video feedback technique to enhance communication skills training. *Med Educ* 38(2):145–57.

Schuh, L.A., Biondo, A., An, A., et al. 2007. Neurology resident learning in an end-of-life/palliative care course. *J Palliat Med* 10(1):178–81.

Serwint, J.R. 2002. The use of standardized patients in pediatric residency training in palliative care: Anatomy of a standardized patient case scenario. *J Palliat Med* 5(1):146–53.

Sheetz, M. J., and Bowman, M.-A.S. 2008. Pediatric palliative care: An assessment of physicians' confidence in skills, desire for training, and willingness to refer for end-of-life care. *Am J Hospice Palliat Med* 25(2):100–105.

Sherman, D.W., McSherry, C.B., Parkas, V., et al. 2005. Recruitment and retention in a longitudinal palliative care study. *Appl Nurs Res* 18:167–77.

Solomon, M.Z., Browning, D.M., Dokken, D., et al. 2003. *The Initiative for Pediatric Palliative Care (IPPC) Curriculum: Enhancing Family-Centered Care for Children with Life-Threatening Conditions*. Newton, MA: Education Development Center.

———. 2010. Learning that leads to action: Impact and characteristics of a professional education approach to improve the care of critically ill children and their families. *Arch Pediatr Adolesc Med.* 164(4):315–22.

Subboard of Neonatal-Perinatal Medicine. 2008. Content outline: Neonatal-perinatal medicine; subspecialty certification and maintenance of certification examinations, 2010. www.abp.org/ABPWebSite/certinfo/subspec/suboutlines/neon2010.pdf (accessed February 10, 2010).

Subboard of Pediatric Critical Care Medicine. 2008. Content outline: Pediatric critical care medicine; certification and maintenance of certification examinations. www.aap.org/Sections/critcare/contentspecs10–04.pdf (accessed January 10, 2011).

Subboard of Pediatric Hematology-Oncology. 2006. Content outline: Pediatric hematology-oncology; certification and maintenance of certification examinations.

www.abp.org/abpwebsite/certinfo/subspec/suboutlines/hemo2011.pdf (accessed January 10, 2011).

Upperman, J.S., Staley, P., Friend, K., et al. 2005. The introduction of computerized physician order entry and change management in a tertiary pediatric hospital. *Pediatrics* 116:e634–42.

Vaidya, V.U., Greenberg, L.W., Patel, K.M., et al. 1999. Teaching physicians how to break bad news: A 1-day workshop using standardized parents. *Arch Pediatr Adolesc Med* 153(4):419–22.

Von Roenn, J.H., Neely, K.J., Curry, R.H., et al. 1988. A curriculum in palliative care for internal medicine housestaff: A pilot project. *J Cancer Educ* 3(4):259–63.

Ward-Smith, P., Linn, J.B., Korphage, R.M., et al. 2007. Development of a pediatric palliative care team. *J Pediatr Health Care* 21:245–49.

Wolfe, J., Grier, H.E., Klar, N., et al. 2000. Symptoms and suffering at the end of life in children with cancer. *N Engl J Med* 324(5):326–33.

World Health Organization. 2002. *National Cancer Control Programmes: Policies and Managerial Guidelines*, 2nd ed. Geneva: World Health Organization.

Zarubi, K.L., Reiley, P., and McCarter, B. 2008. Putting patients and families at the center of care. *J Nursing Admin* 38:275–81.

5

The Art of Advocacy

Devon Dabbs, Lori Butterworth, Mary Jo Gilmer, Ph.D., M.B.A., R.N., Brian Greffe, M.D., and Melody Hellsten, M.S.N., P.N.P.

This chapter features the story of Nick Snow, a teenager from California who rallied to bring about change in the care of children faced with life-limiting and life-threatening conditions, while dealing with his own struggle against brain cancer. Key points in this chapter include the following:

- Advocacy, while taking many forms, is largely about effecting change around a cause.
- Advocacy requires knowledge about the cause, but also about the targeted community.
- Advocacy demands patience and persistence and is effected by addressing methodologies available through the media, the health care industry, and the government.

Nick Snow never expected to be a champion for a cause, a hero in the eyes of many. Like most heroes, he was thrust into the role by circumstance; rather than shrink from the challenge, he confronted it with courage and dignity. Nick wanted to play drums in his room or swim in the river with his brother, not be bothered by a strange growth in his body. At age 6, he was diagnosed with neuroblastoma, a rare cancer of the nerve cells of some children who are usually under 10 years of age. Four years later, doctors told his parents just before Halloween that he probably would die by Christmas; instead, Nick enjoyed those holidays and many more, confounding the dire predictions until succumbing to an infection related to his cancer in 2006, at age 16.

Nick strongly believed that what we do with the life we have is more important than how long we live. His short life is a model for how to handle adversity, how to stand for something bigger than oneself, and how to inject meaning into the brief time that we all have, inspiring people long after our physical presence is gone. Nick's ordeal—84 months of treatment, including chemotherapies, surgeries, four types of radiation, a bone marrow transplant, many experimental therapies, two referrals to hospice, and countless predictions that his time was up—demonstrates that believing you can go on can be healthy and that anyone willing to put his or her shoulder to a solution and get it rolling can generate big change. Through his actions and his enduring spirit, Nick personified the art of advocacy.

Creating Change and Summoning Empowerment

Advocacy is defined as "the act or process of supporting a cause or proposal." In Nick's story, advocacy can be understood as the pursuit of influencing outcomes, which may include influencing the allocation of resources as well as policies affecting families' lives (Cohen, de la Vega, and Watson, 2001). Health care providers view engaging in advocacy as a professional ideal, but implementation is left to the individual. Some may argue that advocacy means defending a child and family's rights or ensuring that a child's immediate needs are met. Others see advocacy as a role-related responsibility of the health care provider.

Realizing that advocacy as a professional ideal has its roots in the field of law may be helpful in understanding practical application of Nick's story. In legal terms, advocacy means the "verbal act of arguing for a person's cause against the cause of an adversary" (Grace, 2009, p. 122). In this manner, an attorney may argue for the cause of an individual, but not necessarily for policy or the rights of a group of people, such as children with life-threatening conditions. Health care providers, however, have simultaneous responsibilities to more than one child and family. Advocacy may then extend beyond an immediate decision and action applicable to the well-being of an individual child to a wider arena of policy affecting a population of patients and their families.

Even in the best of circumstances, the process of change can be difficult and fraught with conflict. But in palliative care, with the prospect of death always present, change may be even more difficult because of the intense emotions, many of which revolve around fear. Both cognitive and behavioral processes need to be addressed when trying to orchestrate enduring change; thus, the advocate's strategy should be to acknowledge and address stakeholders' emotions, values, and understanding and then plan an action

accordingly (Prochaska, DiClemente, and Norcross, 1992). Change is difficult to achieve. People fear change because of the accompanying uncertainty
and potential costs, both emotional and financial. Again, in palliative care
patients bring to the forefront the ever-present specter of death, which often
intensifies feelings and skews behavior. Any substantive effort to foment
change in the organization and delivery of health care, especially as it applies
to palliative care for children, must consider the complexities of the human
elements that are at play—the unimaginable loss of a young life, the associated potentially overwhelming emotions, personal values, often limited
understanding of events, potentially irrational behavior, fear, and attempts
to reason and understand the unfamiliar and unfathomable.

Existing systems of care are mostly sufficient to meet the needs of adults
with life-threatening conditions but are inadequate to meet the needs of children. Enabling consistent expertise and capacity to meet the needs of children
with life-threatening conditions and their families will require profound,
transformative changes in health care delivery in the United States. Such
meaningful change can occur only with the collaborative efforts of caregivers, institutions, and families. The challenge is to educate the public, legislators, researchers, and third-party payers about the needs of patients, families,
and caregivers faced with the unenviable task of enabling a child with a life-
threatening condition to live well and to die peacefully. The families, too,
need to be supported throughout the illness experience and often long afterward. Clinician advocates need to recognize that people respond differently
to change. Fears needs to be addressed proactively and managed effectively,
expectations may not be met for everyone at the same time, and change
inevitably involves loss. For these reasons, compassionate, open communication is essential every step of the way. Those affected by change need an
opportunity to express their concerns. Honest and open interactions, as well
as collection of data to determine the success of the change or the need for
modifications, are essential to creating enduring and well-supported change.

One of the greatest communication challenges in bringing together a
group of individuals or organizations with the goal of creating change is to
give that effort a name. While it seems on the surface a trivial detail, in reality the name attached to an organization communicates its goals and sets
a participatory tone for the members of the organization. Below are some
common labels that are beneficial in enabling such collaborative efforts.

Coalition—a temporary alliance or gathering of competing organizations
for the purposes of joint action toward a specific aim. It typically does not
include sharing or pooling of resources or collaborative project development
(www.merriam-webster.com, www.BusinessDictionary.com). Coalitions are

often associated with political activities. Today, in states across the United States, including California, Pennsylvania, Texas, and North Carolina, coalitions are actively working to increase children's access to community-based palliative care services through community and political advocacy.

Consortium—a group of organizations, each with similar aims, that cooperates to undertake an endeavor that is beyond the resources of any single organization. The term is generally associated with academic or not-for-profit groups and often involves sharing of resources to achieve a common goal (www.merriam-webster.com, http://dictionary.reference.com).

Collaborative—individuals or organizations work jointly toward an identified goal (www.merriam-webster.com). For example, California established regional collaboratives with a goal of improving care for children living with life-threatening conditions through collaboration and sharing of resources. The collaboratives in Northern, Central, and Southern California meet quarterly and communicate regularly via e-mail and Listserv.

Network—an informally interconnected group or association of persons who interact and remain in contact for mutual assistance or support (www.merriam-webster.com, www.thefreedictionary.com).

Strategies for Creating a Community Network of Support

Nick's life reveals the power of attitude: if change is desired and help is needed, then ask for it. Don't be defeated before you start by the odds against success. Nick wasn't; he was committed to making sure that the federal government and the State of California would change their regulations so that a child wasn't denied potentially life-prolonging treatment because a family opted for hospice. Of course, Nick didn't do it alone; no one can. In 2002, Nick met Lori Butterworth, co-founder of the Children's Hospice and Palliative Care Coalition (CHPCC). Never one to mince words, he said, "So you're that hospice lady," quickly adding with his characteristic smile, "You know, I flunked hospice twice." An alliance was born. Nick and his mother Shannon joined forces with Butterworth and co-founder Devon Dabbs, rallying organizations to combine goals, resources, and energies to work toward a shared vision. The result was the passage in California of Assembly Bill 1745 (Chan), the Nick Snow Children's Hospice and Palliative Care Act of 2006.

Success didn't magically happen; it was born of hard work, intelligence, perseverance, and organizational skills. Enhancing the quality of life for children living with life-threatening conditions requires the coordinated effort of numerous providers from a variety of disciplines in and outside of health care. Effective advocacy to improve the availability and quality of palliative and hospice care services for children involves families, health care providers, administrators, and policy makers.

Tackling deep-rooted practices and issues (e.g., the 6-month prognosis qualification for hospice services, the perception of death as failure, or practicing the technologic imperative—all of which may prevent access to pediatric palliative care services) is always more effective when supported by group efforts, but how does one gather the troops or unify the champions? Some guidelines follow.

BUILD A VILLAGE

The diagnosis of a life-threatening condition in a child affects the entire family and quickly ripples out into the community. A good starting place when trying to lessen the challenges for such families is to understand what is working well in your community in the delivery of care to children living with life-threatening conditions. Determine who is already committed to the cause and build your coalition from there. Here are some of the questions to ask yourself in finding allies:

- What home health and/or hospice agencies are currently caring for seriously ill children in your area?
- What community-based organizations currently provide children and their families with emotional, psychosocial, spiritual, practical, and/or financial support?

Consider hosting a forum of potential allies to discuss mutual visions for change and how the assembled community members and organizations can collaborate to improve the support of these families.

REPLICATE, DON'T DUPLICATE

With limited resources and time, it is important for partners in the community (e.g., nonprofits, businesses, and even government agencies) to share efforts and information with one another. Duplicative programs and services are an inefficient use of the community's limited resources, often resulting in confusion and distress among referral sources and community partners. This duplication also is confusing for affected families and can cause stress and additional hardship at the least opportune time.

REMEMBER: COMMUNICATION IS KEY

Effective advocacy is based on good community-based care that is rooted in good communication among all parties. Options include monthly conference calls, e-mail and/or phone chains, and monthly or quarterly gatherings. When establishing a system of communication, make sure that you are factually prepared and comply with current regulations related to patient privacy, such as the Health Insurance Portability and Accountability Act (HIPAA).

UNDERSTAND THE LEXICON

For advocates trying to change health policy who are not employed in the health care field, it is imperative to become familiar with the medical terminology and related language that families are forced to learn as they navigate the health care system. This can include terms describing a multitude of conditions (e.g., genetic, neurological), side effects, clinical titles (intern, primary care physician), medical specialties (e.g., oncology, cardiology), and acronyms like H&P (history and physical). Compile resources to help translate in both directions (visit www.childrenshospice.org/benefit/links-to -resources/ for a list of common medical terms) and consider convening a forum of local clinicians and families to discuss the intricacies of the unique ways children navigate the health care system.

CIRCLE THE WAGONS

When a family is dealing with a serious illness or a death, it is more effective to offer something tangible rather than a vague promise to help if needed. Asking for help is difficult for most people in the best of circumstances. That reticence is exaggerated when the colossal pain of the impending death of a child is involved. Individuals and community members can ease the burden by doing rather than gesturing. Sites such as www.partneringforchildren.org, www.sharethecare.org, or www.projectcompassion.org provide information about how to create a caregiving circle or support team.

KEEP YOUR EYE ON THE GOAL

Establish clear, concise, and measurable goals for your community-based care coordination efforts. Assess the needs of the families in your area and chart unmet or underserved community services and resources. This information will help you establish your goals and delineate the activities necessary to meet those goals. For example:

Goal: build the capacity of traditionally adult-focused palliative and
   hospice care providers to care for children;
Activities: conduct a series of trainings in pediatric palliative care; establish
   a resource library in a local hospice or hospital.

When the inevitable difficulties, conflicts, and disagreements arise, it is wise to return to the original intent of the group—to improve community-based care for seriously ill children and families. To quote Margaret Mead, "A small group of thoughtful people could change the world. Indeed, it's the only thing that ever has." Remind your constituents that together, you can make a significant difference in the lives of the children and families in your community. Extol your successes, however small, to keep the motivation high. For more information about coalition building, go to www.caringinfo .org (under "Community").

Whether you are rallying support within your institution or within your community, it is important to identify existing or natural champions and to provide opportunities for collaboration. A hospital in the southeastern United States invited clinicians interested in improving the care of children living with life-threatening conditions to attend an exploratory meeting. Fourteen physicians, nurses, and social workers attended. At subsequent meetings, members of additional disciplines including chaplains, child-life therapists, ethicists, and pharmacists participated. The organizers of the group then invited families, members of the hospital administration, and legal/ regulatory representatives, expanding attendance to more than 30 interested champions. These leaders then divided themselves into work groups to address clinical, educational, research, and support initiatives throughout the hospital and associated clinics. The most important members in helping the team influence outcomes and enhance quality of life were the families; their experiences, good and bad, created an impetus to help the group focus on practical ways to mitigate physical and emotional pain and other symptoms. This simple model has been successfully developed in multiple communities, whether or not coordinated pediatric palliative care delivery systems exist. The overriding priority is to ensure that the group remains motivated, active, and productive, ever moving toward their joint vision of ideal service delivery.

Know Your Issue

Nick was a natural in terms of exposing the core elements of an issue. At a conference in Newport Beach, California, Nick addressed hospice leaders and held them in silent awe by the poignancy of his cause. He challenged them to defend the right of ailing children to receive hospice care without having to relinquish all hope of surviving by asking, "What kind of condemnation is that to impose on the help-less?" Nick had the power to help people confront issues that had previously been avoided.

The Institute of Medicine (IOM) report *When Children Die* (Field and Behrman, 2003) established several working principles designed to improve the delivery of pediatric palliative, end-of-life, and bereavement care that are germane to advocacy work. These principles include the following:

- Appropriate care for children with life-threatening medical conditions and their families is designed to fit each child's physical, cognitive, emotional, and spiritual level of development.
- Good care involves and respects both the child and family.
- Families must be a central part of the care team.
- Effective and compassionate care begins from the time of diagnosis and continues through death and bereavement (if that occurs).
- Professional education on identification, management, and discussion of the terminal phase of a child's life-threatening illness is crucial.
- Individual and organizational changes are needed to provide consistently excellent palliative, end-of-life, and bereavement care for children and their families.
- There must be more and better research to increase understanding of clinical, cultural, organizational, and other practice or perspectives that can improve palliative, end-of-life, and bereavement care for children and their families.

The IOM also recommended that public and private insurers, including Medicaid, consider restructuring hospice benefits for children to allow hospice care services specific to children, eliminate eligibility restrictions related to life expectancy, substitute criteria based on a child's diagnosis and severity of illness, and drop rules requiring children to forgo curative or life-prolonging care.

In response, many have stepped forward. Children's Hospice International, established in 1983, has furthered pediatric palliative and end-of-life care issues on the national level by working closely with the Centers for Medicare and Medicaid Services in developing the Children's Hospice International Program for All-inclusive Care for Children and their families (CHI PACC). CHI PACC Standards of Care and Guidelines embody many of the principles of the IOM report, most importantly providing for palliative/supportive care services from the time of diagnosis of a life-threatening condition (Lowe et al., 2009).

The Children's Project on Hospice/Palliative Services (ChiPPS), an initiative of the National Hospice and Palliative Care Organization, has released "Standards of Practice for Pediatric Palliative Care and Hospice" to improve access to and quality of pediatric-specific services and is advocating on a national level on behalf of children and their families.

CHPCC developed an active Family Advisory Council and a collaborative program to reassure parents and children of the continued involvement of caring and skilled clinicians, as well as a supportive community during life and after death. This community-based care coordination program is the cornerstone for a comprehensive pediatric palliative care benefit that is being developed in California (Dabbs, Butterworth, and Hall, 2007).

The Ohio Pediatric Palliative and End-of-life Network (OPPEN), in addition to seeking legislative change at the state level, developed and unveiled the Comfort Line, a toll-free number that health care providers and families can call to seek general palliative care advice and resource information in the state of Ohio.

Several other states have released white papers and formed active coalitions, collaboratives, networks, and consortia in support of concurrent pediatric palliative care and disease-modifying or cure-directed therapies.

Rallying and Unifying the Champions

Nick Snow wasn't wealthy. He didn't have friends in high positions. He wasn't a visiting dignitary. Instead, he was an adopted boy of color whose parents had discovered a small lump in his chest when he was 6. That small lump changed Nick's life, just as his short life would change the lives of numbers of people he encountered, including members of Congress. Nick had never been to Washington, D.C., but he went with members of the California coalition to meet legislators to advocate for concurrent palliative/hospice and curative care.

It is often difficult for an individual to feel capable of advocating for change at the level of local, state, or national government. There are a number of ways, both indirect and direct, to exercise influence with elected officials to increase their awareness of an issue.

Indirect Advocacy

While it may sound obvious, being an informed voter is one of the easiest means of having a voice in shaping policy.

Sending a well-crafted letter to the editor of the local newspaper or an informed e-mail to local, state, and federal representatives can be effective.

Joining a professional society or advocacy organization provides funds for the organization to lobby policy makers and other key individuals on issues.

Direct Advocacy

Calling the local or national office of elected officials provides the opportunity to speak to the appropriate legislative aide for the issue of concern. It is helpful to use a talking point sheet to make sure that issues are communicated in an organized and concise fashion. Legislators and aides appreciate callers who share personal experiences with the issues and suggestions for addressing the problem. Another winning strategy is to offer to be available to the staff if they have any further questions after looking into the issue.

Contact your representative's local office or, for federal representatives, their office in Washington, D.C., to schedule an appointment to meet with the legislative aide. Be knowledgeable about the issues and have a brief presentation with compelling talking points, as well as a "leave-behind" packet of information that will provide the aide with information to give the representative when they brief them on the issues.

For nurses, physicians, allied health care professionals, parents, community members, support and donor organizations, and all others involved in healing or relieving illness and/or grief, the focus on improving the health of individuals may necessitate addressing social injustice and unfair practices. Health care providers and patients are on the front line of this battleground and are intimately familiar with what can happen when access to medical care is limited to what individuals can afford or insurance companies are willing to pay. Long-term, fundamental social struggles that confront deep-rooted practices and issues usually cannot be waged by isolated individuals and instead require group efforts. The people who respond to calls for action, either through their professionalism or from their passion, are the champions.

Assessing Your Community

Before launching into any outreach and education efforts, you should assess and understand the issues that children with life-threatening conditions and their families confront. This can be done by getting information directly from key stakeholders, such as parents of seriously ill children, community organizations, and pediatric health care providers. They offer broad, diverse perspectives and information about what children and families need most.

This section includes *specific strategies* and *sample questions* for a needs assessment with each key stakeholder mentioned above.

Overall, assessing your community will help you

- learn what people caring for children believe to be important;
- identify unmet needs for services or information;
- establish your credibility as a collaborator interested in working with the pediatric community; and
- identify potential partners in your outreach efforts.

GETTING STARTED

Attend meetings and support groups where family members talk about caring for a seriously ill child, their personal needs, and what is important to them—*and just listen.*

Familiarize yourself with materials aimed at supporting children and families, such as local newsletters, websites, professional publications, and special interest magazines.

Reach out to other community organizations that can help provide access to more information.

Talk to the families of your pediatric patients and let them tell you what issues are important to them. Tell them about what you've learned through your information gathering and ask if you are on target.

Strive for diversity when talking with families (e.g., varied attitudes, spiritual beliefs, backgrounds, diagnoses, and social and ethnic makeup).

ASSESSING PARENTS' NEEDS

The parents/families your program has served can provide guidance as to how to improve services and community outreach. If possible, gather information from parents or adult family members who are living with a child who is seriously ill and/or families who have had a child die.

Because of the sensitivity of the subject, make sure you do the following:

- Come prepared to listen, listen, listen.
- Approach families with questions, not answers. Let the information you've collected guide your questions.
- Maintain confidentiality. Always assure your respondents that you will never use their names (without permission) or attribute information. *Make sure you check with your organization about specific privacy rules.*
- Pay attention to timing. Before speaking with parents/families, be aware of whether there is a special anniversary or a crisis in the family;

Table 5.1 Sample questions for family members

How have you found your child's health care providers to be in interactions with you and your child?

To what extent do you feel that you have gotten the information you need from your child's health care providers about things like the diagnosis, prognosis, and treatment options?

Was the information provided in a timely manner?

How could the needs of your family be or have been better met?

What services do you wish you had access to that aren't or weren't available to you?

What services did you receive when caring for your child at home?

What other services would have been helpful to your family while your child is/was at home between hospitalizations?

Have you turned to sources other than your child's health care providers for information, advice, guidance, or support?

Is there anything that you know now or recently learned that you wish you'd known earlier?

What do you know about pediatric palliative care?

What do you think your pediatrician/specialist needs to know about pediatric palliative care?

How can we best help you now?

---

the timing of your communication can either help or hinder your efforts.

- Be responsive when talking with parents. Respond to what is happening and to requests immediately, even if the answer is, "I'll find out and get back to you." This can build relationships for future aid and assistance.

- Become familiar with national parent resources. Online resources provide a good deal of information about local, regional, and national disease-specific and topic-specific parent organizations. If questions or concerns arise about talking with family members, parent organizations will be able to refer you to additional resources and information. Table 5.1 provides some sample questions for talking with family members.

ASSESSING COMMUNITY NEEDS

To distinguish between available and needed services in the community for children and families, it can be helpful to answer the following questions:

- What local health care facilities, home health agencies, and/or hospice agencies are caring for seriously ill children?
- What palliative care programs, health care providers, and/or consult services are available?
- What community-based organizations provide children and their families with emotional, psychosocial, spiritual, practical, and/or financial support?

Once you have compiled a list of community resources and contact information, conduct a more formal needs assessment with each organization. Table 5.2 contains some sample questions for community organizations.

ASSESSING PEDIATRIC HEALTH CARE PROVIDERS' NEEDS

Conducting a needs assessment with pediatric health care providers will help outline the services they provide and will identify knowledge gaps concerning pediatric palliative care and hospice (Carter et al., 2004). Also, talking with staff and volunteers will present valuable perspectives that can help shape outreach efforts while simultaneously informing them about your outreach initiatives. Table 5.3 contains sample questions for pediatric health care providers (including physicians, staff, and volunteers).

Table 5.2 Sample questions for community organizations

How many seriously ill children (or children with life-threatening conditions) do you serve?

What are your eligibility criteria?

How is a child referred to your program?

What services do you provide?

How are you reimbursed and/or how do you fund these services?

Where do you get the majority of your referrals?

Do you collaborate with other community agencies, providers, and/or institutions when coordinating care for children? If so, who?

What challenges do you face in providing care for children with life-threatening conditions?

What resources would be helpful to you in providing care for children with life-threatening conditions in your area?

What are the unmet needs or challenges in caring for children with life-threatening conditions in your area?

Source: Adapted from www.partneringforchildren.org.

Table 5.3 Sample questions for pediatric health care providers

Are you currently caring for children with life-threatening illnesses or conditions? If so, approximately how many?

Do you provide palliative and/or hospice care to children?

How do you define palliative care and hospice services? Do you think palliative care is inclusive of hospice?

For providers who are *not* currently providing palliative and/or hospice care to children:

Have any of your pediatric patients ever received palliative care or hospice?

If so, what were your impressions of the care they received?

Would you refer patients/families to a hospice/palliative care program?

Why or why not?

For providers who *do* currently provide palliative and/or hospice care to children:

Are there any constraints that limit you and/or your organization's ability to provide care for children with life-threatening conditions?

Are there any constraints that limit the number of children you are able to serve? If so, what are they?

For *all* providers:

What do you think children with life-threatening conditions most need that you are not able to offer them? What do you think their parents/families most need?

As we begin to talk to people in the community about pediatric palliative care and hospice, whom do you think we need to get to know?

What educational opportunities or training would be helpful for continuing education for your staff and volunteers? What topics need to be addressed?

What are the challenges in caring for children with life-threatening conditions?

In your opinion, how could we improve community-based care for children with life-threatening conditions in our area?

What agencies/providers/institutions do you collaborate with when caring for children with life-threatening conditions?

METHODS FOR CONDUCTING BIDIRECTIONAL NEEDS ASSESSMENTS

Gathering information can be done formally or informally, depending on available staff time and resources.

One-on-one interviews can provide valuable insights from families and/or health care providers. Although time consuming, this may be the preferred strategy given the sensitive nature of the topic. Interviewers need to be sure to ask the same questions in the same way to make it easier to find trends in the information gathered.

Informal focus groups or feedback sessions provide an opportunity to hear families and/or health care providers identify issues and needs in their own words. A good rule is to limit the size of the focus group to a maximum of eight participants (Huddleston, 2009).

Each organization can create a simple, short, written survey to distribute to carefully selected families and/or health care providers. The focus of the survey should be to assess respondents' needs related to their child's/patients' health care and your service delivery. An important key to enhancing response rate is to create a survey that will take no more than 5 or 10 minutes to complete. Surveys can be distributed electronically or by mail. Response rate can be further increased through phone follow-up.

Although primarily a research tool, helpful information can be gained through systematic review of patients' charts, following a standardized chart review tool developed to elicit the desired information and outcomes. In some cases, this will require consent and/or institutional review board approval.

It is strongly recommended to work with research professionals in designing and administering focus groups and formal surveys. Performing assessments, whether informally or formally, is not a one-time event. Ongoing listening and learning will help ensure that outreach and educational efforts are in tune with the needs of children and their families.

Tips for Working with the Media

Regardless of the size, developmental stage, and specific mandate of your initiative, cultivating and nurturing an ongoing relationship with the media will be an essential ingredient to success. As with other forms of advocacy, the key to success with media relations centers on the relationships you have built. The relationship between your organization and the local media is an important aspect of the broader communications umbrella. Building an ongoing relationship with your local media takes place over time and requires ongoing commitment. It's important to reach out to the media proactively and respond quickly when they reach out to you. Time sensitivity is important when dealing with the media, as reporters almost always are under deadline pressure. This investment will reap dividends when you need to promote an issue within the community. If a professional relationship with local media contacts already exists, be sure to maintain it. All relationships require regular attention and consideration.

Here are some basic pointers to assist with media relations in your community:

1. *Develop an internal policy* for how your organization will respond to calls from the media and familiarize all staff and volunteers with the policy.

2. *Identify and prepare a media contact and/or spokesperson.* The spokesperson must be well versed on the subject and available to speak with the reporter on the reporter's schedule and deadline. Post the contact information in all of your media materials and, where appropriate, on your website. Make it easy for the media to reach you.

3. *Be protective of parents.* When it comes to putting reporters in touch with parents who have experience with hospice and palliative care, make sure to speak with the parents first. It helps to identify and prepare a few families who feel comfortable speaking with reporters; offer to sit in on the interviews to serve as a buffer or to intercede if the parent becomes uncomfortable.

4. *Do your research.* Conduct research on reporters; know what they do and what topics they cover. Connect on a personal level or through their blogs if possible. Also, call at the right time—watch their deadlines.

5. *Focus on a few key points when communicating with the media.* Keep it simple and clear, and avoid jargon and acronyms. What is commonly known to you isn't known to everyone; avoid condescension if a reporter requests clarification or explanation.

6. *Emphasize the local angle or hook.* The media are concerned with issues that affect their readers, viewers, or listeners. Be prepared to answer the question clearly that news editors always ask: "Why should I care?"

7. *Use your resources.* Make sure key reporters have the information they need to tell your story—a press release, fact sheet, brochure, web address, ready access to a spokesperson, etc.

8. *Be clear about the story you're pitching.* Make sure that what you tell the reporter is what you want to see in a story. If you are unhappy with the way you have phrased something, stop and rephrase or clarify your original statement.

9. *Don't waste the time of local media.* You will lose your credibility quickly if you continually seek media attention for events or activities

with little if any news value. Be familiar with the news organization's definition of news value. However, the work of your organization is important to the community, so keep the media informed about significant activities. The ability to judge what is important and what is not is critical to successful media relations (www.partnering forchildren.org).

Table 5.4 offers some helpful suggestions and things to avoid in dealing with the media.

Methods of Change

> Nick Snow wasn't an "all talk and no action" kind of person. He saw action in his struggle when he served as plaintiff in a federal lawsuit that challenged the discriminatory components of federal hospice eligibility regulations related to children. The suit was dropped when the California Department of Health Care Services agreed to work with CHPCC to pursue a federal waiver of hospice eligibility requirements for children.

There are a number of ways to create change to address the unique needs of children with life-threatening conditions through the political process. Becoming familiar with policy and legislation that create barriers or interfere with care is the first step to beginning the process of change.

Lobbying involves working to influence elected officials through a variety of methods to vote for particular legislation in a manner that favors the issues of the group.

Change can also occur through the development of new legislation to address an issue or by proposing changes to existing legislation to reflect the issues. This process can be lengthy and requires working closely with people who understand the intent of legislation and can assist in writing the changes desired. A high-profile example of this process is the passage, in March of 2010, of the Patient Protection and Affordable Care Act (PPACA), containing provision 2302. If not repealed, this provision allows for children covered under either Medicaid or the Medicaid expansion State Children's Health Insurance Program (SCHIP) to receive both hospice services and curative treatment concurrently. The PPACA does not change the criteria for receiving hospice services but does require states to make hospice services available without forgoing any other services for which the child is eligible, including pain and symptom management, family counseling, and other services.

Table 5.4 Dos and don'ts to keep in mind in media relations

DO make sure your story is newsworthy and relevant to the reporter and/or outlet. Tailor your pitch to the specific reporter and publication.

DO prepare carefully before contacting the media about an issue: know the facts about an issue and use key messages and materials to shape the discussion.

DO be on time and brief, using short words and simple, declarative sentences.

DO have a list of questions and answers prepared in advance.

DO decide in advance the questions you cannot answer. You don't have to answer every question a reporter asks—steer the reporter to one of your key messages.

DO ask for clarification if you do not understand a question.

DO remember that reporters cover a wide range of issues and might not recognize the importance of a specific issue—it's your job to make the issue recognizable.

DO be prepared to offer additional materials such as pictures, background information, and sources they may need to complete a story.

DO feel free to stop an interview if a parent becomes distressed. Most reporters will be respectful in such a situation.

DO keep a record in your media database of what stories you pitch and to whom. This will provide a log of reporter interests and requirements to facilitate future encounters.

DO retry, re-pitch, but DO NOT harass a reporter. If a new angle or development arises, pitch the story again. Eroding resistance over time is a legitimate strategy for placing a story.

DO offer feedback when appropriate. If a story contains a major error (not simply phrasing that you don't like but that is accurate), bring it to the attention of the reporter.

DO be careful about being overly effusive with a reporter, but if you like a story, send a short thank-you note.

DON'T speak "off the record."

DON'T ask to review a reporter's story prior to publication (but if offered the opportunity, take it and respond promptly).

DON'T mislead reporters with false information.

DON'T answer a question with "no comment." Instead, redirect the reporter to one of your key talking points.

DON'T try to answer hypothetical questions.

DON'T be afraid to say you do not know the answer, but DO say you will try to find out.

DON'T schedule a press conference unless you have breaking news that merits coverage.

DON'T work in isolation from your organization's media relations office; they may be making contacts with media of which you are unaware, and conflicting or overlapping messages will only detract from your power and credibility.

In situations in which the political process is not creating the change that is necessary, it may be advisable to consult legal counsel to determine if it is advisable to pursue a lawsuit on behalf of a child and family.

Available services may differ by state, and knowledge of accessible resources is essential in helping families navigate the health care system. For example, prior to the passage of the PPACA, some states recognized the need to identify pediatric palliative care services available under their individual state plans. Prior to taking further action, and with the knowledge that the hospice regulations for enrollment and reimbursement are federal, several states sought to modify or waive those requirements by submitting a federal waiver to receive federal matching funds.

Added to the Medicaid Act of 1967, the Early Periodic Screening, Diagnosis, and Treatment (EPSDT) Program is sometimes called the child health package of Medicaid. Required in every state, it is a set of services and benefits designed to improve the health of low-income children, by financing appropriate and necessary pediatric services.

The Health Resources and Services Administration (HRSA) website (www .hrsa.gov/epsdt/overview.htm#1) provides information about how EPSDT can be accessed by families, managed care organizations, pediatricians, and other health care providers. EPSDT is available to all individuals under age 21 who are enrolled in Medicaid. According to the program, screening services to detect physical and mental conditions must be covered at established, periodic intervals (periodic screens) and whenever a problem is suspected (interperiodic screens). These services may include pain and symptom management at end of life; in fact, hospice care falls under the EPSDT scope of services. As a specific example, Washington State has used EPSDT to authorize and reimburse concurrent community-based palliative care services for children.

Medicaid Waivers

Medicaid was implemented in 1965 as a means to provide health and long-term care services to low-income families and to the elderly and disabled. It is referred to as Title XIX of the Social Security Act, originally created in 1935. At this writing, Medicaid insures more than one in seven persons (more than 58 million) and accounts for 17 percent of the nation's spending on health care (www.cms.gov). Slightly fewer than 50 percent of Medicaid recipients are children. Because Medicaid partners with states to provide health and long-term care coverage, it acts as a primary source of federal assistance to states. Medicaid initially covered mostly primary/acute health care services but expanded to include other services such as home health care, personal care, and home- and community-based care. Each state is able to structure its own program.

Title XIX allows the Secretary of Health and Human Services, via the Centers for Medicare and Medicaid Services, to waive certain provisions required by the state plan, such as comparability (amount, duration, and scope), geographical extent of services, income and resource requirements, and freedom of choice of all willing and qualified health care providers. As mentioned above, several states, including Florida, Colorado, and California, worked to put in place a 1915(b)(3) Managed Care Waiver or 1915(c) Home and Community-Based Waivers that provide concurrent pediatric palliative and hospice services.

The Section 1915(c) Home and Community-Based Waiver is a section of the act that permits states to provide home- and community-based services to people who otherwise would require a nursing facility, intermediate care facility, or hospital level of care. The major purpose of this waiver is to help meet the rising demand for long-term services and support. The populations that can be served by this waiver include children with life-threatening conditions. Relevant authorized services include case management, homemaker, home health aide, personal care, habilitation, respite, and services for individuals with chronic mental illness. To avoid institutionalization, other services are available through the waiver, such as specialized medical equipment and supplies, skilled nursing, private duty nursing, assistive technology, behavioral support services, and bereavement counseling. In the traditional method, the cost of the waiver services must not exceed institutional costs to a comparable population. This policy decision allows children to maintain waiver eligibility while being served in the community.

The Importance of Funding

The needs of every family of a child who has a life-threatening condition are unique, and any reimbursement structure will fall short of meeting the complexity of needs in many cases. No matter which approach is taken, even the best policy changes in reimbursement for the care of children who have complex medical needs still require support from philanthropy.

In its simplest form, *development* means raising money to support the basic operations and initiatives of an organization. While they're used interchangeably, the term *development* often is preferred over *fundraising* because the success of the process depends largely on developing relationships. While nonprofits often prefer general support or unrestricted gifts because they can be deployed to wherever the need is greatest, or even used to pay salaries and rent, grant-making organizations prefer to make programmatic gifts (e.g., a children's bereavement program).

Three primary sources of funding for pediatric palliative care initiatives are as follows:

1. Individuals, the largest source of funding for nonprofit organizations. Individual giving to nonprofits reached almost $200 million in 2005.
2. Corporations, which often give in order to get—exposure, publicity, community respect, and market share. Most prefer to fund specific programs or projects related in some way to their business interests.
3. Foundations, which come in various sizes and types. Private foundations are nonprofit organizations whose funds come from one source, whether individual, family, or corporation. Independent private foundations typically have large endowments and are governed by an independent board. These foundations usually employ professional staffs and follow carefully developed grant-making strategies and criteria. Corporate foundations are also private foundations, but their boards are often composed of corporate officers and their funding comes primarily from one company with which they're closely aligned. Family foundations are private foundations that receive endowments from and are usually governed by one family or a few individuals. Community foundations pool the assets of many donors and usually serve a specific geographic community.

As relationships are being cultivated and nurtured, it helps to know who the decision makers are in each area and how closely connected they are to the funding source. Motive matters, and it may be easier to make headway with the board member of a family foundation who has a personal interest in pediatrics than with a program officer at a major independent foundation that funds pediatric initiatives as part of a larger portfolio.

Conclusion

In Aesop's fable *The Tortoise and the Hare*, the tortoise appears to be a loser at the start of the race. Yet the tortoise wins because it perseveres in a steady approach to the challenge, while the hare speeds ahead and allows confidence to lull it into slumber. The struggle for justice requires many methods, but history and personal experience show that one of the most successful is the way of the tortoise: steady and methodical, with conviction in the sanctity of the cause.

To the end, Nick Snow never stopped fighting. Regardless of his circumstance, of his pain, of prognostications, or of the odds against his aging into adulthood, he continued sharing his story with anyone who would listen. Even as he knew he was dying, even as he and his family realized that another miraculous escape would not happen, Nick kept his focus. Hours before he succumbed he used the time to talk with his music therapist about his intention to dedicate his life to ensure that kids facing similar ordeals would have access to hospice without forfeiting life-sustaining treatment.

Organizations and individuals who follow in Nick's wake also need to keep their eye on the goal. The fight is long and sometimes hard, and despair always is a threat, but following Nick's legacy of a clear head and a steady step will bring the finish line into view.

Social movements that have improved our human experience are often ignited by the most humble and unassuming among us. Throughout history, there have been those who, because of circumstances, timing, and a willingness to put themselves on the line, have rallied people together to improve the lives of others. Improving conditions for kids like him was Nick Snow's opportunity and his legacy. As professionals in the field of pediatric palliative care, we have an opportunity to partner with children and their families in engaging and mobilizing communities, policy makers, the media, and funders toward this common goal. With a clear and unified message, we can rally the champions and speak out on behalf of those too little or too sick to speak for themselves. This is the true art of advocacy.

References

Carter, B.S., Howenstein, M., Gilmer, M.J., et al. 2004. Circumstances surrounding the deaths of hospitalized children: Opportunities for pediatric palliative care. *Pediatrics* 114(3):361–66.

Cohen, D.R., de la Vega, R., and Watson, G. 2001. *Advocacy for Social Justice*. Bloomfield, CT: Kumarian Press.

Dabbs, D., Butterworth, L., and Hall, E. 2007. Tender mercies. *MCN Am J Mater Child Nurs* 32(5):311–19.

Field, M., and Behrman, R.E. 2003. *When Children Die: Improving Palliative and End-of-Life Care for Children and Their Families*. Washington, DC: National Academies Press.

Grace, P. 2009. Professional responsibility, human rights, and injustice. In *Nursing Ethics and Responsibility*, ed. P. Grace. Sudbury, MA: Jones & Bartlett Publishers.

Huddleston, J. 2009. Health promotion and behavior change. In *Health Education and Health Promotion: Working with Patients, Families, and Communities*, ed. A. Lowenstein, L. Foord-May, and J. Romano. Sudbury, MA: Jones & Bartlett Publishers.

Lowe, P.A., Curtis, C.A., Greffe, B., et al. 2009. Children's Hospice International Program for All Inclusive Care for Children and Their Families. In *Hospice Care for Children*, ed. A. Armstrong-Dailey and S. Zarbock. New York: Oxford University Press.

Prochaska, J.O., DiClemente, C.C., and Norcross, J.C. 1992. In search of how people change. *American Psychologist* 47:1102–14.

PART II

THE CYCLE OF CARE

Decision Making

*Robert J. Graham, M.D., Marcia Levetown, M.D.,
and Margaret Comeau, M.H.A.*

The heart has reasons that reason cannot know.
—*Blaise Pascal*

Key points discussed in this chapter include the following:

- The "right decision" for a given child and family will evolve over time; decision making is a process that accommodates ever-changing facts and perceptions rather than a one-time event.
- Avoidance of advance care planning usually results in less-than-optimal care and long-term outcomes for the patient and family.
- The child, nuclear and extended family, and health care team are all integral members of the decision-making team.

Managing a life-limiting or life-threatening condition in partnership with an affected child and family inevitably requires making choices that vary in complexity, immediacy, and perceived significance; rarely is there a single "right" answer. Through clinical vignettes and focused summary of the literature, this chapter identifies factors involved in decision making for children living with life-threatening conditions and offers practical suggestions to optimize the process.

Three families are each informed that their infant has spinal muscular atrophy type I. The diagnosis was made when upper respiratory illnesses resulted in hospitalization for each child. The infants, Abigail, Bailey, and Carmen, had each been a little "floppy," but nothing serious was initially suspected. After neurologic, pulmonary, and genetic consultations, each family is referred to palliative care services for the purpose of engaging in advance care planning, including a discussion of goals of care and their associated treatment options.

Given the inevitability of death during childhood for the child diagnosed with spinal muscular atrophy, regardless of medical interventions, the following topics should be addressed over time with these families and others whose children have similarly fatal conditions:

1. The name of the condition, how and why it occurs (when known), whether and how it is heritable, reversible, or treatable (*should be discussed in the initial conversations*).
2. The range of usual life expectancy.
3. The anticipated illness trajectory, probable symptoms, associated quality-of-life challenges for the child and family, and likely mechanisms of death.
4. Types of disease-directed treatment available, associated short- and long-term benefits (certain and hoped for), and known and potential burdens. *In the case of spinal muscular atrophy, this discussion must include the pros and cons of various forms of assisted ventilation and artificial nutrition and hydration.*
5. Discussion of illness complications, including their mechanisms, preventive measures, and outcomes. *In the case of spinal muscular atrophy, this includes a discussion of aspiration pneumonitis.*
6. Discussion of means to prevent and ameliorate the child's discomfort and suffering, as well as maximize the quality of life for the child and family. *In the case of spinal muscular atrophy, this includes managing fever, weight loss, and dyspnea, as well as helping families connect with similarly affected families and community-based supports.*
7. Discussion of the impact of the illness on the family and potential means to enhance their quality of life.

Abigail's parents discuss her prospects with their extended family, minister, and other families affected by spinal muscular atrophy that they "meet" online. They decide to pursue a gastrostomy tube during this admission and discuss plans for nocturnal and nap-time BiPAP when needed. They are, however, hesitant about the idea of a tracheostomy tube, stating that they want Abigail to be free of a breathing machine when awake to help her be as "normal" as possible.

Bailey's family feels that their son would suffer unnecessarily by undergoing invasive procedures. If he will never be able to hold his head up or suck his thumb and "death is inevitable," they do not want machines to prolong his life. After discussing their son's diagnosis and their own philosophy with their primary pediatrician, they elect to go home with hospice once he recovers from his acute respiratory decompensation. They do not want a feeding tube, "even the one in the nose," and do not want an oxygen saturation monitor at home. They have no interest in initiating mechanical ventilation.

Carmen's family discusses their realistic options with their social worker and family. They request the placement of a gastrostomy tube now and ask if she can be at home with a breathing tube (i.e., tracheostomy tube) and ventilator when she gets weaker. They are interested in any treatments, surgeries, or technology that will keep Carmen at home with her family and alive as long as possible.

Is it reasonable for these families to come to differing conclusions regarding goals of care, given the same diagnosis? Is it reasonable for a health care provider to promote a plan of care supporting a child's quality of life based on the family's perception, even at risk of that life being briefer? Is this decision wrong if other families in the same situation choose to "do everything" to extend the child's life? What role, if any, do the values of health care providers play in the decision-making process? If there is a conflict of values between families and health care providers, or among the providers themselves, how should these be resolved?

Health care decision making is evolving from the historically paternalistic (Todres et al., 1977, 2000; Todres, 1992) style to inclusive, family-centered paradigms (King, Rosenbaum, and King, 1997; Cuttini et al., 1999; AAP COHC, 2003) ideally built on informed consent and mutual participation (Szasz and Hollender, 1956; Curley, 1988). Decision making is, at its core, a shared experience and a shared responsibility of the child (as willing and able), the family, and the health care team. The child's primary care physician or medical home should be an integral part of this team, particularly when the child is likely to receive care in the community. This physician will be intimately familiar with existing community resources and can serve as the core of information and service coordination. While families still appropriately depend on and desire health care providers to educate and advise them, the expectation is that the family's informed and considered values will direct the ultimate choices (Meert et al., 2008). This is not because families "own" their children, but because children are raised in the context of the family; thus, families are considered the best surrogate decision makers for their minor children. Each child and family possesses a unique set of values, knowledge, and cultural expectations regarding health, health care, and disability. It is the job of the health care team to elicit these values and preconceptions as they relate to the child's health care situation, to provide education, and to discuss options, making recommendations based on the family's priorities and on the knowledge and experience of the team. Further, the provision of support and respect for the child and the family is a critical element of creating a functional decision-making team. It is also important to remember that the family lives with the outcome of the choice forever; to a lesser extent, so does the health care provider.

While advance care planning is not easy and may even be painful, the ultimate goals are improved care outcomes and greater family satisfaction. Studies of families of children who have special health care needs indicate that there are substantial benefits to engaging in a thoughtful and timely process of advance care planning (Wharton et al., 1996; Hammes et al., 2005). Parents in these studies reported that the process of advance care planning

- ensured their child's and family's best care;
- provided time and information to make the best decisions;
- helped them communicate the desired care outcomes;
- provided peace of mind; and even
- prompted them to complete their own advance directives.

Given the same set of medical facts, the "right" advance care plan can vary from patient to patient. In addition to the illness-related factors already discussed, other key factors in health care decision making for children include

- the age, capacity, and maturity of the child;
- the family's values, experiences, concerns, beliefs, and priorities, including cultural and religious perspectives;
- perceptions of mutual respect and acknowledgement of emotions;
- practical factors, including finances and available services;
- pre-existing and illness-influenced family dynamics.

Health care providers' advice is often influenced by "the last patient" phenomenon, their own perspective regarding clinical care and experimental trials, the scope and depth of their clinical experience, and the depth of reflective practice and understanding of ethical principles (Kon, Ackerson, and Lo, 2004). Capacity for compassion and empathy, interpersonal feelings for the patient and family, and the health care provider's educational, social, cultural, and religious background also affect clinical decision making (Christakis and Asch, 1993; Randolph et al., 1999). Similarly, children and their families draw on experiences that occur before and during the illness. Elements affecting decisions shift in relative importance as experience with the illness and life more generally accumulates; this evolution can best be accommodated by revisiting the situation and care goals over time, making modifications of the treatment plan as needed. In other words, the "right answer" for a given child and family will be modified over time; thus, it is essential to understand that decision making is an ever-evolving process rather than a one-time event. Beliefs, prejudices, regrets, and coping skills similarly change, especially in the setting of a long-term, chronic condition. As Mattie Stepanek, a bright young man with a mitochondrial disorder, said, "There are big choices and little choices" (Browning and Rushton, 2002). Even in the setting of an acute, unexpected overwhelming injury or illness, decisions evolve as the severity of injuries or illness becomes clearer, as trust is engendered, and as emotional reactions subside.

Communication

Effective communication and respectful relationships among all parties are central to good decision making (Browning, 2002; Browning et al., 2007). Feudtner (2007) proposes a model of collaborative communication, grounded in repeatedly reframing and reanchoring hopes and goals of care based on the child's illness progression and response to treatment. Open communication enables the identification of concerns and disagreements, allows the resolution of otherwise unrecognized conflicts, and facilitates the creation of a care plan that is acceptable to all. Health care communication is a skill that can be learned, mentored, practiced, and honed over time; it is not innate for most people. Refer to chapter 7 in this volume, "Communication Skills and Relational Abilities," for further discussion of this important topic.

The "Decision-Making Tool," devised by the Pediatric Palliative Care Consulting Service at Children's Hospital and Regional Medical Center, Seattle, is a practical example of an aid to facilitate communication. Having a tangible outline with prompts can guide a conversation or provide a child and family with a framework to posit questions, state fears, and identify goals. Written documentation of the thought process, questions, and factors influencing the decisions allows participants to reflect on and articulate what is important in the palliative care process. Further, this documentation is a crucial step in communicating the thought process behind and associated care decisions to other members of the team, preventing doubts and unhealthy divisiveness.

Extended Family Members and Community Advisors

A nuclear family consisting of one parent and the ill child may be the entirety of the patient portion of the decision-making team, but health care providers must also be open to extended family and community members participating directly or indirectly in the process. Helping the child and parents or guardians recruit their own trusted advisors to make critical decisions can facilitate good decision making. Virtually any member of the health care team can facilitate the involvement of these other important individuals by simply asking the parent(s) and child who has helped them make tough choices in the past, or whom they have depended on in times of crisis; such prompts help families contact their best advocates and advisors when needed. Friends, school or religious leaders, the primary care clinician, home care nurses, and others can provide insight into the context of these decisions, identify support systems, and facilitate the building of trust between the family and the health care team. Some families may initially resist the involvement of their broader social and care circles. Most ultimately appreciate the additional support to help them shoulder not only the burdens associated with decision making but also their pragmatic needs, including food, transportation, work, and child care accommodations (Graham, Pemstein, and Curley, 2009). The benefits of involving the extended family in making decisions affect not only immediate care but also care occurring in the future, such as when the nuclear family returns to their community. There is significant potential for long-term misunderstanding and blame if the larger family is not involved during the illness and the child dies (Meyer et al., 2006).

Adolescent Decision Making

Adolescents and young adults seeking individuation from parents and caregivers may benefit from the counsel of other adults or experienced peers to evaluate and express their priorities and wishes for care (Lyon et al., 2009). Often such patients fear burdening or "letting down" their parents and may choose not to confide in them for that reason, turning instead to others. While parents are legally the child's surrogates (Burns and Truog, 1997), they may recognize the value of working with the child's likely confidantes to gain insight into the patient's views. The process of determining the child's priorities, either directly or indirectly, is critical to truly honoring the wishes of the child with decision-making capacity, although this falls short of informed assent. The latter process adds a discussion of burdens and benefits, answering the child's questions, addressing his or her concerns, and then negotiating preferred goals and an agreed-upon course of action.

Prognostic Certainty

The degree of prognostic certainty is an important factor when exploring care goals. Uncertainty may propel some health care providers and families to continue efforts to prolong life in the face of low odds of success despite the ongoing suffering of the child and family. The uncertainty may reflect the rarity of a condition (lack of an adequate statistical database), lack of a definitive diagnosis (previously unnamed complex of malformations, organ or enzyme failures), the tempo of evolution (commonly, valleys and plateaus leading to doubts regarding the team's accuracy in prognostication), resources available to the team, or the range of potential outcomes, whether disability, chronic illness, or death. Uncertainty is uncomfortable, but it should be enabling, not our undoing.

In their study of barriers to palliative care, Davies and colleagues stated that "an uncertain prognosis should be a signal to initiate, rather than delay, palliative care" (Davies et al., 2008, p. 282). The onus remains on the medical team to provide the most up-to-date and accurate information with respect to the diagnosis and prognosis, to acknowledge uncertainty where it exists, and to explain its clinical relevance. Seemingly important details, such as the ability to name the child's condition, often do not change the decision at hand. For example, many cases of severe neurodevelopmental delay have no named etiology, but when the child has frequent seizures, recurrent aspiration pneumonias resulting in hospitalizations, frequent ICU stays, and recurrent respiratory and cardiac arrests, the exact diagnosis is no longer relevant; the clinical trajectory provides significant prognostic clarity. This must be carefully explained to the family, as they may feel uneasy making decisions in the absence of a clear diagnosis, particularly because it is harder to explain the situation to family and friends. Families often find uncertainty harder to manage than a clear diagnosis of a devastating or fatal condition (Ablon, 2000; Mack et al., 2007).

Sometimes uncertainty will resolve with time and/or test results; letting families know the time frame for resolution provides some comfort. For example, in their review of predictors for outcomes of children who have hypoxic ischemic encephalopathy, Abend and Licht (2008) suggest that time, adjuvant testing, and consultation allow for better prognostication and elimination of confounding factors. When definitive diagnoses are unlikely to be identified, health care providers can support families by reinforcing their insights and observations, as well as reviewing and discussing the evidence for the likely outcomes. Whether there is a nameable diagnosis or not, it is always helpful to affirm the family's choices and to acknowledge the difficulty of making decisions without definitive information. Rather than allowing uncertainty to limit options, prohibit decisions, or create tension in the relationship, health care providers should coach the patient and family regarding the inexact nature of medical science and reinforce that the child, not the disease, is the focus of therapy and decision making. Helping families understand that they will not be abandoned creates the mutual respect and bonds needed when decisions affect life and death.

Managing Other Sources of Information

Families have access to nearly limitless medical information of variable quality through the Internet, as well as through extensive networks of family support groups. Directing families to reliable websites and assisting them to recognize information that may be misleading can avert tragedies. Acknowledging that the family will (and should) seek additional information from a variety of sources is critical to building trust. Open discussion about the information obtained elsewhere also provides the opportunity to correct any misinformation and will ensure that all parties are operating from the same data in making decisions.

When the stakes are high, health care providers should recommend and facilitate second and even third opinions. In the end, however, many decisions are made not based on the facts, but on the emotional response to the situation, including parental desperation to keep their child alive. On behalf of their children, many parents will tolerate a quality of life that they would not allow for themselves. Assisting parents to recognize this double standard of suffering can only occur in the context of a mutually respectful, compassionate, and trusting relationship.

Establish Trust and Reinforce Supportable Hope

Trust is a crucial factor when making care decisions. Even in the setting of diagnostic and prognostic uncertainty, trust can be established by consistent, honest assessments accompanied by nonverbal and verbal expressions of genuine care and concern. Without trust, it is difficult to engender the willingness to engage in difficult discussions and decisions, especially those that precede the death of one's own child. In fact, recent research validates the fact that families derive hope from the ability to trust their health care providers, more so than from being misled to believe their child might survive when it is evident that this will not happen (Mack et al., 2008). With a change in prognosis, or in the face of uncertainty, the trust established between the family and health care providers may allow appropriate validation and timely shifts in goals.

Managing Disagreements among the Health Care Team

Miguel, an infant who had hypoplastic left heart syndrome, underwent a stage I Norwood procedure with a Blalock-Taussig shunt and was discharged home in good condition. He returned for a "routine follow-up" and unexpectedly arrested in cardiology clinic. Rapid response ECMO cannulation was performed during a 45-minute resuscitation and emergent cardiac catheterization identified a shunt obstruction. Over the next several days, it becomes evident that Miguel's heart is severely damaged and his neurologic prognosis remains uncertain. There is impassioned discussion between the surgeons and cardiologists, as well as quiet murmurings and disagreements among other members of the team, about the value of offering Miguel's family the possibility of a longer-term ventricular assist device/ pump and potentially even listing Miguel for cardiac transplantation. Some feel that the likelihood that he has sustained a devastating neurologic injury is too high for these options. Others are concerned about the low likelihood of a heart becoming available before Miguel's death; still others worry about the burden/benefit balance associated with the long-term outcome of newborn heart transplantation.

Many families report that dissension among the health care team is stressful to them, preferring the presentation of a united front, once differences are resolved (Contro et al., 2002; Meyer et al., 2002; Meert et al., 2008). Depending on the nature of the disagreement and the family's preferences, this may be a helpful tactic. A vetting process to determine the collective expert assessment of the likelihood of reversibility or at least the achievement of a stable and acceptable quality of life versus incurability and attendant suffering associated with a child's condition can be extraordinarily helpful. This is best done with all experts participating in person in a facilitated discussion of the case, gathering the input of all concerned to create an integrated likely prognosis.

However, disagreements among health care providers regarding appropriate goals of care cannot always be resolved; they arise as a result of differing personal and professional experiences, priorities, and ethical concerns. It is important to acknowledge the numerous studies that have shown that health care providers project their personal perspectives when considering goals of care, particularly when considering the discontinuation of no-longer-beneficial medical interventions (Christakis and Asch, 1995; Cook et al., 1995; Kelly et al., 2002; Pettila et al., 2002). Points of contention may therefore indicate choices that depend primarily on personal values. Given that families' values may vary as much as those of members of the health care team, these types of disagreements should not always be hidden from the family. Such transparency may, in fact, enable the family to consider the decision from perspectives to which they would otherwise not have been exposed and that, if discovered later, may affect their long-term adaptation.

Decision Making in the Context of an Acute and Unexpected Terminal Condition

Unexpected injuries and sudden overwhelming illness confound the decision-making process. Shock, denial, and other strong emotions may interfere with the family's ability to comprehend the situation, likely outcomes, or therapeutic options. While not all decision making in the acute care setting pertains to end-of-life care, numerous researchers (Heller and Solomon, 2005; Meyer et al., 2006; Mack et al., 2007; Meert et al., 2008) have found that parents value honest and complete information, ready access to staff, communication, and care coordination. Use of lay language, at a pace in accordance with parents' ability to comprehend, is also highly valued. Withholding prognostic information from parents often leads to false hopes and feelings of anger, betrayal, and distrust. Mosenthal and Murphy (2006) discovered that in an emergency situation involving traumatic injury and the likelihood of death, a proper introduction, frequent brief updates, and a willingness to be available to answer questions fostered greater trust and more rapid and peaceful decision making. Families cannot change gears suddenly. Health care providers have the luxury of receiving data as they become available and applying the new information to what is known, allowing the gradual realization of the patient's likely outcome. Families similarly and logically will also likely benefit from such a process and may be better prepared to make decisions based on the facts of their child's condition when given information as it becomes available. Families also identify emotional expression and support by staff, preservation of the integrity of the parent-child relationship, and faith as necessary aids in optimizing end-of-life care (Sharman, Meert, and Sarnaik, 2005; Meyer et al., 2006; Meert et al., 2008).

The provision of palliative care for children and families in the acute care setting can be daunting for health care providers, whether physicians, nurses, social workers, or other professionals (Burns et al., 2001; Browning and Solomon, 2005; Docherty, Miles, and Brandon, 2007). In an arena where resuscitation and "saves" are the focus, one of the greatest challenges is to shift the focus of care from injury- or disease-directed intervention to patient-centered palliative care (Davies and Steele, 1996). Greater attention to the prevention and relief of suffering in these arenas, regardless of the overall goals of care, would be a tremendous benefit to all patients and may also improve the acceptance of palliative goals of care when they are potentially appropriate.

When surveyed, critical care nurses and physicians agreed that patient and parental perceptions of quality of life were important when considering discontinuation of no-longer-beneficial interventions (Burns et al., 2001). However, both physicians and nurses noted that they considered "potential for neurologically intact survival" and "quality of life with a chronic disorder" when evaluating the proper goals of care. Nurses were also significantly less likely to agree that families are well informed and ethical issues are well discussed when assessing actual practice in their intensive care unit (Burns et al., 2001). Ultimately, implementation of an integrated model of disease-directed and palliative care is ideal (AAP COB/COHCC, 2000; Field and Behrman, 2002), but its realization will be difficult, as these objectives are unfortunately still perceived by some as competing and mutually exclusive (Docherty, Miles, and Brandon, 2007).

Decision Making in the Context of Chronic Illness

For children living with chronic conditions and their families, the experience of a prolonged period of stability and the momentum of an unwavering commitment to disease-modifying interventions can be difficult to overcome. Families are often caught off guard when the child experiences anticipated but unpredictable deteriorations in health status (Serwint and Nellis, 2005). Too often, they are unprepared for the "drop off the plateau" of medical stability—either factually or emotionally (Steele, 2000). Health care providers must acknowledge past successes in managing the child's condition, while clearly differentiating the current circumstances for themselves and the family (Graham and Robinson, 2005). In addition, health care providers should acknowledge the emotional upset, fear, disappointment, and grief, as well as the personal sacrifices, love, and dedication provided by families of chronically ill children. In guiding the decision-making team to understand when it is time to reconsider goals of care, health care providers may find answers to the following questions to be of help:

- How does this deterioration differ from previous episodes?
- Are there objective measures (e.g., pulmonary function testing in patients who have advanced lung disease) that can verify that this is the terminal phase of the illness?

Patients and families living with chronic conditions often establish long-term relationships with select health care providers. Forging an alliance with these partners to help answer these questions can be beneficial in numerous ways, particularly in engendering trust with the family and in increasing the accuracy of assessment. Parents lament that the acute care provider does not see the child at his best and does not understand the good quality of life the child is able to enjoy. Therefore, it is critical for acute and long-term health care providers to communicate seamlessly and with mutual respect, to understand both the longitudinal and immediate perspectives, and to attempt to provide consistent messages to the child and family. The importance of honoring the work of previous decision making and advance care planning cannot be overstated.

Exploration of Religious and Cultural Beliefs

Many families draw on and rely on their spirituality, cultural groundings, and understanding of their religious teaching to guide and support them in end-of-life decision making (Robinson et al., 2006). However, "spirituality or religion often presents a foreign element in the clinical environment" (Kuczewski, 2007, p. 4). The dominance of technology and medical discourse is at odds with what many experience as a spiritual journey. A family-centered approach requires health care providers to be explicit and holistic in their hospitality to parents' spirituality and religious faith (Kuczewski, 2007). Caution must be taken, however, not to assume that a common affiliation or tradition among a family and the health care provider will result in a shared interpretation of a given clinical situation (Wicclair, 2007). Similarly, a stated affiliation or ethnic background does not dictate individual beliefs and behaviors. These must be explored on an individual basis, while being aware of potential views unique to the affiliations. Facilitating access to pastoral care providers or encouraging families to seek guidance from their extended family members, usual spiritual guides, and other familiar community supports can be helpful. Simultaneously, health care providers may need to seek spiritual support themselves, as they share the moral burden of decision making (Robinson, Thiel, and Meyer, 2007).

Establishing Goals of Care

The establishment of the goals of care is essential to the task of decision making and care planning. While the task may seem nebulous and even daunting, and some may feel frustrated that the goals of care will inevitably evolve despite good planning and communication, the investment of such effort is critical to high-quality, appropriate care. The working goals of care, which should be altered with any major change in the child's condition, serve an important purpose; when effectively disseminated and understood by direct care providers, they guide all care decisions, providing a firm foundation and reassurance to family and health care providers alike.

As the child's condition evolves, making decisions consistent with the goals of care and the changing facts of a condition can be challenging for families and all team members. Thoughtful and flexible decision making can only occur when team members are valued and treated as partners and collaborators. By inviting all care providers (inpatient or home care nurses, respiratory therapists, social workers, child-life specialists, and chaplains) who consistently work with the patient and family to participate in rounds, family conferences, or outpatient visits during which these goals are discussed, a team approach is reinforced. If this is not feasible, then ensuring a mechanism to report the conversation results and the care plan implications, as well as air any concerns, is critical to maintaining cohesion and consistency. This inclusive strategy makes potential courses of action clearer when unexpected situations arise, enabling the entire team to function seamlessly and in accordance with the goals and resulting plan of care negotiated with the patient and family.

This process also frees the parents of the burdens of the details of every care decision. Instead, they can focus on enjoying their child. The discussion establishing the goals of care should clarify the interface between palliative and disease-directed paradigms, leading to the creation of a viable, practical care plan that honors the integrated whole (AAP COB/COHCC, 2000; Field and Behrman, 2003). With experience, reflection, more information, and the evolution of the child's condition, the goals of care will almost inevitably require recalibration over time.

Abigail has been doing well at home with nocturnal BiPAP for 6 months. However, 2 days ago she began to need increased cough-assist for secretion clearance, oxygen supplementation, and continuous BiPAP. Empiric antibiotics were started. While opposed to permanent ventilator dependence, Abigail's parents wish to explore whether short-term intubation and "invasive" mechanical support would enable a return to her previous baseline well-being.

When confronted with an important benchmark in a child's anticipated illness trajectory, the clinician may find it helpful to return to the values driving the care goals, to determine if there is a need to change the goals based on new information or family capacity for adaptation and to create a revised care plan. It is difficult to predict when and how a child will die; sometimes it is difficult to discern whether the current decline in health is the terminal deterioration, or whether there is an intercurrent acute process that may resolve. If the latter, it may be reasonable to initiate treatment in an attempt to return to the previous baseline. However, before embarking on such treatments, the family should be aware that this change may, in fact, represent the terminal phase of the underlying illness. With that in mind, any limitations of intervention should be agreed on in advance. In addition, it is helpful to set a specific interval after which progress will be evaluated to determine whether a change in plan is needed.

Health care providers should openly ask the parents to reflect on their hopes and expectations, as well as feelings of grief and loss, as these pertain to decisions about pursuing more interventions (e.g., transtracheal ventilation), the nature of the interventions (e.g., starting morphine for relief of respiratory distress), and where care should be provided (home, hospital, inpatient hospice, etc.). Children and families should be encouraged to reengage their supporters, be they friends, extended family, spiritual or religious counselors, or other health care providers, regardless of the perceived gravity of the decision or perceived imminence of death.

Decisions regarding Interventions

Filomena, a previously healthy 8-year-old girl, presents with seizures, headache, and vomiting. She is diagnosed with a supratentorial glioma, carrying a 10–30 percent 2-year survival rate (Broniscer and Gajjar, 2004). Disease-directed treatment options include radiation, chemotherapy, surgical resection, or a combination thereof. These treatments offer minimal survival advantage, although they may offer some solace to parents helplessly watching their child lose function and die. Counterbalancing these benefits, these treatments have significant physical, practical, social, and financial burdens.

When presenting and considering treatment options, clinicians should discuss a number of factors; most important is the likelihood of response to treatment and clarity regarding how success or response to treatment is defined. In addition, all alternative options should be explored. For each option, the following considerations should be explicitly examined:

- Likely duration of survival with and without disease-directed intervention
- Likely burdens of disease-directed intervention, to include pain, nausea, weakness, and other forms of discomfort
- Disfigurement—temporary (such as loss of hair) and permanent (e.g., amputation)
- Likely overall duration of treatment, time away from home, time in isolation
- Potential and likely costs to the family
- When or if a return to baseline function can be expected

In cases in which the treatments have a potential for disproportionate burden in comparison to their likely benefits, the discussion should include the pros and cons of forgoing disease-directed treatments, opting for the greatest comfort possible for the time remaining.

The Use and Limitations of Medical Technology and Interventions

Medical technology has enabled children who have severe acute and chronic conditions to survive; many can maintain an acceptable quality of life (Kirk, 1998; Kirk and Glendinning, 2004; Carnevale et al., 2006; Noyes, 2006). Previous successes in overcoming deteriorations can promote disbelief among family and even health care providers when ultimately faced with the limits of technology. The effectiveness of modern medicine should not forestall planning for the end of life (Graham and Robinson, 2005). When considering integration of a new technology (e.g., gastrostomy tube or tracheostomy tube) into a child's care plan, it is important to reflect on whether the child's clinical deterioration and the potential indication for the use of technology are actually an indication for further discussion of the goals of care, whether the technology helps achieve the goals of care, whether families clearly understand the practical long-term ramifications for the child and family of the use of the technology, and whether they have been apprised of its potential burdens for the child in addition to its hoped-for benefits. In other words, the use of medical intervention should be subjected to open discussion in light of patient and family values and goals of care. When helping patients and families make good decisions, one should specifically discuss the following:

- Will the intervention meaningfully improve the child's prognosis / chance of survival? If so, is it likely to result in the child's return to his or her baseline? If not, is the likely new normal acceptable?
- What is the likely outcome of each intervention (e.g., CPR, surgery, chemotherapy, artificial nutrition and hydration)?
- Will the intervention help achieve the goals of care?
- What is the impact of the intervention on communication with the child, site of care, comfort?
- Is this anticipated to be a short-term process that should resolve with support, or is there a likelihood/possibility that this is a permanent intervention or even the final phase of life? If this is anticipated to be a permanent change, with ongoing use of technology hereafter, additional issues to discuss include the following:
  - Will the technology improve the child's symptom burden?
  - Will it be burdensome to the parents to maintain?
  - Does the new technology require additional supports (e.g., nursing) or preclude care by a neighborhood babysitter or personal care assistant? Does it preclude care at home?
  - Is the intervention itself associated with any morbidity or potential mortality?
  - Does the intervention improve or decrease mobility or medical dependence?
  - What are the noninvasive or temporary alternatives to the proposed technology?

The language chosen to explore these issues may make some choices difficult. For instance, when a physician tells a family, "She *needs* a trach or she will die!" it is difficult for families to choose an alternative course of action.

A reciprocal process of learning about the disease, treatment options, and cultural and religious backgrounds and beliefs and identifying support networks should attenuate potential conflicts and avoid the need for legal action.

If there are ethical concerns or irreconcilable differences between a family and health care providers, consultation with the institution's palliative care service should be pursued, followed by an ethics consult if needed. Involving the legal department is a step that should be taken reluctantly. Empathy, respect, and time are powerful tools to increase understanding and resolve disagreements.

Anticipatory Management of Symptom Distress

When the child and/or family and the health care provider are electing not to pursue the use of medical technology, a plan must be in place to ameliorate the child's anticipated progressive symptom distress. For instance, a plan of care that includes forgoing mechanical ventilation in the face of increasing respiratory failure must include plans to manage dyspnea. From positioning to opioids, nonabandonment, benzodiazepines for anxiety, and soporifics for sleep, all interventions to improve comfort must be considered and a viable plan crafted. Moreover, it is helpful to acknowledge that death is nearing and to discuss the likely events to follow, their probable time course, and the "last dose phenomenon" (worries about giving opioids or sedatives near the time of death and feeling responsible for the death as a result). Reiteration of the basis of the decisions (maximizing comfort and minimizing distress until the last moment of the child's life), that the choices are good and loving choices, and that the child and family are respected can be affirming and may prevent a last-minute change of heart or lasting doubt and regret. Finally, as the time of death nears, families often appreciate the offer of increased support, contact, and care.

Resuscitation Choices and Contemplation of Surgery

Each institution has its own policy regarding resuscitation status for patients undergoing surgical procedures and anesthesia (Truog, Waisel, and Burns, 1999, 2005). Some require the suspension of all limitations during the perioperative period. Others tailor a procedure-directed approach, addressing anticipated potential periprocedural complications. Still others support an outcome- or goal-directed approach, focusing on the goals of care, the reasons to pursue the invasive intervention (usually improved symptom control, ease of care, and improved quality of life), and values. This last approach is more difficult to achieve, as it requires trust, articulation and understanding of care goals, and clinical judgment at the time of a complication (Fallat and Deshpande, 2004).

The Site of Care

Thankfully, not every child death occurs in an intensive care unit. The non-ICU hospital care areas, home, and inpatient hospice settings are often alternative options (Feudtner, Silveira, and Christakis, 2002; Feudtner et al., 2007). Dussel et al. (2009) found that families who planned the location of death as part of their advance care planning were more likely to feel prepared for their child's end of life, were comfortable with the actual location of death, and were less likely to have preferred a different location, regardless of the chosen site. Health care providers should inform themselves about the practical options available given the individual child's condition and then explore and facilitate the actualization of the child's and family's desires, while addressing their fears and preventing them from coming to fruition. In this setting, parents often fear not being able to keep their child comfortable. However, given the proper education and tools, parents and home care providers can do as well as, if not better than, inpatient settings in managing symptom distress at the end of life.

If the child and family decide to return home and to school with formal limitations of resuscitative efforts, the community must be prepared. Public health laws and policy differ jurisdiction to jurisdiction; the reader is encouraged to consult local sources for specific guidance and available comfort care forms. Contacting the school nurse, school administration, and even possibly the school board, as well as local emergency responders (i.e., fire, police, or emergency medical services), regarding the orders and goals can help avoid conflicts, confusion, and suffering. Of note, families should be informed that their resuscitation goals may not be respected in the community, although the physician or care manager should make every attempt to ensure that they are (AAP COB/COHCC, 2000; AAP COSH/COB, 2000; Kimberly et al., 2005).

Ethical and Legal Issues

In describing the concept of medical futility, Burns and Truog (2007) note three different eras in medical ethics. The first era was characterized by efforts to define futility in terms of certain clinical criteria or by the numbers (i.e., therapy was futile if it was only successful in x out of 100 or 1,000 cases); this approach was limited because it proposed limitations of medical interventions based on value judgments for which there is no consensus among a significant segment of society. Further, it did not allow reassessment based on medical progress and innovation over time. The second era saw the emergence of a pragmatic or procedural approach to futility, operationalized through committee. Many institutions and states adopted and still maintain such mechanisms. This approach, however, has proven insufficient, as it provides "hospitals authority to decide whether or not to accede to demands that the clinicians regard as unreasonable, when any national consensus on what is a 'beneficial treatment' remains under intense debate" (Burns and Truog, 2007). In the absence of consensus and certainty, the current era is one of communication and negotiation at the bedside. While not everything that the health care team and family confront involves determinations of futility, the same approach can be applied to the clinical care decision-making process.

Patient Participation in Decision Making

From an ethical standpoint, every child should be given the opportunity to participate in his or her own health care decision making, recognizing that the ability and desire to do so vary substantially with age, condition, and personality (Ladd and Forman, 1995). Legally, parents are the final arbiters of the care goals (in association with the child's care providers) as surrogate decision makers. This fact does not excuse care providers from the obligation to explore the child's preferences and ability to participate. At a minimum, health care providers should inquire if the child or adolescent with capacity has made explicit statements about goals of care; this should invite further direct exploration of the child's wishes. If not, there is still room to explore the child's goals and concerns, whether indirectly, through child life or another vehicle, or more directly. Often, parents need education about the benefits of the child's direct participation, ranging from the assurance that the parents are aware of the child's preferences and then can address and sometimes honor their needs (Goldman, 1994), to lessening the child's sense of being unloved and abandoned (Bluebond-Langner, 1978), to improved bereavement outcomes for the parents (Kreicbergs et al., 2004). In the absence of the child's direct input, substituted judgment based on the child's previously indicated overall beliefs, values, and preferences should be used to make decisions. For younger patients who are unable to communicate or comprehend, health care providers and families rely on an assessment of the "best interests" of the child, attempting to weigh the benefits and burdens of treatment options through this lens (Burns and Truog, 1997). This tactic is laden with pitfalls, and health care providers and families must appreciate that they have biases when making such decisions (Christakis and Asch, 1995; Hardart, Burns, and Truog, 2002).

Few states provide means for a child to officially document his or her preferences in the form of an advance directive. However, such directives merely represent an opportunity for a patient to document the preferences he or she has determined for future medical care so that, in the event of future incapacitation, his or her wishes will be known and honored. Thus, when a child still has the ability to interact, the need for advance directives is moot. State-specific information on advance directives can be found at www.caringinfo.org/PlanningAhead/AdvanceDirectives/Stateaddownload .htm.

Decision-making capacity, informed consent, and assent are essential considerations when making decisions with adolescent or mature pediatric patients (AAP COB, 1995). Competence is defined by law, assigning an age (typically 18 years) that qualifies the individual to be considered an autonomous adult; this can only be overridden in a court of law. However, "capacity," which is not predetermined by age, means that an individual has the ability to understand information relevant to the decision, to communicate with health care providers regarding questions and concerns about the decision at hand, and to reason about relevant alternatives in the context of "reasonably stable" personal values and life goals (Burns and Truog, 1997). When the decision involves life and death, understanding that death is permanent is also required. Controversies often arise when giving adolescents a voice in the decisions because of concerns about the "stability" or the "reasonable nature" of adolescent values and goals (Mercurio, 2007).

Darius, a high school senior who has advanced cystic fibrosis, desperately wants to participate in his graduation ceremony. It is April and he may be called in for a transplant at any moment.

- What are reasonable choices if he were called for the transplant now?
- Is it legitimate to forgo the transplant in favor of the graduation ceremony? According to whose values?
- Who bears the greatest risk in the ultimate decision?
- How is it determined whether Darius has capacity for decision making?

For many adolescents, psychosocial issues and peer acceptance can paradoxically be even more important than life itself. Darius is well aware that his life expectancy is short; he may not be aware that lung transplantation has questionable benefit in his disease process (Liou et al., 2007). Even if he were convinced that transplantation might prolong his life, he may choose to risk that opportunity for the experience of his high school graduation, feeling that this will likely be his crowning achievement and will constitute the legacy that so many adolescents crave. Further, recent studies indicate that children who have cystic fibrosis (or other chronic conditions) are not willing to trade duration of life for improved health (Yi et al., 2003). However, Darius's parents and physicians are dedicated to providing all interventions with any hope of prolonging life. Clearly, resolution of such conflicts requires time and mutual respect.

Steroids, surgical interventions, chemotherapy-related hair loss, nutritional supplementation, immunosuppressive drugs, and other interventions all alter a patient's appearance. Especially if alternative therapies are not an option, it is critical when dealing openly with adolescents in particular to acknowledge the impact of potential treatment side effects, including changes in appearance. Offering peer and adult support and advice regarding clothing and cosmetic choices may allow the young person to understand that his concerns are heard, that his values are respected, and that the goal of remaining socially acceptable is shared. Respect for such concerns can ease decision making, especially for adolescent patients.

If Darius is over 18, he has the legal right to make independent decisions. However, in practice it is always best to negotiate a mutually agreeable plan that respects patients' and parents' perspectives and concerns, regardless of legal status. Recent court cases have highlighted the difficulty of forcing an adult-sized child to undergo complicated and prolonged treatment regimens with which they disagree (e.g., Abraham Cherrix, Daniel Lindberg) and the fracturing of families that can result. Ethicists may disagree about the approach, and the reader is referred to more definitive explorations of this complex issue (Nitschke et al., 1982; King and Cross, 1989; Leikin, 1989; Doyal and Henning, 1994; AAP COB, 1995; Ladd and Forman, 1995; McCabe, 1996; Traugott and Alpers, 1997; Weir and Peters, 1997; Rushforth, 1999; British Medical Association, 2001; Doig and Burgess, 2002; Ross, 2009).

The determination of comprehension, elicitation of preferences, and affirmation of understanding for young adults and children who have developmental disabilities pose additional challenges. For many disabled children, parental or proxy consent suffices, but health care providers must also respect the decision-making abilities and concerns that such a patient may have.

Reflecting on the Decisions and the Process

Following family interactions, whether providing a diagnosis, establishing resuscitation status, determining a course of chemotherapy, or actual discontinuation of no-longer-beneficial interventions at the end of life, documentation and debriefing regarding the decision-making process helps the team evolve and mature. Too often, perceived "lack of time," discomfort with emotion, dissension regarding the decisions, and professional and institutional politics and hierarchies prevent the review of the shared experience, yet these are the very reasons to debrief.

It is essential to recognize that there is no "normal" response or correct answer when confronted with a life-limiting condition. The end-of-life decision-making process can be supported if it is inclusive, bidirectional, and clear; is based on the best information possible; and results in informed decisions that honor family and patient values in the formulation of the resulting goals of care. The unpredictability of diseases, variable efficacy of therapies, and other factors, including the final outcome, may nevertheless alter the ultimate perception of the decisions made.

Postmortem Evaluations and Organ Donations

Will postmortem evaluation help the family answer any unresolved questions and assist them in the grieving process? Many times the answer is "yes" (Feinstein et al., 2007). Thus, the standard procedure of forgoing this final opportunity to better understand what happened and the implications for the family's future childbearing may represent a tragedy. Dealing with the unknown can interfere with healthy grieving. On the other hand, when counseling families, health care providers must acknowledge that the autopsy may not yield "the answer." In addition, factually correct information should be provided regarding associated costs. Health care providers should also be aware of relevant state requirements and the medical examiner's authority in certain situations to perform postmortem examinations, independent of family wishes. Determining whether the medical examiner will require an autopsy or other postmortem procedure before discussing the family's preferences can help avoid unpleasant and potentially damaging consequences. The integrity of the trusting relationship, optimally established before the child's death, is still of significant value and should be protected. Once it has been established that postmortem examinations are an option rather than a requirement, ask the family about cultural and religious beliefs that influence these decisions and explain available accommodations, such as core biopsies rather than organ removal, etc. Consider engaging community and spiritual leaders for guidance on issues such as time factors for burial, concerns for the integrity of the body, need to accompany the deceased's body, or other considerations. Despite their grief, the family may be interested in "the greater good" and "meaning of the death" through postmortem evaluation, as well as tissue or organ donation. When considering organ donation, especially in the context of donation after cardiac death, clinical care providers should avoid conflicts of interest, as they may be simultaneously caring for potential recipients. The health care team should engage their institutional pathologists, local organ procurement organization, and legal/ethics counsel to inquire about options. Follow-up on these decisions also cannot be overlooked; the health care team must coordinate to ensure that postmortem results are explained to the family and that time is taken to check in on bereaved families' well-being (Meert, Thurston, and Sarnaik, 2000).

A PARENT'S PERSPECTIVE ON DECISION MAKING

For the past 22 years, I have lived as the parent of a child (now young adult) with a complex, life-limiting genetic disorder that has associated significant medical, developmental, and behavioral impacts. This experience is fundamental to who I am, not just as a parent, but as a person—it has burned itself into my DNA and I will carry it with me beyond my physical existence. I don't presume to speak on behalf of my husband, but I imagine the same is true for him.

While it is easy to identify and reflect on the sorrow and suffering this experience has brought my daughter, Sarah, and our family, it is equally important to recognize and respect the joy and satisfaction that have accompanied it. Having a daughter with her particular diagnosis combines the mundane (Seriously, are we out of shampoo again? I left it on the counter and she's poured it down the drain because she likes to see the bubbles) with the dramatic (yet another middle-of-the-night emergency room trip). It has influenced and affected every aspect of our lives. Like everyone engaged in raising a child, we hold the ultimate responsibility for her physical, developmental, spiritual, and emotional well-being. Unlike parents of typically healthy, typically developing children, our decision making has often centered on complex medical choices. The consequences of those decisions are weighted differently; they are influenced by the intensity and ongoing nature of Sarah's immediate needs, as well as an awareness that we will not have her forever to enjoy. Unlike the overwhelming majority of parents, we do not have the luxury of assuming that our daughter will outlive us. Mistakes in our decision making have often cost her too much, and we haven't always known if there will be time to fix them.

Time has also been our friend, however. After two decades, I am almost always the person in the exam room or on the inpatient unit with the most medical knowledge about her rare syndrome; I am *always* the one who knows the most about what it means for Sarah as a person, not just as a patient. My husband and I are the knowledge holders of the nonmedical influences (our family's values with regard to quality of life, our cultural background, our views on spirituality and the meaning associated with suffering) that go into our decision making, and we have the responsibility not only of factoring them into our decision making but also of conveying that information to the clinical team. Additionally, we are charged with interpreting and conveying Sarah's ideas and preferences and making sure they are factored into the decision-making process, even if she cannot verbally express them.

All of these factors have influenced our approach to medical decision making. After many years' experience, we can appreciate the evolutionary nature of families' development of complex medical decision-making processes. We've been fortunate to have time to develop a process that feels right for us. As the mother of a newborn in the NICU, I knew nothing of Sarah's diagnosis and only slightly more about who she was as a new person in the world. Through a combination of learning from her over time, as well as from her doctors and nurses, researching her diagnosis independently, and talking with other experienced families, I gained medical knowledge and a corresponding increase in confidence in making good-quality decisions for her care.

The process by which we determine and pursue our goals for her care and make decisions for Sarah has been a developmental one. Over the years, two guiding principles have emerged that have served us well:

1. Have we learned everything we can about what is happening, why it is happening, and what the options are and their likely consequences? In other words, are we making an informed decision with the information we have available at this particular point in time?
2. Have we put her needs and her preferences at the center of the decision-making process, rather than our own?

When the answer to these two touchstone principles is "yes," while there may be negative or unexpected consequences of the decision at hand, we can feel we have done our best for her. Use of these two principles has also allowed us to understand and accept that there are limits to human knowledge. Forgiveness, of both ourselves and the medical world, is sometimes necessary to move forward.

Living this life has given us all an intimate acquaintance with pain, grief, fear, and anger. But we have also learned much we probably would not have about joy, the value of each individual person regardless of ability or disability, and the power of love and what commitment to others means. If given a choice, I would not have chosen to learn these lessons in this way, because they've cost Sarah most. Because we don't have a choice, however, I feel we have an obligation to focus on and celebrate the positive as well as acknowledge and deal with the negative, because this perspective honors Sarah's value and the lessons this experience has taught us. Other families have their own lessons and hard-won knowledge.

In your work, please join us in honoring these lessons by focusing on families' strengths as wells as challenges, in seeing the joy as well as the pain, in celebrating the good times as well as supporting us in the bad, and in sharing the moral burden of the impossible decisions families and children with life-limiting illness or complex disabilities face. I believe that if you do so, like me, you'll find your life, as well as your work, the richer for it.

Conclusion

Decision making is an integral element of pediatric palliative care. It is neither easy nor clear-cut. By sharing the responsibility and experience with patients and their families, health care providers can optimize care. Health care providers need to understand that avoidance of advance care planning usually results in less-than-optimal care and long-term outcomes for the patient and family. A passive approach, or not making decisions, may be less emotionally taxing in the moment but is, in fact, a decision. "Big Choices and Little Choices" have significant consequences; helping the child and family actively make decisions enables them to gain some control of their quality of life and the end-of-life process, when relevant. Health care providers must consider the disease, child- and family-specific factors, availability of resources (medical, social, emotional, community, and financial), and the dynamic interface among these in facilitating good decision making. Such facilitation is a skill that must be taught, learned, honed, and reflected on after each encounter. This skill, accompanied by adequate preparation and empathy, is required for the health care community to optimally serve children living with life-threatening conditions and their families.

References

Abend, N.S., and Licht, D.J. 2008. Predicting outcome in children with hypoxic ischemic encephalopathy. *Pediatr Crit Care Med* 9:32–39.

Ablon, J. 2000. Parents' responses to their child's diagnosis of neurofibromatosis 1. *Am J Med Genet* 93(2):136–42.

American Academy of Pediatrics, Committee on Bioethics (AAP COB). 1995. Informed consent, parental permission, and assent in pediatric practices. *Pediatrics* 95(2):314–17.

American Academy of Pediatrics, Committee on Bioethics and Committee on Hospital Care (AAP COB/COHC). 2000. Palliative care for children. *Pediatrics* 106:351–57.

American Academy of Pediatrics, Committee on Hospital Care (AAP COHC). 2003. Family-centered care and the pediatrician's role. *Pediatrics* 112:691–97.

American Academy of Pediatrics, Committee on School Health and Committee on Bioethics (AAP COSH/COB). 2000. Do not resuscitate orders in schools. *Pediatrics* 105:878–79.

Bluebond-Langner, M. 1978. *Private Worlds of Dying Children*. Princeton: Princeton University Press.

British Medical Association. 2001. *Consent, Rights and Choices in Health Care for Children and Young People*. London: BMJ Books.

Broniscer, A., and Gajjar, A. 2004. Supratentorial high-grade astrocytoma and diffuse brainstem glioma: Two challenges for the pediatric oncologist. *Oncologist* 9(2): 197–206.

Browning, D. 2002. To show our humanness—relational and communicative competence in pediatric palliative care. *Bioethics Forum* 18:23–28.

Browning, D.M., Meyer, E.C., Truog, R.D., et al. 2007. Difficult conversations in health care: Cultivating relational learning to address the hidden curriculum. *Acad Med* 82:905–13.

Browning, D.M., and Rushton, C.H. 2002. *Big Choices, Little Choices. What Matters to Families*. Newton, MA: Educational Development Center.

Browning, D.M., and Solomon, M.Z. 2005. The initiative for pediatric palliative care: An interdisciplinary educational approach for healthcare professionals. *J Pediatr Nurs* 20:326–34.

Burns, J.P., Mitchell, C., Griffith, J.L., et al. 2001. End-of-life care in the pediatric intensive care unit: Attitudes and practices of pediatric critical care physicians and nurses. *Crit Care Med* 29:658–64.

Burns, J.P., and Truog, R.D. 1997. Ethical controversies in pediatric critical care. *New Horiz* 5:72–84.

———. 2007. Futility: A concept in evolution. *Chest* 132:1987–93.

Carnevale, F.A., Alexander, E., Davis, M., et al. 2006. Daily living with distress and enrichment: The moral experience of families with ventilator-assisted children at home. *Pediatrics* 117:e48–60.

Christakis, N.A., and Asch, D.A. 1993. Biases in how physicians choose to withdraw life support. *Lancet* 342:642–46.

———. 1995. Physician characteristics associated with decisions to withdraw life support. *Am J Public Health* 85:367–72.

Contro, N., Larson, J., Scofield, S., et al. 2002. Family perspectives on the quality of pediatric palliative care. *Arch Pediatr Adolesc Med* 156:14–19.

Cook, D.J., Guyatt, G.H., Jaeschke, R., et al. 1995. Determinants in Canadian health care workers of the decision to withdraw life support from the critically ill. Canadian Critical Care Trials Group. *JAMA* 273:703–8.

Curley, M.A. 1988. Effects of the nursing mutual participation model of care on parental stress in the pediatric intensive care unit. *Heart Lung* 17:682–88.

Cuttini, M., Rebagliato, M., Bortoli, P., et al. 1999. Parental visiting, communication, and participation in ethical decisions: A comparison of neonatal unit policies in Europe. *Arch Dis Child Fetal Neonatal Ed* 81:F84–91.

Davies, B., Sehring, S.A., Partridge, J.C., et al. 2008. Barriers to palliative care for children: Perceptions of pediatric health care providers. *Pediatrics* 121:282–88.

Davies, B., and Steele, R. 1996. Challenges in identifying children for palliative care. *J Palliat Care* 12:5–8.

Docherty, S.L., Miles, M.S., and Brandon, D. 2007. Searching for "the dying point": Providers' experiences with palliative care in pediatric acute care. *Pediatr Nurs* 33: 335–41.

Doig, C., and Burgess, E. 2002. Withholding life-sustaining treatment: Are adolescents competent to make these decisions? *CMAJ* 162(1112):1585–88.

Doyal, L., and Henning, P. 1994. Stopping treatment for end-stage renal failure: The rights of children and adolescents. *Pediatr Nephrol* 8:768–71.

Dussel, V., Kreicbergs, U., Hilden, J.M., et al. 2009. Looking beyond where children die: Determinants and effects of planning a child's location of death. *J Pain Symptom Manage* 37:33–43.

Fallat, M.E., and Deshpande, J.K. 2004. Do-not-resuscitate orders for pediatric patients who require anesthesia and surgery. *Pediatrics* 114:1686–92.

Feinstein, J.A., Ernst, L.M., Ganesh, J., et al. 2007. What new information pediatric autopsies can provide: A retrospective evaluation of 100 consecutive autopsies using family-centered criteria. *Arch Pediatr Adolesc Med* 161(12):1190–96.

Feudtner, C. 2007. Collaborative communication in pediatric palliative care: A foundation for problem-solving and decision-making. *Pediatr Clin North Am* 54:583–607.

Feudtner, C., Feinstein, J.A., Satchell, M., et al. 2007. Shifting place of death among children with complex chronic conditions in the United States, 1989–2003. *JAMA* 297:2725–32.

Feudtner, C., Silveira, M.J., and Christakis, D.A. 2002. Where do children with complex chronic conditions die? Patterns in Washington State, 1980–1998. *Pediatrics* 109:656–60.

Field, M.J., and Behrman, R.E. 2003. *When Children Die: Improving Palliative and End-of-Life Care for Children and Their Families.* Washington, DC: National Academy Press.

Goldman, A. 1994. *Care of the Dying Child.* London: Oxford University Press.

Graham, R.J., Pemstein, D.M., and Curley, M.A. 2009. Experiencing the pediatric intensive care unit: Perspective from parents of children with severe antecedent disabilities. *Crit Care Med* 37:2064–70.

Graham, R.J., and Robinson, W.M. 2005. Integrating palliative care into chronic care for children with severe neurodevelopmental disabilities. *J Dev Behav Pediatr* 26: 361–65.

Hammes, B.J., Klevan, J., Kempf, M., et al. 2005. Pediatric advance care planning. *J Palliat Med* 8:766–73.

Hardart, M.K., Burns, J.P., and Truog, R.D. 2002. Respiratory support in spinal muscular atrophy type I: A survey of physician practices and attitudes. *Pediatrics* 110:e24.

Heller, K.S., and Solomon, M.Z., for the Initiative for Pediatric Palliative Care, Investigator Team. 2005. Continuity of care and caring: What matters to parents of children with life-threatening conditions. *J Pediatr Nurs* 20(5):335–46.

Kelly, W.F., Eliasson, A.H., Stocker, D.J., et al. 2002. Do specialists differ on do-not-resuscitate decisions? *Chest* 121:957–63.

Kimberly, M.B., Forte, A.L., Carroll, J.M., et al. 2005. Pediatric do-not-attempt-resuscitation orders and public schools: A national assessment of policies and laws. *Am J Bioeth* 5:59–65.

King, G.A., Rosenbaum, P.L., and King, S.M. 1997. Evaluating family-centered service using a measure of parents' perceptions. *Child Care Health Dev* 23:47–62.

King, N.M.P., and Cross, A.W. 1989. Children as decision-makers: Guidelines for pediatricians. *J Pediatr* 115(1):10–16.

Kirk, S. 1998. Families' experiences of caring at home for a technology-dependent child: A review of the literature. *Child Care Health Dev* 24:101–14.

Kirk, S., and Glendinning, C. 2004. Developing services to support parents caring for a technology-dependent child at home. *Child Care Health Dev* 30:209–18; discussion 19.

Kon, A.A., Ackerson, L., and Lo, B. 2004. How pediatricians counsel parents when no "best-choice" management exists: Lessons to be learned from hypoplastic left heart syndrome. *Arch Pediatr Adolesc Med* 158:436–41.

Kreicbergs, U., Valdimarsdottir, U., Onelov, E., et al. 2004. Talking about death with children who have severe malignant disease. *N Engl J Med* 351:1175–86.

Kuczewski, M.G. 2007. Talking about spirituality in the clinical setting: Can being professional require being personal? *Am J Bioeth* 7:4–11.

Ladd, R.E., and Forman, E.N. 1995. Adolescent decision-making: Giving weight to age-specific values. *Theor Med* 16:333–45.

Leikin, S. 1989. A proposal concerning decisions to forgo life-sustaining treatment for young people. *J Pediatr* 115(1):17–22.

Liou, T.G., Adler, F.R., Cox, D.R., et al. 2007. Lung transplantation and survival in children with cystic fibrosis. *N Eng J Med* 357:2143–52.

Lyon, M.E., Garvie, P.A., McCarter, R., et al. 2009. Who will speak for me? Improving end-of-life decision-making for adolescents with HIV and their families. *Pediatrics* 123:e199–206.

Mack, J.W., Joffe, S., Hilden, J.M., et al. 2008. Parents' views of cancer-directed therapy for children with no realistic chance for cure. *J Clin Oncol* 26:4759–64.

Mack, J.W., Wolfe, J., Cook, E.F., et al. 2007. Hope and prognostic disclosure. *J Clin Oncol* 25(35):5636–42.

McCabe, M.A. 1996. Involving children and adolescents in medical decision-making: Developmental and clinical considerations. *J Pediatr Psychol* 21(4):505–16.

Meert, K.L., Eggly, S., Pollack, M., et al. 2008. Parents' perspectives on physician-parent communication near the time of a child's death in the pediatric intensive care unit. *Pediatr Crit Care Med* 9:2–7.

Meert, K.L., Thurston, C.S., and Sarnaik, A.P. 2000. End-of-life decision-making and satisfaction with care: Parental perspectives. *Pediatr Crit Care Med* 1:179–85.

Mercurio, M.R. 2007. An adolescent's refusal of medical treatment: Implications of the Abraham Cheerix case. *Pediatrics* 120:1357–58.

Meyer, E.C., Burns, J.P., Griffith, J.L., et al. 2002. Parental perspectives on end-of-life care in the pediatric intensive care unit. *Crit Care Med* 30:226–31.

Meyer, E.C., Ritholz, M.D., Burns, J.P., et al. 2006. Improving the quality of end-of-life care in the pediatric intensive care unit: Parents' priorities and recommendations. *Pediatrics* 117:649–57.

Mosenthal, A.C., and Murphy, P.A. 2006. Interdisciplinary model for palliative care in the trauma and surgical intensive care unit: Robert Wood Johnson Foundation Demonstration Project for Improving Palliative Care in the Intensive Care Unit. *Crit Care Med* 34:S399–403.

Nitschke, R., Humphrey, G.B., Sexauer, C.L., et al. 1982. Therapeutic choices made by patients with end-stage cancer. *J Pediatr* 101(3):471–76.

Noyes, J. 2006. Health and quality of life of ventilator-dependent children. *J Adv Nurs* 56:392–403.

Pettila, V., Ala-Kokko, T., Varpula, T., et al. 2002. On what are our end-of-life decisions based? *Acta Anaesthesiol Scandinavica* 46:947–54.

Randolph, A.G., Zollo, M.B., Egger, M.J., et al. 1999. Variability in physician opinion on limiting pediatric life support. *Pediatrics* 103:e46.

Robinson, M.R., Thiel, M.M., Backus, M.M., et al. 2006. Matters of spirituality at the end of life in the pediatric intensive care unit. *Pediatrics* 118:e719–29.

Robinson, M.R., Thiel, M.M., and Meyer, E.C. 2007. On being a spiritual care generalist. *Am J Bioeth* 7:24–26.

Ross, L.F. 2009. Against the tide: Arguments against respecting a minor's refusal of efficacious life-saving treatment. *Camb Q Healthc Ethics* 18(3):302–15; discussion 315–22.

Rushforth, H. 1999. Practitioner review: Communicating with hospitalised children: Review and application of research pertaining to children's understanding of health and illness. *J Child Psychol Psychiat* 40(5):683–91.

Serwint, J.R., and Nellis, M.E. 2005. Deaths of pediatric patients: Relevance to their medical home, an urban primary care clinic. *Pediatrics* 115:57–63.

Sharman, M., Meert, K.L., and Sarnaik, A.P. 2005. What influences parents' decisions to limit or withdraw life support? *Pediatr Crit Care Med* 6:513–18.

Steele, R.G. 2000. Trajectory of certain death at an unknown time: Children with neurodegenerative life-threatening illnesses. *Can J Nurs Res* 32:49–67.

Szasz, T.S., and Hollender, M.H. 1956. The basic models of the doctor-patient relationship. *Arch Intern Med* 97:585–92.

Todres, I.D. 1992. Ethical dilemmas in pediatric critical care. *Crit Care Clinics* 8: 219–27.

Todres, I.D., Guillemin, J., Catlin, E.A., et al. 2000. Moral and ethical dilemmas in critically ill newborns: A 20-year follow-up survey of Massachusetts pediatricians. *J Perinatol* 20:6–12.

Todres, I.D., Krane, D., Howell, M.C., et al. 1977. Pediatricians' attitudes affecting decision-making in defective newborns. *Pediatrics* 60:197–201.

Traugott, I., and Alpers, A. 1997. In their own hands: Adolescents' refusals of medical treatment. *Arch Pediatr Adolesc Med* 151:922–27.

Truog, R.D., Waisel, D.B., and Burns, J.P. 1999. DNR in the OR: A goal-directed approach. *Anesthesiology* 90:289–95.

———. 2005. Do-not-resuscitate orders in the surgical setting. *Lancet* 365:733–35.

Weir, R.F., and Peters, C. 1997. Affirming the decisions adolescents make about life and death. *Hastings Cent Rep* 27(6):29–40.

Wharton, R.H., Levine, K.R., Buka, S., et al. 1996. Advance care planning for children with special health care needs: A survey of parental attitudes. *Pediatrics* 97: 682–87.

Wicclair, M.R. 2007. Professionalism, religion and shared decision-making. *Am J Bioeth* 7:29–31.

Yi, M.S., Britto, M.T., Wilmott, R.W., et al. 2003. Health values of adolescents with cystic fibrosis. *J Pediatr* 142:133–40.

7

Communication Skills and Relational Abilities

Marcia Levetown, M.D., Elaine C. Meyer, Ph.D., R.N.,
and Dianne Gray, B.S.

Jedidiah was born at 26 weeks' gestation. His teenage mother and grandmother were full of hope. Now, after several complications, his prognosis has changed dramatically and the goals of care must be revisited.

Marisol has lived with cancer for 3 of her 9 years and she has had three relapses. Still, she is at a major research center. Her family is told that the "only thing left to do is a phase 1 trial."

David has managed cystic fibrosis for 18 years. He is short of breath, unable to sleep, and afraid of dying. His team encourages him, "Keep your chin up, Buddy, you are at the top of the transplant list!"

Hakim has lived with mucopolysaccharidosis for 16 years. The illness spared his brain, but made him a "progressive cardiorespiratory cripple." He and his family now face the choice of whether to use mechanical ventilation full-time. Hakim is tired and willing to accept a trade for maximal comfort in the face of a possibly foreshortened life span. However, his parents will not acknowledge that Hakim has an opinion about the goals of care.

Good communication is the foundation of trusting relationships among the patient, family, and health care provider. Under ideal circumstances, there is free exchange of information and room for emotions that can be difficult to discuss, such as fears and anxieties on the part of the patient and family or disclosure of a terminal diagnosis on the part of the clinician. Effective, empathic communication is particularly critical in the setting of a child's potentially life-threatening or terminal condition, when the stakes are high and the potential for long-lasting harm is great. Facilitating mutual trust within the clinical relationship is the essential cornerstone of palliative care and has been shown to be the anchor allowing families to maintain hope, regardless of the child's ultimate outcome (Mack et al., 2007).

Communication in the pediatric setting has unique challenges, including the need to assess the child's developing and ever-changing desire and capacity to learn clinically important information. This chapter provides practical information and tools to assist patients, families, and health care providers in communicating in a manner that facilitates the development of trust, conveyance of compassion, and conduct of ethical decision making.

This chapter illustrates the need to

- understand and consider the elements of communication;
- recognize the impact of the role of the person within the family dynamic, the trajectory of illness, and cultural, societal, and legal issues on the conduct of communication in pediatric palliative care;
- be deliberate in teaching the skill of communication to facilitate excellence in the delivery of pediatric palliative care, using "breaking bad news" as an exemplar;
- understand the importance of effective communication with all family members, including the patient and extended family;
- have respectful communication within the care team.

What Is Communication?

THE PURPOSE AND DEFINITIONS OF COMMUNICATION

Street (1991) describes three primary elements of communication among the clinician, parent, and child:

1. Informativeness: the quantity and quality of health information provided by the clinician
2. Interpersonal sensitivity: the affective behaviors that reflect the clinician's attention to, and interest in, the parents' and child's feelings and concerns
3. Partnership building: the extent to which the clinician invites the parents (and child) to state concerns, perspectives, and suggestions

Effective communication is responsive to the needs of the whole patient and the family dynamic; it is essential to patient- and family-centered care, the basic building block of the medical home concept (www.medicalhome info.org) (AAP Med Home, 2002).

Taking time to build rapport and understand the child and family builds trust, an essential ingredient enabling optimal caregiving and promoting informed and effective clinical decision making.

SHOWING EMPATHY, RESPECT, AND COMPASSION

Two broad kinds of patient and family needs must be addressed during the medical interview: the cognitive (the need to know and understand) and the affective (the emotional need to feel known and understood). Cognitive needs focus on information exchange; meeting this need requires the provision of information, followed by responding to questions and concerns and eliciting the child's/family's understanding. Affective needs focus on the child's/family's feelings and emotions, requiring the development of a safe space between the clinicians and patient/family. Such a space enables the recognition, expression, acknowledgment, and understanding of emotional needs. Affective needs are addressed by listening attentively, reflecting feelings, and showing respect, concern, and compassion. Clinicians often demonstrate these feelings through nonverbal means, such as gestures (e.g., nodding in affirmation), body posture (e.g., leaning closer to the patient), and physical touch, as well as the liberal use of silence. Silence allows for the processing and expression of emotional responses. Thus, clinicians need to be comfortable and competent with a repertoire of information exchange, relational skills, and abilities. In general, clinicians are more familiar with and adept at the cognitive information-exchange aspects than the affective, relational aspects of communication.

Patients' concerns are typically best elicited through the use of open-ended questions and attentive listening. In the context of a natural integration of the psychological aspects of the illness, this is followed by summarizing and by clarifying areas of misunderstanding. Using closed-ended or leading questions, offering advice prematurely, and focusing on the physical aspects of disease tend to truncate the exchange, inhibiting disclosure of symptoms and related experiences and concerns.

Patients receiving care from clinicians who have good communication skills and relational abilities report greater satisfaction with care, improved understanding, enhanced adherence to treatment, better outcomes, and decreased litigation (Levinson et al., 1997). In contrast, poor communication and relational competence can derail the partnership between the patient/

family and the health care provider and be devastating for patients and families, affecting their psychological adaptation to illness and bereavement (Johnson, 1972; Lynch and Staloch, 1988; Garwick et al., 1995; Ablon, 2000; Jurkovich et al., 2000).

The quality of the clinician's attention and the therapeutic use of silence are among the essential elements of communication and relational competence. Silence, in particular, can provide the opportunity for the patient and family to process new information intellectually and emotionally, formulate responses, ask questions, and clarify their values and feelings. The traditional imbalance of power and knowledge in the physician/family relationship can be particularly intimidating for young patients and their families. Silence on the part of the physician conveys that the patient and family are welcome and encouraged to speak up. Moreover, research suggests that when clinicians "speak less and listen more" in family conferences, families gain better understanding, are more satisfied with care, and have less conflict with staff (McDonagh et al., 2001; Meyer et al., 2009). The duration of silence needed to create the right conditions and "to coax" the family to speak often feels painfully long to clinicians. Physicians have been found to interrupt patients prematurely, on average within 18 seconds of the clinical encounter, even when they have offered patients the opportunity to speak (Dyche and Swiderski, 2005). In fact, patient satisfaction with communication is inversely proportional to the proportion of clinician speech during family meetings (McDonagh et al., 2001). This is likely due to the fact that when the family's questions and concerns are voiced, there is a greater likelihood that they can be addressed early and effectively.

THE CRITICAL ROLE OF NONVERBAL COMMUNICATION

Little attention is traditionally paid to the topic of communication skills and relational abilities in health care training, yet patient and parent satisfaction with quality of care is substantially influenced by clinicians' interpersonal skills, particularly in the case of anxious parents (Lashley et al., 2000; Young et al., 2003). Nonverbal communication is especially important, as it is estimated to encompass approximately 80 percent of communication (Halpern, 2007). Nonverbal behavior encompasses a variety of communicative behaviors without linguistic content, including facial expressivity; smiling; eye contact; head nodding; hand gestures; postural positions (open or closed body posture and forward-to-backward body lean); paralinguistic speech characteristics such as speech rate, loudness, pitch, pauses, and speech dysfluencies; and dialogic behaviors, such as interruption.

Nonverbal behaviors, such as sitting down, making eye contact, lending one's full attention to the patient or family, and not looking at one's watch, for example, can help create the perception of ample time and convey empathy. Although many clinicians feel empathy toward patients and families, they are often unsure or inhibited about how to convey that caring. Openly expressed empathy and the demonstration of genuine emotions on the part of the clinician can decrease patients' anxiety and convey valuable affective and emotional information. Further, emotions exert a profound influence on the experiencer's cognition and behavior, including prosocial acts, recall, decision making, persuasion, information processing, and interpersonal attitudes (Roter et al., 2006). For example, a patient who is occupied with feeling angry with the clinician owing to a perception of insensitivity is not able to absorb information about a new diagnosis or the proposed treatment plan. However, a patient who feels able to express anxiety and have it respectfully addressed can then clear her or his mind and be encouraged to listen to the important aspects of the diagnosis and proposed treatment plan, posing questions to ensure a mutually agreeable final treatment plan.

TREATING PARENTS AS PARTNERS

Children with life-threatening conditions often have chronic, complex, and rare disorders, some of which have not been well characterized in the medical literature. Their parents are often more expert on the illness and its manifestations than their clinicians and are the best experts on the child's and family's experience of the disorder. These families' day-to-day lives are upended by the child's illness; although they may not follow a theoretically perfect regimen, they are often heroic in their willingness to attempt to balance the needs of their children and to provide the best care they can. Many parents appreciate sincere affirmation of their contributions to their child's health care and well-being:

> A parent, describing her 18-year-old son who was quadriplegic from cerebral palsy but intellectually intact, mentioned that he had graduated from high school, had many friends, and was happy other than the pain from muscle spasms, which persisted despite intensive treatment. The clinician stated, "He sure is lucky to have you and your husband as parents! You have helped him to be so successful!" The mother became tearful, saying her son's neurologist had never told her in the 15 years he had treated her son that he thought she was doing a good job.

In addition, parents want their views and concerns factored into the care plan (Walker et al., 1989; Dragone, 1990; Marchetti et al., 1995; Perrin,

Lewkowicz, and Young, 2000). Showing the family respect by asking them to share information and insights and inviting them to be partners in determining the care goals and care plan enhances the likelihood of creating a successful therapeutic alliance. Families and sometimes patients themselves can troubleshoot the practical issues associated with carrying out the treatment plan.

Even in the intensive care setting with an acute illness or injury, parents may wish to be active participants in information exchange and care provision. Conducting bedside rounds that are open to and inclusive of family members is a controversial yet growing practice in pediatric critical care settings. Clinicians worry that including parents on rounds may breach confidentiality, dramatically increase the time of rounds, confuse the parents, degrade the teaching environment, and undermine respect for junior practitioners who are learning from more senior colleagues. Despite these concerns, units that are committed to patient- and family-centered care practices have moved forward and reported positive experiences and benefits of open bedside rounds (Kleiber, Davenport, and Freyenberger, 2006). Clinicians working in newly constructed units that foster greater parental involvement and provide accommodations for parents will likely need to grapple with issues such as open bedside rounds and establish relevant policy.

In addition to being treated as partners in care, family members want to be recognized as needing care, too. They are affected by a child's health condition, whether it is an overwhelming and sudden problem or a more chronic process. Families desire assistance with and recognition of the need to preserve family solidarity and support, including social support, child care, education, and professional services (Horner, Rawlins, and Giles, 1987; Walker et al., 1989; Bailey, Blasco, and Simeonsson, 1992; Meyer et al., 2006); in some studies, parents of chronically ill children report assistance with family and social support as their greatest unmet need. One proposed solution for such families is to have an annual family meeting to discuss the "big picture." In short, parents of chronically ill children want a "medical home" as envisioned by the American Academy of Pediatrics (www.medicalhome info.org). When appropriate information is not provided and careful attention to communication and relationship building does not occur, bitterness can fester and linger for years (Quine and Pahl, 1987; Nursey, Rohde, and Farmer, 1991; Krahn, Hallum, and Kime, 1993; Ablon, 2000; Jurkovich et al., 2000). Conversely, clinicians who are empathic, well informed, and honest can serve as a trustworthy source of strength for parents, particularly those struggling to adapt to a difficult situation.

A PARENT'S REQUEST LIST: DIANNE GRAY, BEREAVED MOTHER

Please know that we are appreciative of your knowledge and need you. However, it may take us a while to accept your role in our lives, much less absorb what you are saying.

Please know that we are watching you closely: how you breathe, how you stand, whether you are patient with us. We have become accustomed to watching for nonverbal cues in our children and will apply the same skill with you.

Please know that one of the more important conversations you will have with us is the one regarding diagnosis. We will replay this conversation in our minds for the rest of our lives. Therefore, please take care to choose the location of this conversation carefully. Please do not answer your cell, pager, etc., during this time. You are changing our lives. Wouldn't you wish the same of us if we were changing yours?

Please understand that we are awash in emotion; therefore, your words may not sink in. We are not "stupid or ignorant," so please be patient if we ask the same questions over and over. We hope we will get in sync with you regarding the care of our child, but it may not happen today.

Please talk to us out of earshot of our children, if appropriate or possible. The location of our communication is critical. If you talk over or in front of my child, I am probably focusing on protecting my child from the "unknown" information you may share, and I may not hear you at all, which wastes your time and my valuable time with my child.

Please know that your language may not make sense to me. You wish to discuss a "care plan"? I have only one plan of care in mind: "Save my child." The terminology you use is of critical importance to my ability to feel comfortable with you and your suggestions. Let's talk in "real" terms, such as how to make my child comfortable, how to get through today, the next few months. This I can understand and can discuss.

Please know that I am trying my best to be patient with you, as you are trying to be patient with me. My whole world has turned upside down. While I am trying to interpret the information you are giving me, I am also watching all of my lifetime dreams wash away with each passing sentence you are asking me to accept, to understand. The enormity of the situation is overwhelming at times.

Please know that I am probably dealing with other family members delivering their own expectations of the situation, as well. They are sharing their own cultural values, religious beliefs, and wishes with me. It is an enormous amount to deal with.

Please call me by my name. "Mom" is not my name, and while it may seem friendly to you, to me it may seem demeaning. Also, please call my child by name, as well. He or she is not "kiddo" or "buddy." We may see this as an infringement of your role. We are still trying to get comfortable with you becoming an integral part of our lives.

Please do not discuss other patients in front of my child. He or she may not know you are talking about someone else and may think you are talking about him or her.

Know that it helps me to hear you praise me sincerely. I am looking to you for guidance, support, and information. Your input is of the utmost importance to me. If I feel good about my caregiving and decision making, I will also feel better about my role as a parent with other children in my family.

Know that I do hear you; I just may not be able to retain the information you are giving me.

Know that how you treat me and my sick child will affect my well child (children) for the rest of their lives. This time will affect who he or she becomes as a student, a parent, a member of society. This is one of the most important periods of my well child's life, and you have a critical role in our entire family's history.

Know that I appreciate you and your expertise although I may not show it. I have been dealt an incredible blow and am trying my best to cope. I hope I will look back on this time with appreciation for your role in our lives.

Please communicate with me as though I will be in your life for the rest of your life, because you are an indelible part of our life story.

It behooves clinicians to be mindful of the language used every day to describe patients and families. It is not uncommon for families to be cryptically described as "good," "intact," "dysfunctional," or "broken" in clinicians' spoken language and written documentation. It is much more helpful and respectful to describe the composition, circumstances, and interactions of the family. Clinicians should communicate with the expectation of being overheard by the family or of the medical record being read by the family. In addition, some families are characterized as being in denial. Our parent coauthor describes her experience this way:

Looking back, I could've been classified as "in denial" but only because I didn't know what the terms were or what the prognosis actually included. The physicians all told me to carefully consider placing a feeding tube in Austin, as he would suffer tremendously long term from spasticity, dystonia, and it would only prolong his life. "Only?"

They showed me pictures in books that didn't look like my son at all. So I thought, they must be underestimating "my son" or "our case" because we're individuals, aren't we?

My denial was actually a case of not knowing what dystonia could do—how it could torture and contort my son's body enough to crack molars or twist large sections of his body. Is that denial? I think many, many parents are not actually in denial, they are just not experienced in this type of disease process (thank goodness), or the potential outcomes associated with it. So what would you call that?

Thus, denial can be the inability to comprehend what is being said as a result of "emotional blocking" or can be the result of inadequate communication. In many cases, although dysfunctional, denial is the only coping mechanism the family can muster, preventing a complete breakdown. Time, the child's evolving clinical situation, and coaching may enable more effective coping skills; in the meantime, listening to the pain, coupled with gentle, compassionate advice and spiritual assistance, can often enable effective decision making that prevents unnecessary suffering.

Therapeutic Use of Self

In contrast to technological assessment and procedural skills that demand precise adherence to standardized protocols, good communication practices and relational abilities naturally invoke the clinician's own interpersonal qualities and style. These skills and abilities may therefore be considered a therapeutic use of self. That is, conversations with families require neither procedures to be accomplished nor equipment to be operated, but rather rely on the clinician's interpersonal skills and relatedness as the therapeutic instrument. Historically, "bedside manner" was considered to be a special quality that one either constitutionally had or did not. Gradually, this understanding of communication and interpersonal skills has been reconceptualized as a fundamental clinical competency that can be brought forth, learned to some extent, practiced, and nurtured across professional disciplines and at all levels of practice (Fallowfield et al., 2003; Makoul, 2006; Browning et al., 2007). As part of the process of learning and refining their talents in the art of interpersonal communication, clinicians also need to develop self-reflective practices and self-preservation strategies in the face of difficult health care conversations (Beach and Inui, 2006).

Informing parents of a chronic or incurable diagnosis can challenge a clinician's sense of preparedness and competency. It is helpful to remember that parents value the affective engagement and attunement of the clinician more than the ability of the informer to "fix it" (Meert, Thurston, and Thomas, 2001). Parents are able to distinguish the difference between the delivery of the news and the news itself. Clinicians are encouraged to show their genuine feelings, demonstrating that they are concerned about the well-being of the patient and family (Browning, 2002; Strong, 2003; Meyer et al., 2006).

Communicating with families during medical crises and difficult health care situations requires sensitivity; it is not simply a matter of divulging information about everything that is known or suspected (Truog et al., 2006; Epstein and Peters, 2009). The process is better understood as an unfolding series of exchanges and conversations between a team of clinicians and a stressed, sometimes traumatized family. Each of the conversations is highly contextual, requiring sensitivity and attunement of the clinician to the shifting capacity of family members to listen, comprehend, and emotionally integrate new information (Browning, 2002). How much to discuss at any given meeting or informal encounter should be determined based on the clinical situation, the choice of what to communicate, the needs and preferences of the family, timing, and pragmatic considerations (Fallowfield, 1993; Rabow, Fair, and Hardie, 1999; Curtis and White, 2008). Under circumstances of severe stress and emotional overload, families may signal their inability to take in more information by looking down at their laps, shielding their eyes, or physically removing themselves from the situation. The issue of readiness to listen and learn is vitally important; trying to impose too much information too fast on parents is not useful or productive. It is better to say, "We have talked about a lot of things today. I am committed to giving you as much information as you need, but perhaps we should take a bit of a breather and meet again later to talk some more. How does that sound? Let me write down the name of the diagnosis for you now, and we can meet again after you have had a chance to absorb this."

One U.S. study (Greenberg et al., 1984) found that parents of children who have cancer, when hearing the initial diagnosis, desire less information at that time, preferring an emphasis on establishing trust with new caregivers. Parents advise that trust is built by acknowledging the grief, anxiety, and fear the family is experiencing and inviting them to share their feelings and ask questions. Gradually sharing additional illness and treatment information, supplemented by written or taped materials, as well as providing a means to contact the physician when additional questions arise, is also greatly appreciated. Many parents now are asking for e-mail contact, and in some instances, this is a reimbursable service.

When the bad news represents a potential change in goals, such as in Jedidiah's and Marisol's cases, it is important to acknowledge the grieving for the hoped-for outcome that is no longer possible.

> We had all hoped Jedidiah would escape all the potential complications of prematurity. Unfortunately, he has had a lot of problems. Let's sit down and be sure we all understand what has happened, then we can discuss what to do next.

> We all hoped Marisol's cancer would respond to treatments that are known to help. As you know, we have no treatments available that are proven to cure her cancer. So we have a choice to make together—based on what is most important to Marisol and your family. One choice is to do everything possible to maximize the quality of her life for the time she has left, allowing her to choose how and where to spend her time; we would remain in charge of her care and keep in contact with you. Another choice is to consider participating in research about a new medication. Study participation has risks, and the treatment is not likely to benefit Marisol herself. However, some families feel strongly that this is a priority for them. I think either choice is good, and I support you in choosing either option.

Disclosing Unwelcome Information

When hearing bad news, parents value a clinician who clearly demonstrates a caring attitude and who allows them to talk and to express emotions (Sharp, Strauss, and Lorch, 1992). One effective opening to the conversation is to ask, "Can you tell me your understanding of [child's name]'s situation and what is most important to you right now?" Once parents' understanding and priorities are elicited, any misperceptions can be addressed and a joint agenda for the meeting can be established. Asking about previous experiences with illness and whether they know anyone else with a similar diagnosis or situation can also be helpful, enabling the clinician to be aware of the family's fears and expectations. Pointing out how their child's situation is similar to or different from their previous experience contextualizes their situation, helping parents better understand their child's likely course.

If and when parents become emotionally upset during the informing interview, clinicians should pause to acknowledge their responses with a comment such as, "I can see you were not expecting this" or "I can understand that this news is upsetting," lending full presence to provide support, and giving them some time to recompose themselves. Some parents will naturally turn their attention back to the clinician and wish to continue the conversation; others may not. Sometimes, on hearing difficult news, parents become emotionally overwhelmed and cannot continue to take in new information. Under these circumstances, it is recommended that the clinician seek the parents' preference regarding whether to continue or to reconvene at a specified later time (perhaps minutes to hours later) to continue the conversation.

Creating a quiet, private space, free from interruptions and the indignity of public display, is important when conducting difficult conversations with families. Having soft facial tissues available conveys thoughtfulness and an acknowledgment of the painful nature of the discussion. Of course, parents want hopeful and positive news about their child, as well as an opportunity to touch or hold the child, particularly newborn infants or children from whom they have been separated during a transport. Parents need recognition by the clinician of the child's unique value as an individual first and as an ill or injured person second (Krahn, Hallum, and Kime, 1993). Speaking about the child as if he or she "is" the diagnosis is limiting, hurtful, and depersonalizing. Sadly, it is not uncommon to hear, "the crani in room 202," "the CFer," or "the liver" to describe patients, quickly reducing the child to be merely defined by the illness, surgery, or organ system failure afflicting him or her. Referring to the baby who has the congenital diaphragmatic hernia by name, for example, is immeasurably more respectful and dignified than "the diaphragm."

Parental dissatisfaction with the process of learning bad news is not uncommon. Several frameworks and protocols for "breaking" bad news can substantially improve the experience. The language describing this process is unfortunate; it is to be hoped that nothing will be "broken" in the process. A growing body of literature, written by clinicians, offers advice and accumulated clinical wisdom about how best to convey bad news (Buckman and Kason, 1992; Feudtner, 2007; Levetown, 2008; Back, Arnold, and Tulsky 2009). Clinicians can expand their repertoire of skills by consulting this literature.

"BREAKING BAD NEWS" WITH SKILL AND EMPATHY (ADAPTED FROM BUCKMAN AND KASON, 1992; CREAGAN, 1994)

- *Timing of the discussion:* If possible, initiate the discussion of the diagnosis when the appropriate members of the family can be gathered. Speaking with a parent who is alone and unsupported can be devastating. If acceptable to the parent, it can be helpful to invite a social worker and/or chaplain to the meeting to address the family's psychosocial and spiritual concerns and to assist them with identifying sources of support.

- *Physical setting:* Whenever possible, communicate bad news in person rather than over the telephone. Ideally, the physical setting should be private, intimate, quiet, and free of unwanted interruptions. Avoid having a large table between the family and the clinicians because it can magnify feelings of isolation and distance and interfere with natural gestures of physical touch.
- *Time:* Allocate sufficient time to allow information to be exchanged, questions to be answered, and parents' emotional responses to be acknowledged.
- *Communication:*
  - Introduce all present, including their names and roles; try not to overwhelm the family with too many people wearing white coats.
  - Use understandable language rather than medical jargon; begin by asking what they understand and address any misperceptions.
  - Engage trained medical interpreters as needed.
  - Elicit parents' ideas of the cause of the problem; ensure that they do not blame themselves or others.
  - Confirm accurate comprehension by asking the family to explain in their own words what they understand.
  - Proceed at a pace that is conducive to family comprehension; strong emotive responses are likely to interfere with comprehension.
  - Encourage the family to express concerns and fears and to ask questions.
- *Nonverbal expression of concern and support:*
  - Sit at the same level as the parents, rather than standing over them; sitting at the corner of a table, close to the parents, rather than across is also helpful so that a caring squeeze of the parent's hand or shoulder can be given if it seems natural and culturally appropriate.
  - Eye contact is important, but the amount is often culturally determined.
- *Discussing the impact of the diagnosis, potential goals, and treatment plans on the family:*
  - A range of information needs to be shared with families, including
    - the diagnosis and prognosis in terms the parents can understand;
    - potential interventions, including the short- and long-term benefits and burdens (some families prefer to receive this and other information in small doses);
    - potential physical, social, and existential ramifications of the child's condition for the patient and the family;

- values held by the family and derivative goals and types of care that might be appropriate based on those values;
- recommendations of relevant community-based resources, recognizing that these suggestions may be rejected at first;
- provision of contact information for other willing families with a similarly affected child;
- reassurance that care and support of the patient and family will continue despite the bad news (Strong, 2003);
- any other implications of the disease that may be important to the patient and family.

Whether initially conveying a new diagnosis or facilitating a change in the goals of care, clinicians should be prepared to repeat the information several times patiently, as well as to present it in different words and formats. Many families do better with graphic representations of the information, including brief films (Volandes et al., 2009), diagrams, radiographs, and anatomic models. Audiotapes of information-giving sessions are also appreciated, as they provide the family the chance to listen several times and at their own pace, as well as the option to share the tape and associated information with friends and family who may have more experience and knowledge about medical issues than they themselves do. It is always a good idea to write down the correct spelling of the diagnosis and potential main treatments because many families will want to conduct their own search on the Internet, preferably on websites recommended by the clinician as being reliable and accurate.

It is important to respond to the family's expressions of grief as they arise. It may be acceptable to express concern by touching the parents, such as by hugging them or touching their hands or shoulders. It is helpful to be aware of any personal, cultural, or faith-specific dictums about the appropriateness of touching; some of this can be detected by the parents' own body language. In addition to being aware and respectful of patients' and families' needs and expectations regarding physical touch, it is vital for clinicians to reflect on their own comfort level, preferences, and intentions regarding physical contact.

At the end of the discussion, it can be helpful to summarize and lay out the next steps, such as new tests needed or time frames to assess response to treatment, as well as setting a time in the near future to review the situation with the parents and answer their questions. During the interim, the physician should either be personally available or identify someone else who will be available to address any urgent questions or concerns, providing reliable contact information for the appropriate person. The physician should ask the parents who else they would like to know about the situation and offer help in explaining it to them. For example, an extended family meeting might be arranged.

MANAGING UNCERTAINTY, ADDRESSING HOPE

Although clinicians may not expect it, parents are often relieved when a diagnosis is finally determined, and even experience less anxiety when facing a known dismal prognosis than when facing conditions with uncertain prognoses (Ablon, 2000). Of course, medical care is often fraught with at least some uncertainty. There are effective ways to handle uncertainty that can retain good will and trust. In general, it helps to emphasize the common purpose and goals of the care team and family. One useful phrase to prevent surprises is to acknowledge that we are all hoping for the best, but planning for the worst. For instance, in the setting of newly diagnosed acute myelogenous leukemia (AML), it might be appropriate to say:

> This is not the diagnosis we had hoped for. Thankfully, a good proportion of children who have AML are cured of the cancer, and we will do everything we can to make sure Juan is one of them. In addition, I want you to know that we will give you honest information no matter whether good or bad, so we can trust each other and make good decisions together, based on Juan's response to treatment. We will have a better understanding if the treatment is working in _____ weeks. We'll talk about the big picture of how things are going at that time, in addition to our other conversations along the way.

> Regardless of Juan's cancer's response to treatment, I want you to understand that Juan's well-being is our highest priority, and regardless of other aspects of treatment, we will all do all we can to prevent suffering for him and for you. For that reason, I would like to introduce you to our team of caregivers who are expert in helping keep children comfortable and preventing and treating suffering. They are the palliative care team, and they are an essential element of providing the best care possible.

Generally, parents prefer honesty when the prognosis for their child is fatal, rather than to be mollified and cajoled into believing that the child might recover (Meert et al., 2008). In fact, parents report that they have more hope when they are given accurate but negative information than when they feel they cannot trust the information they are being given (Mack et al., 2007). When parents feel they have been misled, they can harbor anger and resentment, because they believe they would have made different decisions with accurate information (Surkan et al., 2006; Meert et al., 2008; Dussel et al., 2009). In the case example, when Juan's AML returned after a bone marrow transplant, his clinician might honestly and empathetically say:

> Now that Juan's cancer has come back, I am sorry to say that the likelihood of curing his disease is slim—almost zero. Another bone marrow transplant may lengthen his life by perhaps _____, but this will mean more time in the hospital, along with the associated discomforts you are all too familiar with. Another approach is to focus even more on how to help Juan enjoy his time remaining, ensuring that he receives treatments as needed to help him have energy and minimal symptoms. Regardless of your goals, the people you have depended on throughout his illness will remain part of his care team.

When children are initially diagnosed with a serious illness, they and their parents are thrown into an unfamiliar health care world where bewildering technology and medical vocabulary dominate, and they can find themselves at the mercy of unfamiliar care providers. Parents typically have a steep learning curve to master and may be unsure of their values with respect to health care interventions. Moreover, they may not recognize the need to advocate on behalf of their child or assert themselves in the determination of treatment goals and the care plan. However, when parental concerns remain unaddressed, parents can experience considerable role-related stress and are often disappointed, if not resentful. Therefore, it is best for all involved to coach the family and child to express their concerns from the beginning. Encourage family input by making statements such as:

> We need to work as partners in this journey. So when you have concerns or questions, it is important for you to ask. When we talk to each other, we often use technical terms and abbreviations. While we try hard to use clear language when talking with families, sometimes we don't succeed—so please let us know when we are not being clear. It is critically important that we understand each other.

> It is particularly important that you understand the choices that we face together. So if there is anything that is unclear or confusing, please ask questions. We want you to understand both the likely short-term and long-term outcomes of each choice, before we make any decisions.

COMMUNICATION IN THE SETTING OF UNEXPECTED
LIFE-THREATENING ILLNESS OR INJURY

In situations of sudden fatal illness or traumatic injury, the child may be under the care of the team only mere hours or days, yet the depth and significance of the therapeutic relationship may be profound for both the family and clinicians (Truog et al., 2006). Establishing rapport, professional credibility, and trust quickly and solidly is absolutely vital under these circumstances, because time is so precious. Clear introductions, the provision of honest information in understandable language and portions, and seamless interdisciplinary collaboration that addresses the sometimes-urgent psychosocial needs of families are important. Parents appreciate and value clinicians' genuine expression of emotions and concern for their child and circumstances. Among a sample of 150 bereaved parents whose children died traumatically after automobile accidents, the emotional sensitivity and interpersonal skills of the informant were more important than having had previous contact or professional position (Finlay and Dallimore, 1991). Interestingly, police officers were rated as more sympathetic and supportive than either physicians or nurses. Some parents reported feeling more supported when the informant also appeared emotionally distressed, suggesting the value of shared human experience and humanity in times of extraordinary sorrow.

AUTOPSY AS AN OPPORTUNITY FOR COMMUNICATION

If an autopsy is performed, it is advisable to hold a postmortem conference with the parents (and sometimes siblings as well) approximately 6 to 8 weeks after the death (Riggs and Weibley, 1994; Meert et al., 2007). As parents reflect on the whirlwind events of their final days with their child, numerous questions can arise and complex emotions can surface; the conference can provide a forum to address these concerns. If an autopsy is performed and there is no opportunity to hear and discuss the results, parents may become suspicious that the medical establishment was "experimenting" on their child. Moreover, in the case of illness (compared to trauma), parents may have requested the autopsy to assist in family planning to determine the need for screening procedures on close relatives; thus, they may be anxiously awaiting the results. A face-to-face meeting enables the treating physician to respond to the family's questions, translate the autopsy findings into understandable lay language, and, importantly, check on the well-being of the parents and siblings. It is helpful to coordinate the timing of this meeting so that all important members of the care team can attend. Social workers and chaplains may be helpful in assessing complications in the bereavement process, offering psychosocial support and education, and making needed referrals to assist the family. (See chap. 11 for further information on grief and bereavement.)

Family Dynamics

SOME ADVICE FROM A PARENT

Please know that family issues we negotiated as a well family are now under review as a family with a sick child. This is draining and difficult to handle. Therefore, please show patience with us as we struggle to manage an enormous amount of emotional turmoil on many fronts.

Please know that communicating with both parents (if possible) is always far better than each parent separately. Not only does it save you tremendous amounts of time, but even more importantly, it eliminates the he said / she said issues that can further complicate these emotionally fraught situations.

Please know that we are generally trying our best. Most of us understand the stakes and the issues and are doing our best to deal simultaneously with family issues that have often been problematic for some time.

Please remember that our family communication process may have been ineffective for years and will not improve overnight, even if we recognize that our child needs us now more than ever.

Please know that you are an instrumental part of our family dynamic now and can be of enormous assistance in helping us to heal years of emotional damage due to poor communication.

Please know that we may also be accepting new family members into our lives at this time: stepparents, stepbrothers, and stepsisters, who are also trying to cope with an extraordinarily sensitive situation.

Please know that our difficult family situation may also include issues that do not involve you professionally, but that will affect the care of our child, such as divorce, visitation, child support, and custody disputes.

ENABLING EFFECTIVE CHILD PARTICIPATION

At its core, child health communication is family-centered communication. In the past, children of any age were rarely consulted about their own health concerns. In current Western culture, children are highly valued, yet attention to their autonomous needs, especially when the child is not yet an adolescent, remains challenging (Levetown, 2008). Children can be coached to effectively assume the role of a health partner, to raise concerns, ask questions, note information, and participate in the creation of and troubleshooting of potential problems with the care plan. This active engagement of the child has the potential not only to improve health outcomes but also to bolster the child's sense of self-efficacy, mastery, and self-esteem.

The importance of the child's possessing effective health communication skills becomes evident when trying to assess and treat a child's subjective symptoms, including pain. In the absence of the child's input, it is difficult to understand the nature and severity of the pain; thus, it is nearly impossible to relieve the discomfort effectively and safely. It is well known that the use of patient-controlled analgesia assists with the resolution of pain beyond the dose of medication. The message that the child knows his pain, is in control of his therapy, and is trusted is in itself a powerful therapeutic intervention. Children as young as 4 years of age have used patient-controlled anesthesia effectively (Dunbar et al., 1995).

Children often understand more than has been assumed. Through a process of education and participation in self-care, children can increase their understanding and create a stable framework on which to promote the integration of increasingly complex information. Children need to have usable information, to be given choices (including their desired level of involvement), and to be asked their opinion, even when their decision will not be determinative (AAP COB, 1995; van Dulmen, 1998). It is important to let children know that their opinion matters deeply, and that their opinion and preferences will be elicited and considered throughout the health care decision-making process; it is equally important to stress that the burden of decision making does not rest solely on their young shoulders. Enhanced understanding provides a sense of control, mitigating fear and reducing the harms associated with illness and injury. A child who asks about his or her condition may be ready to learn and know more. Children who do not ask about their illness should be given the opportunity to receive information; if they refuse it, information should never be forced on them.

Parents and children report greater satisfaction with care and better adherence to treatment regimens when the child is included in information gathering as well as in creation of the treatment plan (Lewis, Pantell, and Sharp, 1991; McCabe, 1996; Tates and Meeuwesen, 2001). Parents, however, do want to be involved in the decision regarding whether and how their children will be informed about their health conditions. It is, therefore, important to understand the preexisting parent-child relationship, the family's cultural and idiosyncratic values (Krauss-Mars and Lachman, 1994; AAP COPACFH, 2000; Flores et al., 2000), and the developmental needs of the child, including the desire to participate in his or her own care plan. Simultaneously, determination of the parents' perspectives on providing information to the child is imperative.

Because Hakim is a smart young man, and no one knows better than he what it is like to live with this illness, I think it is important and respectful to ask if and how he would like to participate in determining the goals of care and helping design his care plan. How do you feel about including Hakim in this way? Do you have concerns about doing that? Do you have thoughts about how we can best communicate with him about this?

Parents should be educated that research demonstrates improved health outcomes when the child is treated as a partner (Rushforth, 1999; Tates and Meeuwesen, 2001). Pediatric health care quality will improve if the child is recognized to have his or her own individual cognitive and emotional needs, is taken seriously, and is considered to be capable and have an important perspective that needs to be understood. Parents and clinicians should decide together whether the child will be present at the informational consultations, whether parents would prefer to tell the child themselves or have another person tell the child, and whether the informing interview will occur with or without the parents present. Children 7 years or older are more accurate than their parents in providing health data that predict future health outcomes, although they were less accurate at providing accurate past medical history (Dixon-Woods, Young, and Heney, 1999). Thus, significant attention to the child's input should be routine practice. Enabling the child to achieve gradually increased capacity to take responsibility for the maintenance of health and the treatment of illness is a crucial task, especially in the face of a chronic condition; this task is specific to pediatric physicians and practitioners. Table 7.1 lists helpful strategies to accomplish this goal.

THE NEED FOR HONEST COMMUNICATION WITH THE CHILD

Sometimes, springing from their protective instincts, parents believe that not informing the child about the illness is best. Similarly, some professionals argue that paternalistic decisions (primarily on the part of the family) to withhold "harmful" information from the child can be justified (Lantos, 1996). This position is not supported by the literature that examines the child's preference for information. One of the most striking was Bluebond-Langner's (1978) landmark study of terminally ill children indicating that children as young as 3 years of age were aware of their diagnosis and prognosis without ever having been told by an adult. She found that adult avoidance of disclosure and denial of difficult information led the child to feel isolated, abandoned, and unloved. At the same time, the child's response is often to "protect" the "unaware" adults, despite great personal cost; this situation is referred to as mutual pretense and can harm both parties. Using whatever

Table 7.1 Strategies to engage children in the outpatient setting

Speak *with*, not *at* or *to*, the child.
Speak in a private setting.
Determine whom the child would like to be present (younger children usually prefer parents to be present; abused children may need privacy to facilitate disclosure; most adolescents prefer privacy).
Begin with a nonthreatening topic.
Listen actively.
Pay attention to body language and tone of voice.
Use drawings, puppets, games, or other creative communication tools.
Elicit fears and concerns by reference to self or a third party (e.g., "Some kids who have cystic fibrosis worry about their coughing. Does that worry you?").
Ask the child what he or she would do with three wishes or a magic wand.

Source: Adapted from Lask, 1992.

information they have, children will continually try to make sense of their situations. An incomplete ability to understand does not justify a lack of discussion with a child who desires involvement in his or her care and decision making.

Until the patient is 18, parents can insist that medical information be withheld from the child or adolescent. A reasonable initial approach is to listen to the family's preferences and rationale for information sharing and withholding and to affirm that the parent is making this choice out of concern and love for the child. Thereafter, engage parents in discussion to better appreciate their perspective about the child's understanding; one technique to accomplish this is to ask if they think the child knows that having blood tests and spending a lot of time in clinics and the hospital is not normal and is a sign of being sick. Finally, educate parents that it is likely that the child already knows that something is problematic about his or her health status, and that lack of information and constrained partnership with the child can disrupt the trust essential to the relationship between patient and clinician. Most parents will reconsider and agree to permit the child to receive age-appropriate information as he or she needs and prefers. Rarely, parents remain insistent that the child not be told about the condition. In these cases, one approach is to let parents know that you will honor their request to the point of the child's asking a direct question, but will honestly respond to any question the child poses.

By virtue of their status as patients, children are often more aware of the day-to-day demands and burdens of ongoing treatment intervention than the adults around them. Ideally, children's perspectives on the burden and "cost" of treatment preferences and their ideas of what is important and preferable will be elicited and factored into decision making. Moreover, when children are informed of their approaching death, they are more likely to die at home. Of note, open communication with their dying child enhances parents' bereavement outcomes (Kreicbergs et al., 2004; Sharman, Meert, and Sarnaik, 2005; Surkan et al., 2006). A study of bereaved parents in Sweden indicates that 100 percent of parents who spoke openly with their children about the impending death had no regrets, whereas 27 percent of those who did not speak to their children about dying not only regretted their decision but also suffered from an increased incidence of depression and anxiety (Kreicbergs et al., 2004). Thus, counseling parents about the benefits of honesty and open communication should be invoked when they are reluctant to speak with their child about illness or death.

Clinicians have a moral and ethical obligation to discuss health and illness with the child patient, supported by a number of U.K., Canadian, and U.S. laws, policies, and court decisions, indicating an expectation that children will be active participants in their care. The principle of self-determination applies to children as well as adults. Involving children in communication about their health and in decisions regarding their health care demonstrates respect for their capacities, hones their skill to make future health decisions, and enables their essential input into decisions in which there is no "right answer" other than the one that best meets the needs of the individual child and family. Older children and adolescents should have a significant role in such cases. When the patient and family disagree, the clinician should treat with due respect the cultural and family values, roles, and structure that have always governed the relationship.

COMMUNICATION WITH THE EXTENDED FAMILY

Even if the persons present at clinic visits, hospital stays, and even home hospice calls are primarily the patient and parent(s), other family members have an investment in health care communication, in terms of both providing and receiving information. Members of the extended family and social support network can be key participants in the decision-making process; therefore, as desired by the parents and child patient, efforts should be made to include them in the communication stream. Communication should be interactive, enabling responses to concerns and negotiation of care goals and plans as needed. The health care team is well served when creative means of communication are employed, enabling efficient and accurate dissemination of medical information. Some of these tools include tape recorders, web cameras via secure Internet connections, and conference calls, as well as less technically sophisticated means of communication. The latter may include arranging formal family meetings in advance or using a communication notebook to communicate with family members who are not present. Families and commercial vendors have recognized the need for such communication and have devised and used products such as CaringBridge (www.caring bridge.org), allowing the parent or patient to communicate their experiences to select invited friends and family efficiently.

CULTURAL CONSIDERATIONS

Minority and non-English-speaking families often have cultural expectations and nuanced understandings of language that, if not understood and attended to, can substantially interfere with effective medical care and may lead to a decrease in health status for their children. The American Academy of Pediatrics identifies the responsibility of the clinician to be aware of and accommodate the needs of such families (AAP COPW, 1999). It is a good idea to be aware of the general cultural norms and taboos of the dominant subcultures attending the practice. Although there are general guidelines for what is "culturally competent," none describe any particular family. Rather than assuming that a family will identify itself a certain way or follow cultural "norms," it is safer to ask family members about their preferences and etiquette for communicating with them. "How should I give your family medical information about Mary?" "With whom do I share information?" "Who makes decisions?" "Are there topics that should not be directly discussed in your family?" Offering to wait until the relevant persons are available is culturally respectful. Assuming a posture of cultural humility and accommodating the family's cultural preferences whenever possible is a good rule.

Certain issues can arise among minority cultures that require attention, including passivity with authority figures, distrust and/or fear of health care professionals, decision making that emphasizes the group over the individual, and low educational, English-language, or medical literacy levels. Helpful strategies include offering invitations to ask questions, using silence during discussions, accommodating large groups for information dissemination and health-planning discussions, and providing sufficient time to consult with others when important decisions are to be made. Table 7.2 suggests prompts to elicit culturally related health beliefs, concerns, and practices.

Table 7.2 Prompts to elicit medically relevant, culturally important information

What concerns prompted you to bring your child (use the child's name) for health care?

What behaviors and symptoms are of greatest concern to you?

What do you think caused this problem?

How do you think the illness affects your child?

What have you tried to do to make the illness better? Have you tried any traditional remedies?

Are there any specific dietary, religious, or cultural practices that need to be accommodated?

THE USE OF MEDICAL INTERPRETERS

As the pediatric population across the country diversifies culturally and linguistically, there is a pressing need to serve patients and their families who have limited English-language proficiency. Inadequate communication with health care providers and inability to effectively negotiate the health care system places young patients at a considerable disadvantage and higher risk for poor health care outcomes. These complex situations are rife with potential for miscommunication, compromised care, stress, and preventable errors. When treating such patients, clinicians often order additional tests and diagnostic procedures to mitigate the fear of missing a diagnosis when a thorough history would have sufficed. Effective clinical care and education for patients and their families typically require repeated verbal and written communication and reinforcement of detailed information, often under circumstances of heightened stress. The challenges are even more daunting when language barriers exist. Poor understanding or the inability to advocate on behalf of their child as a result of language limitations exacerbates parents' emotional strain.

The Joint Commission requires the availability of trained medical interpreters. Medicaid partially reimburses for such services. Well-trained interpreters not only possess language proficiency but also bring an awareness of cultural norms to the health care arena and can serve as cultural brokers. Effective use of interpreters as part of the team includes the establishment of a framework for collaboration, according them customary professional courtesies such as updates before meetings and debriefings after meetings. Before the consultation begins, acknowledge the potential for and the desire to prevent cultural missteps. "I may ask you to say some things that you think are not culturally acceptable. If that happens, please let me know and guide me to more appropriately approach these topics." Use of untrained translators, such as bilingual children or other family members who are trying to absorb information and transmit it while emotionally upset, is inappropriate. Nonprofessional hospital employees are also a common source of "translation," but this practice is fraught with problems and is not recommended.

EFFECTIVE ADVANCE CARE PLANNING: A COLLABORATIVE AND EVOLUTIONARY PROCESS

Some family members cope with difficult situations by wanting to know only what will happen day to day. However, most want to understand where their journey is leading; these individuals feel more comfortable when given a context for considering treatment options, goals of care, and how to best prepare for what is ahead (Meyer et al., 2006). At least one person among the decision makers should have a good idea of the "big picture" to accomplish the goal of informed and ethical decision making.

No clinician, even one who has experienced a life-threatening condition him- or herself, can truly understand the feelings and priorities of another patient or family. Therefore, in considering plans of care, the clinician must give honest information and elicit an understanding of patients' and families' priorities in determining the goals of care that inform that plan. Most people have not stopped to consider their health care priorities and values in this fashion. One means of assisting them is to ask about another person they know who has a chronic or terminal condition, what happened to the person, and what the family thinks about it—what was good and what was bad, what they might regret or want to avoid, and what they hope can be their child's outcomes. Clear information and conversation about what we wish could be but cannot, what is likely, and what can realistically be hoped for are helpful in this process.

Research indicates that parents want and need to engage in advance care planning (Wharton et al., 1996; Hammes et al., 2005) and that, when possible, most families want their child to be involved as well (Sharman, Meert, and Sarnaik, 2005). Advance care planning is a process that evolves as the child's response to treatment informs the child's likely future. When either cure or life prolongation is a realistic option, these goals are generally pursued. However, when the burdens of treatment begin to outweigh the benefits, from the patient's, family's, and team's perspectives, it is time to reevaluate the goals and processes of care. Clinicians are encouraged to be ever mindful of the patient's and family's cues and leanings in this regard. In the context of a trusting, open, therapeutic relationship, children, families, and/or clinicians can be free to raise concerns and explore the redirection of care. A child, for example, may declare, "I have tried my best, but now I want to stop this medicine," or a parent may initiate a conversation by asking, "Is it time for us to look into hospice and go home?"

CONTINUITY OF CARE AND THE
ENGAGEMENT OF COMMUNITY RESOURCES

In some instances, community-based pediatricians and religious support personnel remain involved in the care and support of children facing life-threatening conditions. Too often, these sources of support are challenged by geographic distance and the realities of new health care provider relationships (Meyer et al., 2002). However, the primary care physician can serve as a familiar and knowledgeable resource in the decision-making process; can provide ongoing care and counseling for the ill child, siblings, and parents; can suggest realistic care options within the community; and can be an effective facilitator of healthy bereavement if he or she remains involved in the care (Heller and Solomon, 2005). Familiar, trusted religious support personnel can serve as spiritual care providers by performing sacraments, rituals, and prayers; offering consultation in medical ethics within the family's chosen tradition; and serving as a link between the patient/family and the faith community and its prayers, social resources (transportation, meals, respite care), and financial assistance (Meert, Thurston, and Briller, 2005; Robinson et al., 2006). Additionally, they can assist with memorial and funeral planning and provide long-term follow-up for spiritual distress and bereavement. Cultivating relationships with community care providers is invaluable in terms of continuity of care and bereavement support. Successful development of these relationships requires mutual respect as well as communication, cooperation, and effort by the family, specialists, and community-based care providers.

If a hospitalized child is discharged to community-based hospice care, the previous involvement of the primary care pediatrician can be an exceptional source of support and confidence, as well as a vital link in maintaining the involvement of the specialist team throughout the final phase of the child's life. If a pediatric palliative care team was involved with the child at the referral center, that team may be able to guide the ongoing palliative care if community hospice resources are not familiar with the care of children. Commitment of all caregivers to the best outcome of the child and family, regardless of care setting, will take a significant effort on the part of all to forge and maintain relationships.

Abandonment is one of the greatest fears of patients and families; it is a major cause of suffering for the dying and the bereaved. Therefore, "turning their care over" to new caregivers as death nears is not acceptable. Patients and their families need to know that they were cared about as individuals, that they were not just seen as "an interesting case" that is no longer interesting when they are not able to be cured. Adolescents, in particular, fear being forgotten. For these reasons, it is important to introduce the palliative care team early, to facilitate their full integration and optimize continuity of care. In addition, the team primarily involved in disease-directed care is encouraged to find creative means to meet the needs of children who have been discharged to outlying facilities or home, including ongoing contact— by webcam, Facebook, e-mail, telephone, in person, or by other means—to demonstrate that they have not forgotten the child and that they remain invested in and committed to the child's well-being.

END-OF-LIFE COMMUNICATION

When it is clear that the child will not survive the illness or injuries, the clinician must communicate this information clearly and directly to parents and, in some instances, to the child as well. The use of euphemisms can lead to misunderstandings and is discouraged. As with the discussion of other unwelcome news, privacy, empathy, and pacing are important elements of the disclosure. Implying that there is doubt or uncertainty can create unnecessary distress; parents need to hear the clear message that their child will die no matter what else is done.

> Hakim has endured many treatments for his illness, and unfortunately we did not succeed in overcoming the disease. No surgery, no medicine, no forthcoming research, nor all the love you clearly have for him will cure his condition. We want to help him and you live as comfortably as possible for the time he has remaining.

Describing not only what cannot happen but also what can realistically be hoped for or accomplished is important in preventing feelings of abandonment. Parents or the patient may ask about how long the child is expected to live. It is helpful to give them as close an estimate as is reasonable, whether minutes to hours, hours to days, days to weeks, or weeks to months. This enables families to plan their remaining time well and to invite family and friends to support them through their most challenging experience (see box 7.1).

Box 7.1 Insights from a Parent regarding Communication
as the End of Life Approaches

As the child's illness progresses, it is important to understand that the family dynamic and structure may have changed as well. With this in mind, it is imperative to alter communications with the family and to remember a few things:

- Our family is probably stretched to its limits financially, emotionally, and physically, limiting our tolerance for ignorance, insensitivity, and callousness.
- We may have gone through divorce and there may now be additional family members in the mix, which only adds to the possible frustration of the situation. Therefore, please respect biological parents for their roles while also being aware of new "family members." If possible, meet with parents at the same time so as to limit the possibility of "he said / she said," which only muddles the family communication process.
- Please consider giving us a few written sentences on our child's latest condition so we can share it directly with other family members. This limits the possibility of misinterpretation or miscommunication. While it may seem time-consuming to a physician, it is far less time-consuming than several phone calls from various family members.
- Please stay in contact with our family even though we may go to hospice. You have become an important member of our extended family, and losing our child and our connection to you only adds to our emotional loss.

EFFECTIVE WAYS TO TEACH AND NURTURE
COMMUNICATION SKILLS AND RELATIONAL ABILITIES

The growing recognition of the central value of communication and relational abilities in health care has fostered a range of training opportunities and programs. Training approaches vary considerably with regard to their purpose, duration and intensity, participants, teaching methods, composition and role of faculty members, and outcome evaluation methods (Meyer et al., 2009). Typical teaching methods include didactic literature review, role-playing, simulation with professional actors, videotape review and feedback, narrative inquiry and reflective exercises, and group debriefing. A review of communication interventions aimed at clinicians and patients (see Rao et al., 2007) concluded that interventions employing a wide variety of teaching methods were associated with improved physician and patient communication behaviors, although further investigation and more nuanced examination of the communicative interchange between patients and clinicians is needed. At present, most programs target physicians as learners and focus on high-stakes conversations (e.g., communicating a serious diagnosis, discontinuation of no-longer-beneficial medical interventions, relapse, traumatic death) that occur in high-intensity clinical settings, such as critical care, oncology, and emergency departments. There is a relative dearth of educational efforts aimed at typical everyday health care conversations (Greenberg et al., 1999; Fryer-Edwards et al., 2006; Back, Arnold, and Tulsky, 2009). Briefer educational programs typically focus on first-time encounters between physicians and patients, whereas longer, more intensive training efforts address communication skills and relational issues across the disease trajectory. In addition, in day-to-day care, there are many opportunities for senior clinicians to instill the value of and to mentor effective communication skills and relational abilities.

Conclusion

Ensuring effective communication and relationship building among child patients, families, and clinicians in the setting of life-threatening illness or injury, whether acute or chronic, is an essential task. Critical elements of such communication and relationships include honesty, openness, respect, empathy, attention to environment, nonverbal communication, cultural concerns, word choice, pacing, emotional responses, and bidirectional comprehension. Silence is a powerful and underused tool for enabling families to reflect on and respond to difficult information, including the emergence and acknowledgment of emotional concerns. Individuals who should be included in the communication "loop" include the ill child, immediate and extended family members chosen by the parents and child, all members of the health care team, and, in some situations, members of the family's home community—particularly the primary pediatrician. Creative mechanisms for such communication may need to be invoked.

References

Ablon, J. 2000. Parents' responses to their child's diagnosis of neurofibromatosis I. *Am J Med Genet* 93:136–42.

American Academy of Pediatrics, Committee on Bioethics (AAP COB). 1995. Informed consent, parental permission, and assent in pediatric practices. *Pediatrics* 95:314–17.

American Academy of Pediatrics, Committee on Pediatric Workforce (AAP COPW). 1999. Culturally effective pediatric care: Education and training issues. *Pediatrics* 103:167–70.

American Academy of Pediatrics, Committee on Psychosocial Aspects of Child and Family Health (AAP COPACFH). 2000. The pediatrician and childhood bereavement. *Pediatrics* 105:445–47.

American Academy of Pediatrics, Medical Home Initiatives for Children with Special

Needs Project Advisory Committee (AAP Med Home). 2002. The medical home. *Pediatrics* 110:184–86.

Back, A., Arnold, R., and Tulsky, J. 2009. Mastering communication with seriously ill patients. New York: Cambridge University Press.

Bailey, D.B., Blasco, P.M., and Simeonsson, R.J. 1992. Needs expressed by mothers and fathers of young children with disabilities. *Am J Ment Retard* 97:1–10.

Beach, M.C., and Inui, T. 2006. Relationship centered care research network. Relationship-centered care: A constructive reframing. *J Gen Intern Med* 21:S3–8.

Bluebond-Langner, M. 1978. *The Private Worlds of Dying Children*. Princeton: Princeton University Press.

Browning, D.M. 2002. To show our humanness: Relational and communicative competence in pediatric palliative care. *Bioethics Forum* 18:23–28.

Browning, D.M., Meyer, E.C., Truog, R.D., et al. 2007. Difficult conversations in health care: Cultivating relational learning to address the hidden curriculum. *Acad Med* 82(9):905–13.

Buckman, R., and Kason, Y. 1992. *How to Break Bad News: A Guide for Health Care Professionals*. Baltimore: Johns Hopkins University Press.

Creagan, E.T. 1994. How to break bad news—and not devastate the patient. *Mayo Clin Proc* 69:1015–17.

Curtis, J.R., and White, D.B. 2008. Practical guidelines for evidence-based ICU family conferences. *Chest* 134(4):835–43.

Dixon-Woods, M., Young, B., and Heney, D. 1999. Partnerships with children. *BMJ* 319:778–80.

Dragone, M.A. 1990. Perspectives of chronically ill adolescents and parents on health care needs. *Pediatr Nurs* 16:45–50, 108.

Dunbar, P.J., Buckley, P., Gavrin, J.R., et al. 1995. Use of patient controlled analgesia for pain control for children receiving bone marrow transplantation. *J Pain Symptom Manage* 10:604–11.

Dussel, V., Kreicbergs, U., Hilden, J.M., et al. 2009. Looking beyond where children die: Determinants and effects of planning a child's location of death. *J Pain Symptom Manage* 37(1):33–43.

Dyche, L., and Swiderski, D. 2005. The effect of physician solicitation approach on the ability to identify patient concerns. *J Gen Intern Med* 20:267–70.

Epstein, R.M., and Peters, E. 2009. Beyond information, exploring patients' preferences. *JAMA* 302:195–97.

Fallowfield, L. 1993. Giving sad and bad news. *Lancet* 341:476–78.

Fallowfield, L., Jenkins, V., Farewell, V., et al. 2003. Enduring impact of communication skills training: Results of a 12-month follow-up. *Br J Cancer* 89:1445–49.

Feudtner, C. 2007. Collaborative communication in pediatric palliative care: A foundation for problem-solving and decision-making. *Pediatr Clin N Am* 54:583–607.

Finlay, I., and Dallimore, D. 1991. Your child is dead. *BMJ* 302:1524–25.

Flores, G., Abreu, M., Schwartz, I., et al. 2000. The importance of language and culture in pediatric care: Case studies from the Latino community. *J Pediatr* 137:842–48.

Fryer-Edwards, K., Arnold, R.M., Baile, W., et al. 2006. Reflective teaching practices: An approach to teaching communication skills in a small-group setting. *Acad Med* 81:638–44.

Garwick, A.W., Patterson, J., Bennett, F.C., et al. 1995. Breaking the news. How families first learn about their child's chronic condition. *Arch Pediatr Adolesc Med* 149:991–97.

Greenberg, L.W., Jewett, L.S., Gluck, R.S., et al. 1984. Giving information for a life-threatening diagnosis. Parents' and oncologists' perceptions. *Am J Dis Child* 138: 649–53.

Greenberg, L.W., Ochsenschlager, D., O'Donnell, R., et al. 1999. Communicating bad news: A pediatric department's evaluation of a simulated intervention. *Pediatrics* 103:1210–17.

Halpern, J. 2007. Empathy and patient-physician conflicts. *J Gen Intern Med* 22: 696–700.

Hammes, B.J., Klevan, J., Kempf, M., and Williams, M.S. 2005. Pediatric advance care planning. *J Palliat Med* 8:766–73.

Heller, K.S., and Solomon, M.Z. 2005. Continuity of care and caring: What matters most to parents of children with life-threatening conditions. *J Pediatr Nurs* 20: 335–46.

Horner, M.M., Rawlins, P., and Giles, K. 1987. How parents of chronically ill children perceive their own needs. *Am J Matern Child Nurs* 12:40–43.

Johnson, J.E. 1972. Effects of structuring patients' expectations on their reactions to threatening events. *Nurs Res* 21:499–504.

Jurkovich, G.J., Pierce, B., Pananen, L., et al. 2000. Giving bad news: The family perspective. *J Trauma* 48:865–73.

Kleiber, C., Davenport, T., and Freyenberger, B. 2006. Open bedside rounds for families with children in the pediatric intensive care units. *Am J Crit Care* 15(5): 492–96.

Krahn, G.L., Hallum, A., and Kime, C. 1993. Are there good ways to give "bad news"? *Pediatrics* 91:578–82.

Krauss-Mars, A.H., and Lachman, P. 1994. Breaking bad news to parents with disabled children—a cross-cultural study. *Child Care Health Dev* 20:101–13.

Kreicbergs, U., Vladimarsdottir, U., Onelov, E., et al. 2004. Talking about death with children who have severe malignant disease. *N Engl J Med* 351:1175–86.

Lantos, J.D. 1996. Should we always tell children the truth? *Perspect Biol Med* 40: 78–92.

Lashley, M., Talley, W., Lands, L.C., et al. 2000. Informed proxy consent: Communication between pediatric surgeons and surrogates about surgery. *Pediatrics* 105: 591–97.

Lask, B. 1992. Talking with children. *Br J Hosp Med* 47:688–90.

Levetown, M., AAP Committee on Bioethics. 2008. Communicating with children and families: From everyday interactions to skill in conveying distressing information. *Pediatrics* 121:e1441–60.

Levinson, W., Roter, D.L., Mullooly, J.P., et al. 1997. Physician-patient communication: The relationship with malpractice claims among primary care physicians and surgeons. *JAMA* 277:553–59.

Lewis, C.C., Pantell, R.H., and Sharp, L. 1991. Increasing patient knowledge, satisfaction and involvement: Randomized trial of a communication intervention. *Pediatrics* 88:351–58.

Lynch, E.C., and Staloch, N.H. 1988. Parental perceptions of physicians' communication in the informing process. *Ment Retard* 26:77–81.

Mack, J.W., Wolfe, J., Cook, E.F., et al. 2007. Hope and prognostic disclosure. *J Clin Oncol* 25(35):5636–42.

Makoul, G. 2006. Communication skills: How simulation training supplements experiential and humanist learning. *Acad Med* 81(3):271–74.

Marchetti, F., Bonati, M., Marfisi, R.M., et al. 1995. Parental and primary care physicians' views on the management of chronic diseases: A study in Italy. *Acta Paediatr* 84:1165–72.

McCabe, M.A. 1996. Involving children and adolescents in medical decision-making: Developmental and clinical considerations. *J Pediatr Psychol* 21:505–16.

McDonagh, R., Elliott, T.B., Engelberg, R.A., et al. 2001. Family satisfaction with family conferences about end of life care in the intensive care unit: Increased proportion of family speech is associated with increased satisfactions. *Crit Care Med* 29(2 Suppl):N26–33.

Meert, K.L., Eggly, S., Pollack, M.M., et al. 2007. Parents' perspectives regarding a physician-parent conference after their child's death in the pediatric intensive care unit. *J Pediatr* 151(1):50–55.e2.

———. 2008. Parents' perspectives on physician-parent communication near the time of a child's death in the pediatric intensive care unit. *Pediatr Crit Care Med* 9(1):2–7.

Meert, K.L., Thurston, C.S., and Briller, S.H. 2005. The spiritual needs of parents at the time of their child's death in the pediatric intensive care unit and during bereavement: A qualitative study. *Pediatr Crit Care Med* 6(4):420–27.

Meert, K.L., Thurston, C.S., and Thomas, R. 2001. Parental coping and bereavement outcome after the death of a child in the pediatric intensive care unit. *Pediatr Crit Care Med* 2(4):324–28.

Meyer, E.C., Burns, J.P., Griffith, J., et al. 2002. Parental perspectives on end-of-life care in the pediatric intensive care unit. *Crit Care Med* 30(1):226–31.

Meyer, E.C., Ritholz, M.D., Burns, J.P., et al. 2006. Improving the quality of end-of-life care in the pediatric intensive care unit: Parents' priorities and recommendations. *Pediatrics* 117(3):649–57.

Meyer, E.C., Sellers, D.E., Browning, D.M., et al. 2009. Difficult conversations: Improving communication skills and relational abilities in health care. *Pediatr Crit Care Med* 10(3):352–59.

Nursey, A.D., Rohde, J.R., and Farmer, R.D.T. 1991. Ways of telling new parents about their child and his or her mental handicap: A comparison of doctors' and parents' views. *J Ment Defic Res* 35:48–57.

Perrin, E.C., Lewkowicz, C., and Young, M.H. 2000. Shared vision: Concordance among fathers, mothers, and pediatricians about unmet needs of children with chronic health conditions. *Pediatrics* 105:277–85.

Quine, L., and Pahl, J. 1987. First diagnosis of severe handicap: A study of parental reactions. *Dev Med Child Neurol* 29:232–42.

Rabow, M.W., Fair, J.M., and Hardie, G.E. 1999. A failing grade for end-of-life content in textbooks: What is to be done? *J Palliat Med* 2:153–55.

Rao, J.K., Anderson, L.A., Inui, T.S., et al. 2007. Communication interventions make a difference in conversations between physicians and patients: A systematic review of the evidence. *Medical Care* 45(4):340–49.

Riggs, D., and Weibley, R.E. 1994. Autopsies and the pediatric intensive care unit. *Pediatr Clin North Am* 41:1383–93.

Robinson, M.R., Thiel, M.M., Backus, M.M., et al. 2006. Matters of spirituality at end of life in the pediatric intensive care unit. *Pediatrics* 118(3):e719–29.

Roter, D.L., Frankel, R.M., Hall, J.A., et al. 2006. The expression of emotion through nonverbal behavior in medical visits: Mechanisms and outcomes. *Gen Intern Med* 21:S28–34.

Rushforth, H. 1999. Practitioner review: Communicating with hospitalised children: Review and application of research pertaining to children's understanding of health and illness. *J Child Psychol Psychiatry* 40:683–91.

Sharman, M., Meert, K.L., and Sarnaik, A.P. 2005. What influences parents' decisions to limit or withdraw life support? *Pediatr Crit Care Med* 6(5):513–18.

Sharp, M.C., Strauss, R.P., and Lorch, S.C. 1992. Communicating medical bad news: Parents' experiences and preferences. *J Pediatr* 121:539–46.

Street, R.L. 1991. Physicians' communication and parents' evaluation of pediatric consultations. *Med Care* 29:1146–52.

Strong, C. 2003. Fetal anomalies: Ethical and legal considerations in screening, detection, and management. *Clin Perinatol* 30:113–26.

Surkan, P.J., Dickman, P.W., Steineck, G., et al. 2006. Home care of a child dying of a malignancy and parental awareness of a child's impending death. *Palliat Med* 20(3):161–69.

Tates, K., and Meeuwesen, L. 2001. Doctor-parent-child communication. A (re)view of the literature. *Soc Sci Med* 52:839–51.

Truog, R.D., Christ, G., Browning, D., et al. 2006. Sudden traumatic death in children: We did everything, but your child did not survive. *JAMA* 295(22):2646–54.

van Dulmen, A.M. 1998. Children's contributions to pediatric outpatient encounters. *Pediatrics* 102:563–68.

Volandes, A.E., Paasche-Orlow, M.K., Barry, M.J., et al. 2009. Video decision support for advance care planning in dementia: Randomized controlled trial. *BMJ* 338:b2159.

Walker, D.K., Epstein, S.G., Taylor, A.B., et al. 1989. Perceived needs of families of children who have chronic health conditions. *Child Health Care* 18:196–201.

Wharton, R.H., Levine, K.R., Buka, S., and Emanuel, L. 1996. Advance care planning for children with special healthcare needs: A survey of parental attitudes. *Pediatrics* 97:682–87.

Young, B., Dixon-Woods, M., Windridge, K.C., et al. 2003. Managing communication with young people who have a potentially life threatening chronic illness: Qualitative study of patients and parents. *BMJ* 326:305–9.

8

Psychosocial Needs of the Child and Family

Stacy F. Orloff, Ed.D., L.C.S.W., A.C.H.P.-S.W.,
Barbara Jones, Ph.D., M.S.W., and Kris Ford

> "The day our child was diagnosed, the world changed. Nothing looked the
> same; even the colors of the sky and grass looked different. Our family was
> shaken in a way we did not know was possible. I didn't think we'd survive."
> —Parent of a child with a life-threatening condition

Families with seriously ill children have begun on an uncharted journey with few road maps; despite our best efforts, families often feel they are traveling alone. Potentially life-altering decisions must be made, often quickly. The impact of a child's chronic or sudden life-threatening condition on the nuclear family, extended family, and community is great. One role of the health care team is to provide effective psychosocial support to the family as they are able to accept it.

All health care providers will have greater capacity to be therapeutic with families in crisis if they are aware of common psychosocial themes relevant to the function of family systems in such situations. Further, knowledge of some psychosocial aspects of child development germane to chronic or catastrophic illness may be of benefit to avoid unintended conflicts and harm.

This chapter describes the most common and important psychosocial factors that members of the palliative care team need to be aware of and potentially address with patients and families. Helpful interventions and additional resources are also provided. The most significant psychosocial factors to consider in caring for children living with life-threatening conditions and their families include the following:

- Understanding and assessing the role of the immediate and extended family and greater community during the course of the child's illness, death, and in bereavement

- The evolving nature of psychosocial needs during the diagnostic, disease-directed, palliative, and end-of-life phases of care
- The impact of the experience of illness on the siblings and marital relationship
- Strains on communication styles and strategies within the family and between the family and others
- Decision-making strategies

What is meant by "family"? In today's society, there are many different kinds of families. A common definition accepted by many family therapists is "a group of individuals interrelated so that a change in any one member affects other individuals and the group as a whole: this then affects the first individual in a circular chain of influence" (Walsh, 1982, p. 9). From this definition, it follows that care teams may need to attend to a broader circle of people than just the child's parents/guardians and siblings. Ideal palliative care offers services to the child's larger family, including grandparents, other caregivers (including paid caregivers), and any other people identified by the child or child's parents/guardians as family members. Comprehensive palliative care intake assessments include questions regarding the importance of other community resources (such as schools and service groups like Boy/Girl Scouts) as part of the family's larger system. The child's care plan should also include information about out-of-town family members, so that palliative care team members can engage them as both resources for and beneficiaries of the treatment process.

Equifinality is a family therapy term that describes the fact that two families experiencing the same stressor will likely have different outcomes. Palliative care professionals understand that each family is unique and that a thorough psychosocial assessment is a precursor to developing an individualized plan of care that has the greatest potential for good outcomes. It would be a mistake to assume that each family will experience the same stressors in an identical fashion or that illness-associated problems are the only psychosocial concerns affecting the plan of care. Psychosocial assessments should be ongoing and open ended and can be elicited simply by asking families to share their concerns with the care team at each encounter.

Mark, a 16-year-old, was diagnosed with Duchenne muscular dystrophy when he was 5 years old. His mother informed him of his diagnosis when he was 10, with the assistance of the pediatric palliative care program of the local hospice. The palliative care counselor continued to work with Mark and his family thereafter. When Mark was in seventh grade, he required the use of a wheelchair. He underwent heel cord lengthening surgery that same year in an attempt to preserve his ability to stand and walk a bit longer. By eighth grade, Mark was unable to bear weight at all. Two years later, he underwent posterior spinal fusion, but was not consulted in the decision-making process. Mark was confined to bed postoperatively and was admitted to the home health care program of the same local hospice. Thereafter, his functional decline was unrelenting; he developed difficulty swallowing and lost more than 13 percent of his pre-operative weight, leading to feeding tube placement and feedings. One month later, he developed an upper respiratory illness, choked on thick mucus, and landed in the emergency room. Breathing treatments were begun and a suction machine was ordered for the home.

Mark's younger and older sisters live in the home; both have had many school problems. Mark is homebound; just before he became incapable of attending school, he had an episode in which he was left unattended in a restroom, was incontinent, and wet himself.

Mark's parents frequently struggle to pay bills. Because of federal requirements for income eligibility, Medicaid coverage is withheld for a few months every year, creating severe economic hardship for the family. Mark's mother, a petite woman who has depression and back and neck problems, has limited ability to lift Mark. The palliative care counselor has provided family and individual support to each family member. Mark's younger sister is a regular participant in the monthly sibling support group; his older sister has thus far refused to participate in the group.

The Stress of a New Diagnosis

The new diagnosis of a child's life-threatening condition is devastating for any family. As the child and family move through the different phases of care—diagnosis, disease-directed and supportive treatment, cure, survivorship, or death and subsequent bereavement—they require substantial support from an array of professionals. The sooner these resources are marshaled, the greater the likelihood that the family can be helped to strengthen coping abilities. The American Academy of Pediatrics (AAP), International Work Group on Death, Dying and Bereavement, Children's Project on Palliative and Hospice Services (ChiPPS), and other expert bodies all advocate an integrated model of palliative care for children living with life-threatening conditions, *beginning at the time of diagnosis* and continuing throughout the course of the illness, regardless of outcome (AAP COB, 1995, 1997; Davies, 1998; AAP COB/COHC, 2000).

The needs of the family during the diagnostic phase can differ to some extent, based on a number of sociocultural and medical factors. Many times, the diagnosis is made after only a brief period of illness and abbreviated clinical investigations. When parents have little warning that their baby or child has a problem before diagnosis, they most commonly express feelings of shock and disbelief, describing the experience as similar to being hit by a lightning bolt. Examples of this situation include an ultrasound revealing a brain malformation during a seemingly normal pregnancy, or an unexpected severe congenital heart condition being discovered at birth. A child may be playing T-ball one day and then be diagnosed with leukemia or muscular dystrophy the next. A physician, a stranger to the family only moments before, may have to inform them about the unwelcome diagnosis, prognosis, and treatment options.

An uncertain diagnosis and prognosis can be particularly difficult for both the family and health care provider. When the family is presented with a list of potential diagnoses, they may focus on one or two familiar diseases or may search the Internet to obtain as much information as they can. They may even seek out world experts and centers of excellence for their child's presumed condition before a firm diagnosis is established. This sense of uncertainty adds to the family's roller coaster of emotions, often creating tension in their relationship with health care providers. For some, unrealistic expectations can lead to disappointment and doubt regarding their caregivers' competence. Offering reassurance and support while a firm diagnosis is sought can be beneficial to such stressed families.

Even when the diagnosis is certain, the entire family experiences many stressors throughout a child's illness. Parents/guardians are confronted with their own grief as they grapple with the reality of the child's condition and the impact on their hopes, plans, and dreams for the future. Such anticipatory grief begins at the time of diagnosis. Parents can be prepared for the grief and loss associated with their situation if they are educated about the following (NHPCO, 2000):

- The nature of day-to-day losses over the course of the illness
- How to stay connected to their ill child as well as their healthy children
- The unique nature of grief for the mother and the father (as well as other family members)

- How to negotiate needed changes in the family routine and family communication, while maintaining healthy marital and parent-child relationships
- How to ensure effective communication between and among the family and health care providers
- How to identify and connect with resources in the community for support (financial, emotional, spiritual)
- How to engage in funeral preplanning as appropriate and as they may wish to do
- How to recognize the manifestations of grief in the other children in the family, both during the illness and after the death

Helpful interventions during this diagnostic phase include creating opportunities for all members of the family to ask questions in a safe and nurturing environment. It is not unusual for adults to attempt to withhold information, with the intention of protecting the ill child, regardless of age. Even families who have exhibited open styles of communication in other realms often become much more closed in the face of "bad news." The ill child and healthy siblings often know about the illness and want to ask questions and express fears and concerns, but try to protect the adults around them and thus avoid the topic. Social workers and child-life specialists are trained in techniques to assist children to express their concerns and communicate with loved ones and health care providers.

Supporting Families during Disease-Directed Treatment

Once a diagnosis is confirmed and disease-directed treatment begins, most families move past the shock and disbelief phase, throwing their emotion and energy into the treatment phase. They attempt to reestablish some measure of equilibrium and normalcy in their lives. Armed with information about the disorder and its treatment, they cling to hopes for a cure (realistic or not) and endeavor to put their lives back in order. Hopes and dreams are often vital to their continued daily functions, such as eating and sleeping. Professional caregivers can help families evolve to have realistic hopes about the best possible and most likely outcomes, which may include cure, prolonged life, or an improved quality of life. Hope may also focus on maximizing the time remaining by concentrating on milestones, such as having a good family holiday, finishing seventh grade, or whatever goals help the child and family feel complete. Psychosocial team members may assist the family in redefining hope and in finding meaning and purpose in living and dying. Preserving the language of hope is a vital expression of the spiritual and psychosocial experience of children and families (Hinds, 1984; Groopman, 2004; Feudtner, 2005; Feudtner et al., 2007; Mack et al., 2007).

Psychosocial staff offer support by helping families recognize their sources of strength, build on these supports and resources, and strengthen and enhance enduring relationships. Specifically, providing psychosocial support in decision making, effective communication, and coordinated care with third-party payers has been shown to increase family satisfaction and quality of life (Hays et al., 2006).

Understanding the family and their strengths and challenges is critical. Questions that may elicit family strengths include the following:

- What are your sources of support?
- Who can provide concrete support to you (e.g., taking care of pets, child care arrangements, transportation, activities of daily living)?
- How has your family coped with challenges in the past?
- Who or what community has helped you?
- How do you help each other get through tough times?
- What are the ways that you support each other? (Strengths can be further elicited by asking specifics about emotional support, concrete tasks, organizational skills, capacity for self-reflection, humor, and expressions of love.)

Easing the Transition to Exclusively Palliative Goals of Care

For many conditions, a point is reached when disease-directed treatment becomes unduly burdensome given that either cure or life extension is no longer a possibility. Regrettably, some families are told at this point, "There is nothing else we can do for your child." This is at best a poor choice of words and, at worst, simply not true. There is *always* something that can be done for a child and family, including being there for the family and expressing care. Often there is much more than this that can be done to ease the child's suffering and symptoms and to help the family cope with this devastating experience.

Ideally, palliative care services have been integrated into the child's care from the point of diagnosis, but, in reality, this is rarely the case. Thus, the concept of palliative care is often only introduced when it is clear that the child will die in the near future. Most families and professional caregivers find this to be a difficult discussion. For families, this transition may include giving up the team of health care providers they have come to trust and feel comfortable with for a new set of caregivers, such as the hospice team. The child's physician may continue to direct care if he or she is comfortable in the provision of palliative care, but the family almost always faces losing contact with the child's other caregivers, including clinic, hospital, and home health nurses; social workers; child-life specialists; and various therapists who are not likely to be involved in the child's care from this point on. Because this is such a socially difficult transition, it is often delayed until the child is hours to days from dying. Such delays in the initiation of palliative care can result in care that is crisis oriented, exacerbating the family's sense of vulnerability, isolation, and helplessness. Establishing a framework for proactive decision making is made much more challenging with late palliative care referrals.

The case study exemplifies the benefit to the family when an early referral to palliative care is made. In Mark's case, the hospice and palliative home care program was initiated early in the diagnostic phase, making it much easier for the family to accept additional help as Mark's condition began to deteriorate. Social workers and other mental health counselors are trained to assist families in decision making. Through a series of guided conversations, often accompanied by the use of expressive arts, psychosocial staff can assist the family in redefining their goals of care. Using expressive arts allows even young children to give "voice" to their feelings, worries, and concerns, which can then be factored into the decision-making process as appropriate. Art, music, and movement are often used as clinical interventions as well. See the reference section at the end of this chapter for some suggested resources.

Many children's hospitals have begun inpatient palliative care programs so that children and their families have access to additional services while hospitalized. Children who receive palliative care while hospitalized may then be referred to community-based hospice programs as their symptoms increase and their condition deteriorates, particularly if the family prefers to return home to receive care for the child's final phase of life. Continued work is required to develop effective and seamless partnerships between inpatient palliative care services and outpatient or home-based options, to prevent unnecessary jarring and disruptive transitions for the child and family.

In addition to having reservations about giving up their established team of caregivers, parents also resist the transition to hospice care because they equate "hospice" with "giving up." Even if the parents recognize that the chances of cure are slim, they may still need to hang on to the slight hope for full recovery or at least a prolonged life. A Children's Hospice International survey indicated that one of the leading obstacles to providing hospice services to children is the association of the hospice concept with death rather than with life enhancement (Children's Hospice International, 1998). In the last several years, many more children's hospitals have deepened their collaborative relationships with local, community-based hospice and palliative care programs. Through such partnerships, often introduced much earlier in the treatment process, families have been able to grow to know and trust the community-based care team, care planning is conducted jointly and more proactively, and the hospice or palliative care social worker might additionally participate, alongside the hospital staff, in conversations with the family about transitions in care goals and locations.

Although it is beyond the scope of this chapter to discuss new and innovative concurrent models of palliative care, it is helpful to know that some states have successfully developed such programs. The psychosocial assistance provided to the entire family unit does much to ameliorate the challenges in transitioning care to other providers (Knapp et al., 2008; Lowe et al., 2009). For additional information, see http://nhpco.org/i4a/pages/index .cfm?pageid=3409.

Addressing the Child's Psychosocial Needs

Children frequently express the need to have some control over their illness and treatment. They have both the desire and the right to participate in their own treatment decisions in developmentally appropriate ways. Determining how much to tell children and involving them in their care decisions can be difficult for the family and health care team. Most professionals feel that it is important to tell children the "truth" and to help them participate to the best of their abilities. But in real-world practice, decisions about what is the right amount of knowledge and involvement are influenced by many factors, including the child's personality, preferences, and developmental stage; the family's cultural and spiritual beliefs and preferences, as well as previous experiences with the health care system; the support system available to both the child and family; and the health care team's comfort with disclosure and child involvement.

Palliative care team members can offer considerable guidance about communicating with children and understanding their developmental needs. For example, team members can let parents and the other health care providers know that children need honest, brief, factual information that is geared to their cognitive and emotional level. Concrete examples and explanations are helpful. Providing small bits of information and then checking in with the child allow the assimilation of new knowledge and provide the child the opportunity to ask questions. Palliative care team members can routinely check in with patients by asking them to explain what is happening. This will allow the team members to clarify misconceptions, provide reassurance, and continue to offer compassionate support.

Seriously ill children are most likely to talk with professionals and family members who display an open and comfortable communication style. Health care providers don't need to have answers to all of the child's questions; supporting the child's needs can consist of engaging him or her in conversation and listening as the questions, fears, and feelings are explored. When children understand their illness, they frequently want to participate in the planning and delivery of their health care. The primary care team can work with the ill child and family to provide age-appropriate ways for the child to have a voice in the care planning process. For example, children can be asked to talk about, draw, or demonstrate what they would like in their treatment plan. Children can usually easily be engaged to make lists and draw pictures of what they love to do. This will help the team know what is most important to the child's quality of life.

Children may protect their caregivers from their feelings; they therefore often need a "safe adult" with whom they can discuss concerns and ask questions (Jones and Weisenfluh, 2003). This person can be a health care professional, trusted family member, or friend. Children may have questions when their health care providers are not present. Not all children will feel comfortable asking questions of parents or other family members; providing options can help allay anxiety. One way to do this is to say, "Sometimes a kid just needs someone safe to talk to. If you ever have something you want to ask or say, but you feel uncomfortable talking to your family or other caregivers, I am willing to listen and help you find safe ways to be heard."

Children are more likely to experience anxiety about their treatment and illness when they feel unsure about what is happening. Children who are ill become adept at sensing changes in affect in their family and care providers and may worry about what is happening to them. Very young children may also be concerned that they are responsible for the feelings of those around them or for the illness itself (Jones and Weisenfluh, 2003). Open communication and compassion are key elements to help the child. Health care providers can frequently assess the child's level of understanding of the treatment process with questions for both the child and family. Many children living with life-threatening conditions understand much more about their illness and health care in general than their peers and understand changes in their health well before adults tell them. It is important to evaluate their specific level of understanding about diagnoses, tests, procedures, and treatments. Medical jargon and whispered or veiled communication may cause the ill child to become anxious. Health care providers can help children feel empowered to ask questions and obtain developmentally appropriate answers using the following strategies:

- Provide ample time and a safe environment.
- Ask children directly what they understand and whether they have any questions, assuring them that they have permission to ask anything.
- Help the child design a "question box" into which any question may be placed. Make it fun by providing shaped question cards. When health care providers are present, the child can direct them to the question box.
- Play a role-reversal game in which the child is the doctor and an adult is the child. The "doctor" explains to the "child" new developments in his or her illness and treatment options. In this way, adults can assess the child's level of understanding.

Children can be offered choices about where to receive treatment and who will be with them, as well as larger decisions such as when to stop no-longer-beneficial treatment. Older children are most likely to have the cognitive and affective ability to make decisions about further disease-directed versus exclusively palliative treatment approaches. In the hospital, child-life specialists have a unique opportunity to assist the child in this capacity. In home/community-based programs, hospice social workers and counselors can do the same. Questions addressed to the parents that can guide the clinician include the following:

- What is the best time of day to ask the child what he or she wants?
- Is the child providing clues regarding his/her interest in or knowledge about prognosis?
- How does the family want to incorporate the needs and desires of the child in the decision-making process?
- How will the family and palliative care team determine the child's understanding of and willingness to participate in the treatment plan (assent)?

It is also important for the treatment team to decide how to address differences between the child's and family's desires regarding information disclosure, if they arise. Knowledge of the better outcomes associated with open disclosure for both the child and family and the ability to impart this information respectfully to team members and the family, while addressing their doubts, can be an invaluable service to all (Beale, Baile, and Aaron, 2005; Domek, 2010).

It is important to realize, however, that children often understand that their health is failing before the adults and caregivers have acknowledged the child's prognosis. Moreover, children who have faced a recurrent or chronic illness, in particular, learn to read the faces and emotions of their parents and caregivers. Children who do not talk with caregivers about their illness are left to wonder, interpret, and imagine what is happening to them and therefore are at increased risk for anxiety and fear. The child's need for a sense of control can be eased as he or she is given the opportunity to share in the treatment discussion and illness trajectory (Jones and Weisenfluh, 2003; Sourkes et al., 2005).

The palliative care team can offer a number of effective interventions to enhance the child's ability to ask questions. One is to provide children with tape recorders or notepads to record their questions. The tapes or notes can be brought to the child's next appointment so the health care provider and child can listen to the tape or read the questions together. Answers can be recorded on the same tape or written down so that the child and family can review the answers as necessary. Therapeutic games that allow the child to express feelings while playing can be helpful. Clinicians can use puppetry, imaginative play, and expressive arts to draw out the child's feelings (Malchiodi, 2005, 2007; Darley et al., 2007).

Expressive arts interventions are useful in helping children and adults express feelings. Art activities provide an opportunity to take an intangible or inchoate feeling and make it more formed, accessible, and defined. Art also provides a safe outlet for negative thoughts and feelings and is frequently cathartic. Clinical art interventions include the following:

- Create a feeling mandala.
- Design a CD jacket (could also ask an older child to create song titles that reflect a particular feeling).
- Draw an anger container, collage, or mask with inside/outside feelings.
- Trace the child's hands and prompt the family member to write something on each finger (social worker will determine what prompt to use based on the therapeutic intention).
- Using a large art tablet, invite the child to draw a large tree using up most of the space on the paper. This is a "worry tree" that can be used to express concerns and worries by writing the worry on a leaf-shaped sticky note and then placing it on the tree. Talk about the worries that can be controlled and those that cannot.

- Using recycled materials of all kinds, invite the child to construct a "pain buster" (or leukemia buster, etc.) machine. Invite the child to explain exactly how this machine will work to eliminate or reduce the "pain."

Despite its advantages, transparent communication is not the norm. Physicians in particular report experiencing internal and external tensions about how much information to give to families when communicating about the potential death of a child (Parker-Raley, Jones, and Maxson, 2008). Open communication, however, has the potential to help both the child and the family. In a recent Swedish study, parents reported no regrets about talking to their children about their impending deaths. Indeed, parents who did not speak openly with their child expressed regret (Kreicbergs et al., 2004). Bereaved parents report wanting health care providers to give them honest and timely information so that they may best assist their child in understanding what is happening (Meyer et al., 2002). Thus, it is incumbent on the palliative care team to empower health care providers, children, and families to engage in open dialogue whenever possible.

When children are dying, teams can help families build legacies and make memories. Working together, the family and team can develop an appropriate plan for how to inform the child about changes in treatment, illness, and prognosis. This communication may include informing the child of his or her own impending death, when culturally and age appropriate. In fact, older children may wish to make plans for the distribution of their belongings after they are gone and may have specific ideas for the conduct and content of their funeral.

Children who are ill may feel isolated from peers and siblings as lengthy or frequent hospital stays may keep them far from home, out of school, and prevent them from participating in their usual social activities. Care providers can help by identifying ways to enable ongoing interactions with the child's peer group. Health care teams can engage the school community and family in creating opportunities for communication between the child and his or her healthy peers. Child-life specialists and social workers can work with the child's classmates and encourage them to visit as appropriate and able. Internet communication can be encouraged if the distance is too great to travel or there are other reasons why a face-to-face visit is not appropriate. Access to the Internet allows Facebook, iChat, Skype, and other forms of video and Internet communication.

Increased socialization with other children who are ill may also help the ill child decrease his/her isolation and talk about issues of concern. Such peers are often better able to instill a sense of hope, as they may have actually experienced similar situations. Self-esteem and self-image can be enhanced through these interactions. Support through informal and activity-based group meetings can be important. Hospitalized children might want to access the Starlight Foundation, through which they can communicate with other ill children (www.starlight.org).

Many national organizations and local groups offer camp retreats for children facing illness. In the case study, Mark's condition deteriorated to the point where he was not able to attend school. Understanding that Mark still desired to socialize with peers, the hospice team arranged for hospice teen volunteers to visit with him at home.

Easing the Parents' Experience

In recent years, more has been written about the differences in the way men and women, fathers and mothers grieve. Some would say there are clear differences dictated by gender. Others explain the differences in terms of the impact of personality, culture, and gender on the grieving patterns of men and women. The reason for the difference may be less important than is the lesson that it is not helpful to assume how a particular person will respond to a given loss; it is particularly nonbeneficial to judge the way in which an individual chooses to move through his or her personal experience of loss. It is often the case that mother and father have very different experiences before and associated with their child's illness that may inform their way of expressing the grief. Chapter 11 will provide a greater discussion about parental grief, particularly some of the unique and less well-known needs of the father.

Mothers and fathers frequently speak of feeling guilty, as they are unable to significantly affect the trajectory of the illness that is bringing turmoil to their entire family. Most often, there is nothing that could have been done to prevent the onset of the illness; however, because it is the responsibility of parents to protect their children from harm, guilt is sometimes the strongest feeling expressed.

As treatment unfolds, feelings of parental guilt may be magnified as the child is subjected to physically and psychosocially painful procedures and experiences and may even be left with long-term pain and disability. Parents of children born with metabolic or genetic disorders often express guilt for having transmitted the disease. It is especially common for one of the parents to express a great deal of anger stemming from feelings of guilt and helplessness.

Both parents must also carry the burden of trying to attend to needs of the other children in the family while focusing time and energy on the ill or dying child. The impossibility of being fully present to the needs of everyone compounds parental guilt and helplessness. Financial stressors are common as well. Taking time off from work to care for the ill or dying child, to communicate with the medical care team, to investigate treatments, or to obtain treatments in a distant location results in loss of pay and sometimes the loss of a job and associated insurance. Further, there are numerous out-of-pocket expenses that compound the financial strains, including expensive hospital food and parking, out-of-pocket prescription and medical supply costs, and travel and housing when receiving care away from home. The palliative or hospice care team can provide a tremendous service by helping families identify and access resources to reduce these burdens, or by intervening with an employer to facilitate flextime options or other solutions to retaining employment where possible.

There are various reasons why parents might be motivated to work through strain that may develop in the marital relationship. Most parents don't want to further add to their healthy children's burgeoning stress. Many parents also find that discussing the stress of their situation with each other is helpful, as they often find ways to "lighten each other's load." One parent may find a particular issue or task burdensome while the other may feel it is not as difficult to do and be willing to take on the task or problem. Tolerance increases as feelings are shared aloud. Too often, however, the last item on the list of parental priorities is attending to the marriage or committed relationship itself. If the relationship cannot support the differing expressions of grief, loss, and general stress, the marriage will become severely strained. When one person places a judgment on the way the other is grieving, this strain will be magnified greatly. Isolation and withdrawal responses create environments where emotional and sexual intimacy is not perceived as safe, causing further strain on the marriage. Couples are wise to seek out support groups where their common struggles can be shared. Hospitals, hospices, and faith-based communities offer such support groups for parents who have a child who is seriously ill or dying. Other nonprofit organizations dedicated to grief, loss, and trauma often exist within the community as well and offer support groups; however, finding the time and energy to attend a group in the midst of all that is happening may be a major barrier. See the reference section of this chapter for a list of online support groups and resources.

It is common for couples to hear that when a child dies there is a high chance that the marriage will fail. There is no definitive research on this. It is true that marriages that are troubled before the illness and death of a child will be more likely to dissolve than a marriage that is strong and healthy (Shudy et al., 2006). The loss of a child amplifies all that is weak and troubled in a marriage. However, many couples work through this difficult time, using the crisis as an opportunity to grow and work on the issues in the marriage (Klass, 1986; Schwab, 1992; Najiman et al., 1993; Shudy et al., 2006). Hospice and palliative care team members can assist the parents/ guardians in learning how to focus on their marital relationship rather than solely on their role as parents. There are many community resources available to help couples work on this. For mothers and fathers who are grieving amid caring for a very ill or dying child together with surviving family members, the best suggestion may be for each to focus on his or her own grief and healing process. In other words, if parents focus on their own grief process and needs, while allowing each other to grieve individually, the likelihood of a good outcome is increased.

Attention to one's own grief journey models a healthy way of responding for other family survivors, too. Parents might want to consider journaling or blogging during this time. Involvement in service to others is also meaningful and therapeutic for many grieving parents, although it is wise to wait until the intense hurt has subsided.

Addressing Siblings' Psychosocial Needs

Recognizing the often parallel experience of the sibling is the first crucial step toward providing needed support and care throughout the trajectory of diagnosis, treatment, survivorship, or death and bereavement. Siblings must share the time, attention, and affection of their parents. During the diagnosis and treatment process, parental attention will necessarily focus predominantly on the ill child, resulting in the healthy sibling(s) often feeling left out. Children's hospitals may be far from home for families who live in rural areas, necessitating leaving healthy children at home with caregivers while the ill child is hospitalized. Hospital visitation protocols vary around the country, making it difficult for families to be together when the ill child requires hospitalization.

Psychosocial concerns are similar for all children. How these concerns will be acted out behaviorally and psychologically will vary according to the age and personality of the sibling and accepted behavior within the family. Although magical thinking is often associated with younger children, the palliative care counselor should explore these concerns with all siblings. Magical thinking can result if the child is not given age-appropriate information regarding the illness, symptoms, and possible causes of the disease. It is not unusual for a sibling to feel guilty or responsible for the illness. Siblings frequently argue with each other, and one child may have said at some time in the past something such as, "I hate you and wish you were dead." School-age children may worry about "catching" the illness. In the case study, Mark's younger sister, Jane, had a difficult time as Mark's condition deteriorated. She benefited from attending the monthly sibling support sponsored by the local hospice care provider. At this group, Jane was able to meet other children who have ill siblings. She stated that it was the first time she felt that someone, other than her counselor, understood what she was going through, particularly in regard to worrying that she might "catch" the condition her brother had. Careful assessment and accurate information will help decrease many sibling concerns.

Siblings may reasonably feel anger toward the ill child and parents. Healthy siblings frequently feel as though the ill child is receiving an overabundance of attention—attention that could be given to them. Siblings frequently express anger regarding the additional losses that they face as a result of the illness. Such losses include no longer being able to participate in many outside activities or not having family present to watch and support them in their events and games. Even if parents are physically present, they may seem emotionally distant. Well children don't often understand why their parents are acting different and may erroneously interpret the parents' emotional distance as a reaction to something they did. Many palliative care programs provide specially trained volunteers to serve as mentors and companions to siblings. Although the volunteers cannot take the place of the child's parents, they can be a consistent adult presence in the child's life.

Some children also describe feeling ashamed or embarrassed. Children may feel uncomfortable being out in public with a neurologically impaired sibling who looks and acts different from others. Often these children don't know anyone else who has a sibling with a similar condition. Introducing children who have siblings with similar diagnoses to each other helps with these feelings. Sibling support groups also provide opportunities for children to talk about their siblings without feeling ashamed or embarrassed.

The uniqueness and significance of the sibling relationship portends the profound effect that a child's death can have on brothers and sisters. "The physical, emotional, and spiritual care given to the dying child becomes part of the immediate and enduring effect on the bereaved survivors" (Hinds et al., 2005, p. S70).

Children who have complex chronic conditions die a different kind of death, resulting in a different kind of suffering for siblings. Communicating with the sibling (at a developmentally appropriate level) about the efforts to diminish symptoms and related suffering is critical. Allowing siblings opportunities to talk about and express their "suffering" is also critical. Validating the difficulty of witnessing the suffering of a loved one can help to build a trusting relationship between members of the health care team and the sibling who may feel forgotten or left out. Inviting the sibling to express him- or herself through drawings, music, and other projects can assist the child to regain a sense of being important, in control, or powerful.

The patient and sibling may write a story or book together to help other children going through this difficult experience. The sibling might create a book of comforting drawings containing images the sibling finds to be calming and healing. When face-to-face visits are prohibited or severely limited, the use of technology for e-mail, conference calls, and video conferencing will ease the sense of isolation and help keep the lines of communication open as well. Many people are aware of Skype, a free Internet-based means of video chatting. Other computers have built-in cameras and come with software enabling video chatting. Setting a regular time for the family to visit or "have a meal together" via technological assists can bring a fragment of the old family routine back into the picture.

Communication with the siblings should be thoughtful and tailored to the child's needs. In this context communication consists of the interactions among family members, medical personnel, involved friends, and the family's social networks. Ongoing, truthful, and developmentally sensitive conversation about all the various aspects of the dying child's medical condition, treatment, and prognosis ideally will include parents and siblings. Conversations tailored specifically for younger children should take place as soon as possible after the rest of the family has received information. The presence of the parents during these conversations is important, as it signals to the sibling that the information is trustworthy and that he or she is valued and truly included. Structured time for the siblings to be given the opportunity to ask questions of a physician, nurse, social worker, or child-life specialist without parents present is extraordinarily valuable as well. Often siblings will withhold questions they deem to be "sensitive" if the parents are in the room. Communication with siblings related to their grief as the process of dying unfolds is also important. The progressive nature of the illness or the unpredictability of the dying process will likely trigger a myriad of feelings and thoughts. Having someone with whom the sibling can "brief and debrief" before and after visits will assist him or her in managing the "long haul" of the process; see table 8.1 (Taub, 2003).

Giving explicit permission for the sibling to opt out of visits and partici-

Table 8.1 Briefing and debriefing siblings of ill children

Briefing the sibling before a visit might include such questions as:

- What about this visit are you looking forward to the most?
- What are you expecting (if anything) may be different since your last visit?
- What about you and your life activities do you want to share with your sibling?
- Let's talk about anything you are worried about or dreading.

A debriefing chat with the sibling might be helpful after the visit as well. Questions might include:

- How was this visit for you today?
- What did you notice (if anything) about your sibling that may have been a little different?
- Was there anything you were thinking or worrying about but did not know whether to talk it or not?
- What do you want to remember about this visit?

pate in his or her normal day-to-day routines is also important, as long as the options offered can be supported by parents or other responsible adults. Parents and other adults should never assume knowledge of the preferences of the sibling in this process. Merely having a choice is an experience of empowerment much needed by the sibling of a dying child. Another helpful suggestion is to offer the sibling the opportunity to participate in a support group with other children who are living in similar circumstances or seek out appropriate online groups or chat rooms for siblings of terminally ill children.

The inclusion of siblings in the decision-making process can be a difficult choice to negotiate. It is only in the most recent years that the needs and desires of the seriously ill or dying child have been taken into account in decision making, let alone the needs of siblings. However, inclusion of siblings in discussions of various treatment options can be of value in some circumstances. While the sibling may not have "voting power," he or she may offer input regarding thoughts and feelings about a particular path of treatment. In addition, in some circumstances, the ill child may have confided in the healthy sibling; imparting this knowledge may demonstrate the importance of the sibling in the decision-making process and better guide the family and health care providers. After all, in most cases the sibling will be affected both directly and indirectly as the family maneuvers through the treatment process. Knowing this and having an "up-front" investment may increase sibling cooperation and decrease the sense of being out of the communication loop. Further, it will be helpful to work with the siblings to create a plan for the family during the treatment phase. Specifically, the palliative care team can help the family work together to develop a "family treatment team" comprised of friends, other family members, and school and faith community contacts.

Prognostic ambiguities and the participation of the whole family in considerations about research present significant additional challenges. Perhaps the most obvious intervention, communication, is also the most difficult, as emotions and fatigue may peak at this point of the illness experience. However, repeated explicit acknowledgment of the ambiguous nature of the course of the illness and treatment is crucial. Children and even, at times, adults may have the mistaken belief that doctors have all the answers and can always "fix" the situation. The obvious result of such a distorted belief is unrealistic expectations and a greater "fall" when these expectations cannot be met. Helping children to talk about the experience of having questions that have no answers is often really helpful. Letting children know that adults must also tolerate unanswerable questions may be a comfort to the sibling. Use of the metaphor of a "journey" can be a concrete way of visualizing and talking about the time and process involved as the seriously ill or dying child is diagnosed and engaged in various treatments. Consider the following options:

- Invite siblings to draw a picture (can give them many different prompts). While drawing, ask them about this journey. Often the distraction is helpful and encourages the child to talk. Also drawing provides a concrete way to make an abstract concept such as illness more "real."
- If possible and appropriate, the dying child and his or her sibling might share their perspectives with one another.
- Offer the sibling an opportunity to research various treatment paths (as is developmentally appropriate). This task will empower the sibling and bring him/her into the family treatment team experience.
- Ask the sibling to become the "recorder" at a family consult meeting, if appropriate for age.

Ensuring that there are empathic and involved adults available to listen to the siblings debrief afterward is critical to the success of these techniques.

Of course, it would be tragic to ignore the needs of the sibling after the death. The multilayered losses that affect a sibling who has lived through a lifetime or even "just" a few weeks of intense hospital stays must be recognized. As is true for the parents, the sudden loss of contact and relationship with the medical personnel who have been key players in the sibling's life can be devastating. Providing several opportunities for members of the family to meet and interact with the doctor, child-life specialist, primary nursing staff, and social workers can be an important part of the healing process for the grieving family. Logistically, this is difficult to accomplish and is therefore often ignored. However, the impact on health care providers, siblings, and parents of continued contact with and evidence of caring for the bereaved family can be tremendous.

Families

Families who are caring for a seriously ill or dying child often describe their family as a building with a shaky foundation. Some crumble under the strain of caring for a sick child, others plod on, barely surviving, while still other families not only remain standing but also find inner resources of strength, unity, and resolve that they didn't know existed. Families in the midst of the 24-hour-per-day turmoil of caring for a child with a life-threatening condition need some means of stepping away from these pressures, lest they overwhelm their own resources (Diehl, Moffitt, and Wade, 1991). Chauffeuring one of the healthy siblings to a soccer practice, walking the dog, doing the dishes, or going on a family vacation can be challenging—if not impossible—for a family with a seriously ill child. Parents' days can be filled with trips to various subspecialists' offices, hospital stays, ordering supplies and equipment, coordinating with home nursing agencies, and dealing with insurance or Medicaid case managers. A division of labor frequently occurs in two-parent families, with one parent, usually the mother, serving as the ill child's primary caregiver. This parent often stays home with the ill child while the other parent attends to the family's business. This makes it difficult for a family to be a family. Parents must often function, by default or of their own choosing, as their child's nurse, home health aide, social worker, mental health counselor, spiritual counselor, case manager, and health care system advocate.

Often, families urgently need respite assistance. Respite care is designed to give families a break from these intense caregiving obligations. Respite care is defined as the provision of care for the ill child by alternate care providers, enabling parents to take time off from the exhausting care these children require. Some families are able to marshal their own resources, coordinating a cadre of caregivers including their extended family and friends, to provide respite care. In fact, as much as 90 percent of respite care may be provided informally by families (Shantz, 1995). This usage pattern may be borne of necessity rather than choice, as the availability of respite services varies considerably from community to community. Children with life-threatening conditions often have complex care needs, requiring the respite care provider to have specific training regarding that child's care. This further limits the availability of respite care services.

The families that have the greatest need for respite care are usually the families who "fall through the cracks" in terms of existing programs. Their child's care may be too complex for a lay caregiver program, but not complex enough to be granted 24-hour-per-day nursing care. The burden of the child's care then usually falls almost entirely on the parents' shoulders. Without adequate respite, these families can crumble under the chronic stress of ongoing caregiving obligations. Respite care is consistently identified by families as a needed priority (Cohen and Warren, 1995). For many families, "respite care becomes a vital service—a necessity, not a luxury" (National Information Center for Children and Youth with Disabilities, 1996). It is intended to prevent parent burnout and allow the child living with a life-threatening condition to remain at home. The provision of such services by tertiary children's hospitals and community hospitals with pediatric units, reimbursed through state-sponsored support programs, may be an area for improvement in the next few years. In 2004, Florida initiated "Partners in Care: Together for Kids," a pediatric palliative care Medicaid waiver demonstration program for children and their families. Respite care is the second most used service across the state (Knapp et al., 2008; Lowe et al., 2009).

Children living with life-threatening conditions are cared for in many settings, including home, community hospitals, pediatric or specialty hospitals, nursing homes, medical day care facilities, foster homes, and hospice inpatient facilities. Primary care physicians, home health nurses, school nurses and teachers, hospice personnel, Medicaid and insurance case managers, and often a multiplicity of pediatric subspecialists are frequently involved in the care of such children. A technology-dependent child may have as many as seven people designated as "case managers." The dilemma so many families face is trying to coordinate all the coordinators.

Often, depending on the treatment regimen or acuity of the child's illness, the child moves from one care setting to another with regularity and frequency. In these diverse settings, the child's treatment goals can vary substantially as a result of poor communication between caregivers and settings. This can be disturbing and stressful for the child and family. Parents may also find it necessary to provide *supervision* of their child's outpatient caregivers, including home health aides; in-home shift nurses; physical, occupational, and speech therapists; medical day-care personnel; and school nurses and teachers. Parents often directly observe the care rendered by these caregivers and can be best positioned to make judgments about the quality of the care provided. They frequently find this an undesirable responsibility to assume, fearing that any negative feedback they provide about a particular care provider may place their relationship with him/her in peril and put their child in danger of potential retaliation or abandonment.

It is a rare parent who is suited to wear all these "hats"—advocate, direct care provider, coordinator, and supervisor. Infrequently, a parent will relish the role of the child's health care system navigator. Most parents, however, find it to be a demanding and draining experience. Innovative programs are being developed to provide such a key-worker for families, which will serve to simultaneously reduce the family's stress level and improve outcomes for children with life-threatening conditions.

Some families face potential discrimination and disenfranchisement in the health care system. Palliative care teams should be alert to the specific needs of ethnic minority, immigrant, and lesbian, gay, bisexual, and trans-gendered (LGBT) families, among others. For example, it is well known that health care disparities exist for members of ethnic minority families and therefore they may face poorer prognoses owing to later diagnosis, lack of health insurance, or concerns about health care parity (Fiscella et al., 2000; Field and Behrman, 2003). Immigrant families may be at specific risk for not receiving health care for fear of citizenship battles and sometimes owing to extreme language and cultural barriers (Cowles, 2003). LGBT families also face unique barriers of misunderstanding and/or lack of health care or health care decision-making powers (Bonvicini and Perlin, 2003; Harper and Schneider, 2003; Barker, 2008). It is crucial for health care providers to ensure that all families have equal access to, and support to receive, good-quality palliative care. And when that is not the case, clinicians must pay special attention to the unique barriers faced by disenfranchised families.

Conclusion

Children living with life-threatening conditions and their families should be able to expect the highest quality of care from palliative care providers. This includes the availability of competent staff members who can guide them as they embark on their difficult and unpredictable journeys through a cure-oriented health care system. Well-trained palliative care staffs are extremely capable and skilled in assessing the emotional and psychosocial needs of the entire family. Further, they are able to identify the most appropriate psycho-social interventions to assist each family member.

Much can be done to alleviate physical pain. We can use our collective power and skill to reduce psychosocial suffering as well. Helping suffering souls find hope, comfort, and peace in the face of death is a privilege to which few have access.

References

American Academy of Pediatrics, Committee on Bioethics (AAP COB). 1995. Informed consent, parental permission, and assent in pediatric practice. *Pediatrics* 95:314–17.
———. 1997. Religious objections to medical care. *Pediatrics* 99(2):279–81.
American Academy of Pediatrics, Committee on Bioethics, Committee on Hospital Care (AAP COB/COHC). 2000. Palliative care for children. *Pediatrics* 106:351–57.
Barker, M.R. 2008. Gay and lesbian health disparities: Evidence and recommendations for elimination. *J Health Disparit Res Practice* 2:91–120.
Beale, E.A., Baile, W.F., and Aaron, J. 2005. Silence is not golden: Communicating with children dying from cancer. *J Clin Oncol* 23(15):3629–31.
Bonvicini, K.A., and Perlin, M.J. 2003. The same but different: Clinician-patient communication with gay and lesbian patients. *Patient Educ Couns* 51(2):115–22.
Children's Hospice International. 1998. *Survey: Hospice Care for Children. Executive Summary Report.*
Cohen, S., and Warren, R.D. 1995. *Respite Care: Principles, Programs and Policies.* Austin, TX: Pro-Ed.
Cowles, L.F. 2003. *Social Work in the Health Field: A Care Perspective,* 2nd ed. Binghamton, NY: Haworth Press.
Darley, S., Heath, W., Darley, M., et al. 2007. *The Expressive Arts Activity Book.* London: Jessica Kingsley Publishers.
Davies, B. 1998. *Shadows in the Sun.* Philadelphia: Brunner/Mazel.
Diehl, S., Moffitt, K., and Wade, S. 1991. Focus group interview with parents of children with medically complex needs: An intimate look at their perceptions and feelings. *Children's Healthcare* 20(3):170–78.
Domek, G.J. 2010. Debunking common barriers to pediatric HIV disclosure. *J Trop Pediatr* 56 (published online ahead of print). http://tropej.oxfordjournals.org/cgi/reprint/fmq013v1 (accessed April 23, 2010).
Feudtner, C. 2005. Hope and the prospects of healing at the end of life. *J Altern Complement Med* 11(Suppl 1):S23–30.
Feudtner, C., Santucci, G., Feinstein, J.A., et al. 2007. Hopeful thinking and level of comfort regarding providing pediatric palliative care: A survey of hospital nurses. *Pediatrics* 119(1):e186–92. http://pediatrics.aapublications.org/cgi/content/full/119/1/e186.
Field, M., and Behrman, R., eds. 2003. *When Children Die: Improving Palliative and End-of-Life Care for Children and Their Families.* Washington, DC: Institute of Medicine, National Academies Press.
Fiscella, K., Franks, P., Gold, M.R., et al. 2000. Inequality in quality: Addressing socioeconomic, racial, and ethnic disparities in healthcare. *JAMA* 283:2579–84.
Groopman, J.E. 2004. *The Anatomy of Hope: How Patients Prevail in the Face of Illness,* pp. xvii, 248. New York: Random House.

Harper, G.W., and Schneider, M. 2003. Oppression and discrimination among lesbian, gay, bisexual, and transgendered people and communities: A challenge for community psychology. *Am J Commun Practice* 31(3–4):243–52.

Hays, R.M., Valentine, J., Haynes, G., et al. 2006. The Seattle pediatric palliative care project: Effects on family satisfaction and health-related quality of life. *J Palliat Med* 9(3):716–28.

Hinds, P.S. 1984. Inducing a definition of "hope" through the use of grounded theory methodology. *J Adv Nurs* 9(4):357–62.

Hinds, P.S., Schum, L., Baker, J.N., et al. 2005. Key factors affecting dying children and their families. *J Palliat Med* 8(Suppl 1):S70–78.

Jones, B., and Weisenfluh, S. 2003. Pediatric palliative and end-of-life care: Spiritual and developmental issues for children. *Smith College Studies in Social Work: Special Edition on End of Life Care* 78(1):423–43.

Klass, D. 1986. Marriage and divorce among bereaved parents in a self help group. *Omega* 17:237–49.

Knapp, C., Madden, V., Curtis, C., et al. 2008. Partners in care: Together for kids: Florida's model of pediatric palliative care. *J Palliat Med* 11(9):1212–20.

Kreicbergs, U., Valdimarsdóttir, U., Onelöv, E., et al. 2004. Talking about death with children who have severe malignant disease. *N Engl J Med* 351(12):1175–86.

Lowe, P., Curtis, C., Greffe, B., et al. 2009. Children's Hospice International program for all-inclusive care for children and their families. In *Hospice Care for Children*, 3rd ed., ed. A. Armstrong-Dailey and S. Zarbock, pp. 398–438. New York: Oxford University Press.

Mack, J.W., Wolfe, J., Cook, E.F., et al. 2007. Hope and prognostic disclosure. *J Clin Oncol* 25(35):5636–42.

Malchiodi, C. 2005. *Expressive Therapies.* New York: Guilford Press.

———. 2007. *Art Therapy Source Book.* New York: McGraw Hill.

Meyer, E.C., Burns, J.P., Griffith, J.L., et al. 2002. Parental perspectives on end-of-life care in the pediatric intensive care unit. *Crit Care Med* 30:226–31.

Najiman, J., Vance, J., Boyle, F., et al. 1993. The impact of child death on marital adjustment. *Soc Sci Med* 37:1005–10.

National Hospice and Palliative Care Organization (NHPCO). 2000. *Compendium of Pediatric Palliative Care.* Alexandria, VA.

National Information Center for Children and Youth with Disabilities. 1996. *Respite Care.* NICHCY News Digest, June.

Nouwen, H. 1984. *Out of Solitude.* Notre Dame: Ave Maria Press.

Parker-Raley, J., Jones, B., and Maxson, T. 2008. Communicating the death of a child in the emergency department: The negotiation of dialectical tensions. *J Healthcare Quality* 30(5):20–31.

Schwab, R. 1992. Effects of a child's death on the marital relationship: A preliminary study. *Death Studies* 16(2):141–54.

Shantz, M. 1995. Effects of respite care: A literature review. *Perspectives* 10(4):11–15.

Shudy, M., de Almeida, M.L., Ly, S., et al. 2006. Impact of pediatric critical illness and injury on families: A systematic review. *Pediatrics* 118(3):S203–18.

Sourkes, B., Frankel, L., Brown, M., et al. 2005. Food, toys, and love: Pediatric palliative care. *Curr Prob Pediatr Adolesc Health Care* 35:350–86.

Taub, S. 2003. Learning to decide: Involving children in their health care decisions. *Virtual Mentor* 5(8). http://virtualmentor.ama-assn.org/2003/08/pfor3–0308.html (accessed April 23, 2010).

Walsh, F., ed. 1982. *Normal Family Processes.* New York: Guilford Press.

Additional Resources

ACT for Children: www.act.org.uk

American Academy of Pediatrics: www.medicalhomeinfo.org

Canadian Hospice Palliative Care Association: www.chpca.net

Caring Connections: www.caringinfo.org/index.cfm?page=610

Centering Corporation: www.centering.org

Center to Advance Palliative Care: www.capc.org

Children's Hospice and Palliative Care Coalition: www.childrenshospice.org

Children's Hospice International: www.chionline.org

Children's Project on Hospice and Palliative Care Services (ChiPPS): www.nhpco.org/ i4a/pages/index.cfm?pageid=3409&openpage=3409

National Children's Cancer Society: www.children-cancer.org/NetCommunity/Page .aspx?pid=448

National Hospice and Palliative Care Organization

Partnering for Children: www.partneringforchildren.org

Online Chat Rooms / Websites

www.bereavedfamilies.net (Ontario, Canada)

www.beyondindigo.com

www.caringbridge.org

www.genesis-resources.com

www.grieflossrecovery.com

www.griefnet.org

www.griefwork.org

www.grievingforbabies.org (Perinatal Loss)

www.livingwithtrisomy13.org

www.starlight.org (Starlight Children's Foundation)

www.tchin.org (Congenital Heart Information Network)

www.thecompassionatefriends.com

9

Spiritual Dimensions

Dexter Lanctot, M.Div., B.A.Ph., Wynne Morrison, M.D., M.B.E.,
Kendra D. Koch, and Chris Feudtner, M.D., Ph.D., M.P.H.

Some of the most profound encounters with dying children and their families center on questions of spirituality and faith: Why? What happens? How will we survive? For many clinicians, responding appropriately to utterances of such transcendent gravity is perceived as extremely challenging. How, for example, should one react when a parent declares to the bedside nurse, "I can't stand it when people say this is all part of God's plan!" or when a young adolescent boy says quietly to a physician, "I wonder whether I am good enough for God," or when a teenage girl struggles, in a time of crisis, to decide whether she feels more at home in the faith community of her mother or her father, who come from different religious backgrounds?

We hope in this chapter to encourage clinicians to engage children and families in discussions about matters of spiritual or religious importance, and to do so by providing some concrete guidance. Our suggestions and the suggestions of the experts we cite regarding these conversations are not the only possible questions and responses, but rather a starting point to allay the fears of clinicians who are hesitant to begin such discussions: a gentle inquiry from a concerned clinician is almost always preferable to leaving a child and family alone in their distress. By entering into these conversations, we trust that dedicated clinicians over time will develop their own repertoire of tactful queries concerning spiritual issues, as well as certain common heartfelt responses to the difficult questions that inevitably arise for anyone confronted with the possibility of a child's death.

Acknowledging Spirituality and Engaging in a Spiritual Journey

> Crossing the threshold of the patient's room and walking toward the broad window seat, the physician approached the mother and father who held in their arms their son, who had taken his last breath just minutes ago. The doctor crouched next to the parents, who were crying quietly. After a few moments, the mother said: "Right before he left us, the sunlight broke through those clouds and came down and shined on him. I never knew that someone dying could be so beautiful."

Broadly speaking, both religious and spiritual beliefs and practices help human beings to mediate between worldly and transcendent concerns (fig. 9.1) (Feudtner, Haney, and Dimmers, 2003). Said somewhat differently, the conversations we have with ourselves and others about the meaning of life, the nature of our faith or devotion, feelings of awe and sacredness, the relationship we have with God or a higher power, beliefs regarding morality, and questions about mortality, death, and the afterlife are often (but not always) couched in religious or spiritual terms, as are thoughts and feelings of how these transcendent issues are connected to our everyday lives. If we want to enter into this conversation with our patients and families, we need

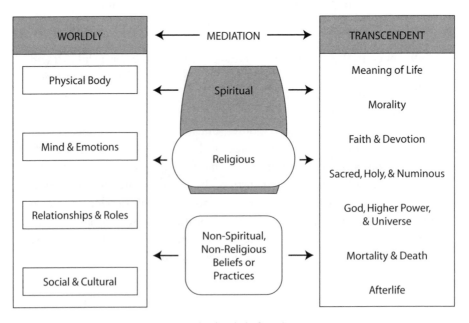

Figure 9.1. Spirituality, religion, and other beliefs and practices

to gain a certain comfort and fluency in talking about spiritual and religious concerns.

We should maintain as wide and inclusive an understanding of the terms "religion" and "spiritual" as we can. Religion usually implies specific structures, doctrines, narratives, beliefs, practices, and rituals that connect an individual or community in its day-to-day life with ultimate or transcendent concerns such as ultimate meaning, purpose, ground of being, God, creator, or the supernatural. The term spiritual, while also embracing the many nuances associated with questions of ultimate meaning and transcendence, is broader in scope than the term religion because spiritual includes those who do not necessarily belong or subscribe to a formal, structured belief system involving doctrines and rituals (Stuber and Houskamp, 2004). Spirituality has been more broadly defined as "that which brings significance, purpose, and direction to people's lives" (Cohen, Wheeler, and Scott, 2001) or "one's relationship with the transcendent questions that confront one as a human being and how one relates to these questions" (Sulmasy, 2006). For young children in particular, however, there may be few distinctions drawn between more global spiritual concerns and specific religious practices (Houskamp, Fisher, and Stuber, 2004).

One final point to emphasize: for children with life-threatening illness and their families, spirituality is progressive and dynamic, not a singular destination but a journey. From diagnosis to death, this journey may deliver hopes one day and disappointments the next. Sometimes the setbacks are swift and substantial; other times, gradual and incremental. As a patient's physical status ebbs and flows, the spiritual outlook and perspective often (but not always) shift in parallel. As a trusted companion on the journey, a clinician should be alert to recognize spiritual changes within the patient and family, as questions once answered may resurface, and doors once closed may open.

Being Present

For 3 weeks, the chaplain had honored his promise of silence, visiting the room in which the mother sat with her comatose daughter, who had a malignant brain tumor. The mother had felt harassed by a hometown pastor, and had made the chaplain promise that he would not talk about God, religion, or anything deep. Then, after the daughter died, the chaplain received a phone call from the mother, asking: "Will you preside at the burial ceremony? My daughter and I counted on you, and you didn't let us down, and that meant so much to us."

Presence and listening are among the most valuable actions that a clinician, accompanying a family through a child's life-threatening illness and possible death, can engage in. Time and again, the "mere" act of being present proves to be of fundamental importance in offering spiritual care. One study of spiritual care at the end of life stated, "Being present was a dominant theme among participants, defined as . . . care that went beyond medical treatment, giving attention to emotional, social and spiritual needs" (Daaleman et al., 2008). Being present and open, actively listening to what patients and family members say, engages us fully in their perspective about what is happening—and this alone has great value. To be simply and utterly present, many clinicians likely have to resist their urge to "fix" every problem; if this urge is not quelled, some clinicians may never inquire about what is bothering a child or family most because they are afraid of bringing issues to the surface that they may not know how to address (Lo, Ruston, and Kates, 2002). Not all difficult questions will be answered, but fear of not being able to answer them should not hinder us from acknowledging and validating the concerns, and letting the child and family know that they are not alone (Nelson, 2005).

Assessing and Facilitating Spiritual Care

Two weeks have passed since the 8-year-old boy was struck by a car while riding his bike and suffered a massive brain injury. He still requires the ventilator to breathe and has not shown signs of consciousness or response to painful stimulus. His family, trying to decide whether to continue mechanical ventilatory support by proceeding with a tracheostomy, asks if they can bring in holy water from their mosque to give him to drink.

Many clinicians at the bedside are intimidated when a child or family brings up questions of a spiritual nature. The doctor or nurse may feel a lack of expertise or education regarding spiritual matters and, consequently, may hesitate to respond to questions or to make an initial inquiry into what concerns a child or family has. A useful analogy in such situations is to consider how, in many other areas of clinical practice, competent "front-line" clinicians need only make an initial assessment of needs and then consult with the appropriate experts or specialists when specific issues have been identified. More specifically, consulting with a chaplain who has formal clinical pastoral education could be thought of as similar to consulting a cardiologist who is trained to take care of cardiac problems—the bedside clinician only needs to be comfortable identifying issues and seeking appropriate help (Nelson, 2005; Puchalski et al., 2009). Just as one should not avoid all questions about the heart in a medical history because one does not yet know if a cardiologist's assistance will be necessary, one should not avoid questions about spirituality just because of uncertainty about what issues will be raised.

Many clinicians worry that they will offend if they ask a patient or family about their spirituality. Studies in adult patients have shown that although a majority of patients would welcome physician inquiries about spiritual or religious beliefs, there are a minority who would rather not be asked (Cohen, Wheeler, and Scott, 2001; Morrison and Nelson, 2007). How can a clinician inquire in a nonjudgmental fashion about what is important to a family without implying an expectation that everyone should have a religious affiliation? Ehman et al. (1999) suggested phrasing that would help patients understand why asking such questions might help a clinician: "Do you have spiritual or religious beliefs that would influence your medical decisions if you became gravely ill?" This phrasing makes it clearer that the clinician is inquiring about such beliefs because he wants to know what values might affect the patient's medical decisions, and not because the clinician is hoping the patient shares his own religious affiliation (Cohen, Wheeler, and Scott, 2001). A similar phrasing in pediatric palliative care could be: "Are there particular spiritual or religious beliefs or rituals that are important to your family that you think the team should know about in their care of your child?" This family-centered approach allows the family the option of deciding whether they think it is important to bring up these issues.

If the family is keen to discuss spirituality, various experts have published formats for clinicians to use in taking initial "spiritual histories" (table 9.1). These various assessment approaches explore spiritual beliefs, affiliations, and support systems. They examine how these influences shape an understanding of the illness and what implications they have for medical treatments, determine if there are moral or ethical concerns, attend to how people's beliefs help them cope, and explore what effect they have on end-of-life concerns. While each of these systematic approaches will lead to a fairly thorough background assessment, they may not necessarily encourage focused attention on the most immediate concerns of a child and his family. Questions of a spiritual nature will likely be at the forefront of the minds of any family caring for a child facing death, so it may be easier and more natural to simply start with exploring what issues have been weighing on them. These questions could be as basic as "Are there concerns or questions that have been on your mind a lot recently?" The conversation can then be directed

Table 9.1 Various schema for taking a spiritual history

Mnemonic acronym	Items
FICA (Puchalski and Romer, 2000)	Faith and belief Importance Community Address in care
III (Matthews, 1998)	Important Influence Interaction
SPIRIT (Maugans, 1996)	Spiritual belief system Personal spirituality Integration within a spiritual community Ritualized practices and restrictions Implications for medical care Terminal event planning
HOPE (Anandarajah and Hight, 2001)	H—sources of hope O—organized religion P—personal spirituality and practices E—effects on medical care and end-of-life issues

Note: The items are typically phrased as questions; see individual references for suggested wording.

to exploring their support systems, coping strategies, beliefs about illness, and values that might affect medical decision making. The range of responses to these spiritual assessments is vast and varied. In a medical crisis, faith and belief systems may be sustained, deepened, or gravely challenged. Any combination of strong feelings such as guilt, hope, or anger can generate inner conflict. In some circumstances, unexamined spiritual beliefs or practices might even become an obstacle rather than a resource in providing care.

In addition to personally held beliefs and emotions, many religious communities have traditions and rituals that are important to the members of the community at the time of a life-threatening illness or a death (table 9.2). Familiarity with the typical rituals of the various traditions can help the palliative care provider understand what might be important to a particular child or family, but should be treated only as a starting point (Davies et al., 2002). Every patient is an individual, and one should never assume that just because the family belongs to a particular religious or ethnic group their views will necessarily align with others within the same group (Kagawa-Singer and Blackhall, 2001).

Table 9.2 Examples of end-of-life practices or rituals from various religious traditions

Religious tradition	End-of-life practices or rituals
Buddhism (Keown, 2005)	No specific hygiene, purification, or dietary requirements. At the end of life, mindfulness and alertness may be valued more than the relief of suffering.
Catholicism (Markwell, 2005)	Traditional distinction between "ordinary" measures, which must be provided at the end of life, and "extraordinary" measures, which should not be. Baptism for infants and sacrament of the sick (extreme unction) for the dying, performed by a priest when possible.
Hinduism (Firth, 2005)	Dead traditionally cremated. Particular dates may be seen as more auspicious for a death. May wish to be placed on the ground (preferably at home) at the time of death. Water from the Ganges placed on the dying person's lips.
Islam (Sachedina, 2005)	Possible resistance to discontinuing therapies unless impending death is certain. May want the bed to face Mecca. Ritual washing of body after death by family. Rapid preparation of body for burial desired and may want family member to stay with body until burial.
Judaism (Dorff, 2005)	May wish to consult their own rabbi and have physician speak with rabbi regarding application of Jewish law to end-of-life decisions. Obligation of relatives and friends to visit the sick. Goal is to have burial within 1 day of death. Family observes 3- to 7-day period of mourning "sitting shiva" together after a death.

Note: Individual assessment should always be made of a patient's/family's wishes, as these generalizations do not apply in all communities and to all individuals.

In general, it can be helpful to a family if the health care team tries to facilitate particular practices that are important to them (Kobler, Limbo, and Kavanaugh, 2007). Being willing to help do so may also help the team build an alliance with the family, which may lead to a more collaborative process around end-of-life decision making. Some requests may be readily accommodated, such as turning a bed to face a certain direction or pinning written prayers to a patient's clothes. Some may be impossible in certain settings, such as lighting candles in an inpatient room where hospital policy prohibits open flames. Other requests, such as placing a child's body directly on the floor rather than a bed at the time of death, may stretch the flexibility and ingenuity of the hospital or hospice personnel but are still possible. In the case that opened this section, the health care team had been uncomfortable placing holy water directly into the child's mouth because of the risk of aspiration, but offered to mix it in with the feeds being given via nasogastric tube. The family was happy with this compromise and felt that they were doing everything possible in both the physical and spiritual care of their child.

Respecting a Child's Spirituality across the Age Spectrum

A 6-year-old child who has relapsed leukemia is working with an art therapist in her home. She turns to the art therapist and asks, "Will my mommy go with me when I go to heaven?"

Children progress through a somewhat predictable developmental understanding of death or the possibility of death as they age (Davies et al., 2002; Stuber and Houskamp, 2004). For infants and toddlers, there is no understanding of what illness or death means, but there may be an acute awareness of a change in routine or lack of contact with a usual caregiver. Children at this age can benefit most from physical contact with their family members and the maintenance of as much of a routine as possible. If they are old enough to understand speech (and young children are usually able to understand far more words than they can speak), they will benefit from being reassured that they will not be alone.

Preschool and young school-age children may be able to talk about death or dying but do not yet usually have an understanding of death as a permanent state. They may ask about where someone goes after death. They may have magical thinking such as believing that someone will come back after death or believing that their own actions have somehow caused an illness or a death. Children at this age often need to talk through their questions, have straightforward answers provided in simple language, and again be reassured that they will not be left alone. They will process many things through play and may seem oddly able to move rapidly from talking about a distressing or sad topic to playing happily, only to then return to the difficult topic at a later time when it feels safe to do so.

Older school-age children will have a better understanding that the death of a loved one or their own impending death is permanent and represents a serious loss. They may experience more overt sadness, grief, or withdrawal.

At this point friends are becoming more important in a child's life, and difficulties doing things with friends or feeling different than others may become more pressing issues. Children at this age may also start trying to "protect" their parents from discussion topics that they think might distress them.

Adolescents have a rational understanding of death but emotionally may feel like death cannot really happen to them. They struggle with illness and having to rely on others at a time in their lives when they would normally be beginning to assert their own independence and self-identity. They will also be acutely aware of physical changes in their bodies or anything else that makes them not fit in, such as having to miss school or not being able to go out with friends at night.

Just as the understanding of death changes over time, spiritual questions likewise take different forms as children age (Miller, 2006). A young child may worry most about being abandoned, whereas an adolescent may rage against the unfairness of having the disease. The spirituality of a child is almost always grounded within the spiritual framework of the family, so coming to an understanding of the values of the family unit as a whole is invaluable in working with a child facing a life-threatening illness (Davies et al., 2002). A child who has experience with a serious illness may also deviate somewhat from the usual developmental patterns. A preteen may have an unusually mature understanding of life's difficult questions because of a long experience with illness, or alternatively could revert back to a perspective more typical of a younger, more dependent child as a potential coping mechanism.

Responding to Questions and Statements

Only 18 months separated the sisters. Soon after the older sister's 13th birthday, the younger sister expressed that she had only recently realized how close they could have been, if the older sister had been born "normal" and not with the numerous brain anomalies that had caused profound neurological impairments. In subsequent conversations, the younger sister expressed sadness, that she was "disappointed," that she felt "anger" for her sister, and finally through tears she said simply: "Why did it have to happen to her?"

When a child is given a serious medical diagnosis with a life-limiting prognosis, spiritual issues emerge. The illness will disrupt the lives of the patient and family. Their sense of self, meaning, and purpose will be rattled. Amid this upheaval, profound questions pour forth, such as: Why am I here?

Why did this happen to me? Did I do something to deserve this? What kind of God would let an innocent child suffer? Will our child die? Is there a life after death? Children, whether the affected child or the siblings, will ask these questions in their own way, just as the adults in their lives do.

Precisely how clinicians can best respond to such questions cannot be prescribed in any detail—because each child, family, clinician, and situation is different—yet some practical guidance is still possible. When young children ask questions about meaning or the future, a useful first step is often to explore with them what made them ask that question or what it means to them. They may already have answered the question to their own liking and are only looking for affirmation that their thoughts on the matter are acceptable. To do this effectively, however, one should not lead the child to think you are avoiding answering: the question is a serious one and should be addressed as such. A response that allows such exploration could be: "That is an important question. I am going to try to give you the best answer I can, but first I want to know what you are thinking and why you are asking." Also important when talking to a child, avoid using religious- or culture-specific references, such as talking about angels, unless the family or the child first used these terms and you know that such references are consistent with the family's worldview.

A clinician may also be able to help a family explore the full range of their hopes when their initial hopes, such as for a cure, are no longer possible. Although premature or false reassurances are not usually helpful and may cut conversation off too quickly (Lo, Ruston, and Kates, 2002), steering conversation away from hope (for fear that such conversation could only be about false hope) is often not the best therapeutic strategy either, because many families are deeply engaged in discussions among themselves and others about what they are hoping for, and hopefulness is vital for sustaining motivation in such difficult times (Feudtner, 2005). A useful way to enter into this dialogue is to say, "I'll be better able to take good care of your child if you can share with me, given what your child is up against, what some of the things are that you are hoping for." The experienced clinician will expect that the first hope offered up may be for a miraculous cure or for the parent to awaken from a bad dream, and on hearing this hope, the clinician need not judge it, but instead only softly say, "I wish that could happen, too. Can you tell me what else you are hoping for?" The subsequently mentioned hopes may be quite different, focusing on relief from physical pain or a remit of suffering or going home from the hospital. With the range of hopes more explicitly spelled out in this conversation, the family and clinician can still hope for the best while also planning to accomplish the other hoped-for goals (Feudtner, 2007).

Providing Spiritual Care in the Midst of Grief and Bereavement

> Lying in bed together, the mother held her daughter for the long hour from the time that mechanical respiratory support was ceased to the moment when the physician pronounced death. Throughout this time, the mother averted her gaze from her daughter's face, too scared to look. After a few minutes, the mother said, "I still feel her, here with me, it's okay"—and turned her eyes to see her child's body.

Ritual and memory making may become extremely important for a family at the time of their child's death and afterward. The most common spiritual need reported by parents after a child's death in one study was the need to maintain a connection with their child (Meert, Thurston, and Briller, 2005). At the time of the child's death, this was manifest as a need for a physical connection with the child, whether holding him, lying in bed together, or providing for his physical needs and comfort. Some parents also deeply desired to maintain their role as caregivers, even when they have to rely on others for some of their child's medical needs. After the death, this need to maintain a connection was met by keeping mementos of the child, recalling events in her life, and attending memorial services.

A palliative care team can help the family at the time of a child's death by encouraging such connections and memory making (Klass, Silverman, and Nickman, 1996; Worden, 2009). Sitting quietly with a family as you make sure a child is comfortable is a perfect time to encourage them to tell you stories about the child. As mentioned above, there may be rituals specific to the family's religious tradition that become important at this time. Inquiring about what they would like, and whenever possible giving them some control over the circumstances and environment of the death, can be helpful.

Parents may benefit from follow-up contact with a health care team after a child's death. They may have unanswered questions or may simply want to be able to see someone who was there with them during their child's last days. They may also benefit from being able to connect with other parents and families who have also lost children through support groups or other such gatherings. Some families may require specific counseling to find meaning or come to peace with what has happened (Humphrey and Zimpfer, 2008).

Managing Boundaries

> A physician is visiting an 8-month-old child who has severe cardiomy-opathy and is now home with hospice. Extended family members are gathered in the home to support the parents and the 7-year-old sibling. After the physician addresses symptom and pain control issues, the baby's grandmother takes the doctor's hand and says, "Doctor, are you born again? Will you lead us in prayer?"

Many clinicians are confused about how to respond if a patient or family member asks them about their personal faith or asks them to participate in a religious ritual important to the family. Some clinicians fear that it may be inappropriate to answer or that the family will be disappointed if they do not share the same religious background. Yet the family is likely asking because they trust and feel close to the health care provider and because the ritual is something important to them to help them cope or make meaning out of a difficult situation. Clinicians must be responsive to such questions but also give an honest answer that does not misrepresent their own beliefs. An appropriate response might be, "I would be honored to join you in prayer, but would feel more comfortable if you would lead us," if the physician is indeed comfortable participating in this fashion, or "I would be honored to stand in silence as you pray, but think that you should lead the prayer" if the physician is more reluctant.

Are there any responses that would be inappropriate? Koenig said, "Physicians must remember that any activity in this area should be patient-centered; it is about the patient's beliefs, not the physician's, and no attempt should be made to change the patient's religious beliefs or to introduce new ones" (Koenig, 2007, p. 933). Published guidelines have suggested that a clinician participating in prayer initiated by the patient or family is acceptable, but that it is not acceptable for the clinician, unless specifically trained to do so, to be the first to bring up the issue (Davidson et al., 2007; Puchalski et al., 2009). The clinician should always remember that the family is in a vulnerable state, and a family might feel uncomfortable refusing if an authority figure offers to pray with them, even if it is not an activity in which they would normally participate (Cohen, Wheeler, and Scott, 2001).

Should the clinician answer when a family asks what he or she believes? There is no right answer: each clinician needs to decide whether sharing this personal information is appropriate or not. Respectfully turning the conversation back to the patient's or family's values is acceptable (Lo, Ruston, and Kates, 2002). Alternative responses that also divert the attention away from the clinician could be, "Well, I am Jewish, but even though I don't come from your religious tradition, I know how much faith can help us all through times like this," or even simply, "My background is not in your tradition, but I understand how important your faith is to you," followed by encouraging the family to talk about what helps them and their values (Sulmasy, 2006). Clinicians should avoid getting into theological discussions or arguments with families that are beyond their expertise; seeking help from someone with training in addressing such questions when they arise helps to avoid confusing the family about the appropriate roles of each member of the health care team.

Confronting Situations When Spiritual Beliefs May Not Be Helpful

The health care team wants to make a hospice referral for a 2-year-old boy who is hospitalized with a relapsed cancer that is resistant to all available treatments. The mother resists being told there are no other cancer-directed therapies and about the possibility of going home with hospice, saying, "It's not time to give up yet." A nurse is in the room when the family's minister comes to visit and overhears the minister tell the mother: "Have faith. If you only have faith, God will not let him die."

Many observational studies of adults have shown that formal religious affiliations are associated with improved medical outcomes and better coping skills in a variety of illnesses (Koenig, 2006). "Spirituality" is more difficult to measure than attendance at religious services, but it has been associated with resilience in children and their parents facing difficulties (Houskamp, Fisher, and Stuber, 2004). Every palliative care practitioner has met families who draw unexpected strength from their faith at a time of crisis.

Strong faith within a family, however, should not be assumed to be unequivocally helpful. For some children and families, faith may lead to greater struggles when confronted with a life-threatening illness. For example, families who believe that prayers are answered may experience mounting doubt or guilt when confronting an illness that progresses despite exhortations to God for a cure: either God is unable to answer prayers, contrary to their most dearly held beliefs, or they have somehow not been found worthy or have not had a strong enough faith to have their prayers answered. Both the child and parents may believe that they are being punished through the illness. Strong faith may also become difficult for the health care team if a family is "waiting for a miracle," particularly if they therefore insist on continuing invasive medical interventions that the team does not believe offer any chance of long-term survival or other form of benefit. Although a family's spiritual advisors from their community can be an incredible help in times of crisis, they may also (as illustrated in the case above) reinforce beliefs that lead to greater distress or conflicts.

Trying to "talk a family out of" beliefs that the clinician may not see as rational is almost always unhelpful (Sulmasy, 2006). Attempting to do so will usually lead to entrenched positions and a lack of trust that will neither help the family through the turmoil they are experiencing nor help the health care team feel they are providing appropriate care for the child. Having patience, building an alliance with the family, and treating any pain and suffering that the child is experiencing will be much more helpful to the family, child, and health care team. One could say to a family, "I know that we are all waiting to see how things will go now that the oncology team says that they don't have any more medications that can cure the cancer. While we are waiting to see what happens next, I want to make sure that we treat your child's pain and that he is as comfortable as he can be under the cir-cumstances." Only the rare family would object to those goals (and then, usually because of a fear that the use of "morphine" or some other drug implies imminent death, or "giving up," or will hasten death—all notions that can be perhaps remedied with better information). Involving a hospital staff member with training in clinical pastoral education, such as a chaplain, may also be helpful. The chaplain may have more experience counseling families of dying children than the community religious leader, and although he should never try to replace or undermine the family's minister, he may be able to help a family work their way through such a crisis of faith.

Promoting Holistic Care for the Child and Family

In their own fashion, the 6-year-old brother related well to his 11-year-old sister, who had a severe seizure disorder and profound impairments. The sister's most recent battle with aspiration pneumonia, however, greatly distressed her brother: his distress was not over her life or death, but over the gastrostomy tube that was placed because of the aspiration. Sitting with his mother while she fed his sister through the tube, he said he was sad, and when asked why, he said, "If I couldn't eat, that would make me sad."

Good spiritual care of an ill child and her family can—and should—involve much more than just addressing questions about God or existential concerns. The importance of good symptom management to help a child and family have the energy and attention to focus on spiritual concerns cannot be overemphasized; thus, advocacy for better control of pain and other bothersome symptoms is also spiritual advocacy. Holistic spiritual care may involve finding a way to help a lonely child get to see friends or a beloved pet despite a long hospitalization, or helping the family find ways to balance caring for other siblings who are at home with the time they need to be with the child who is ill. Families may also benefit from other "soul work," such as writing, meditation, mending broken relationships, memory making, or helping others (Davies et al., 2002; Miller, 2006). The possibilities here, in this domain of total care that unites worldly and transcendent concerns, are bounded only by our creativity and compassion, calling us to participate in the physical and spiritual journey of life and death with our patients and their families.

Conclusion

Acknowledging that chronically ill or dying children and their families share remarkable spiritual encounters and insights to existential meaning, purpose, and faith can help clinicians working with them to pause, reflect, and respond—in silence or in presence—to their often sacred utterances. The opportunities and considerations revealed in this chapter should help the clinician move past bewilderment or feeling challenged toward engagement with these children and families and a working facility in assessing the spiritual dimensions of excellent care across all care settings and even beyond death in working with family and caregiver grief and bereavement.

References

Anandarajah, G., and Hight, E. 2001. Spirituality and medical practice: Using the HOPE questions as a practical tool for spiritual assessment. *Am Fam Physician* 63(1):81–89.

Cohen, C.B., Wheeler, S.E., and Scott, D.A. 2001. Walking a fine line. Physician inquiries into patients' religious and spiritual beliefs. *Hastings Cent Rep* 31(5):29–39.

Daaleman, T.P., Usher, B.M., and Williams, S.W. 2008. An exploratory study of spiritual care at the end of life. *Ann Fam Med* 6(5):406–11.

Davidson, J.E., Powers, K., Hedayat, K.M., et al. 2007. Clinical practice guidelines for support of the family in the patient-centered intensive care unit: American College of Critical Care Task Force 2004–2005. *Crit Care Med* 35:605–22.

Davies, B., Brenner, P., Orloff, S., et al. 2002. Addressing spirituality in pediatric hospice and palliative care. *J Palliat Care* 18(1):59–67.

Dorff, E.N. 2005. End-of-life: Jewish perspectives. *Lancet* 366(9488):862–65.

Ehman, J.W., Ott, B.B., Short, T.H., et al. 1999. Do patients want physicians to inquire about their spiritual or religious beliefs if they become gravely ill? *Arch Intern Med* 159(15):1803–6.

Feudtner, C. 2005. Hope and the prospects of healing at the end of life. *J Altern Complement Med* 11(Suppl 1):S23–30.

———. 2007. Collaborative communication in pediatric palliative care: A foundation for problem-solving and decision-making. *Pediatr Clin North Am* 54(5):583–607, ix.

Feudtner, C., Haney, J., and Dimmers, M.A. 2003. Spiritual care needs of hospitalized children and their families: A national survey of pastoral care providers' perceptions. *Pediatrics* 111(1):e67–72.

Firth, S. 2005. End-of-life: A Hindu view. *Lancet* 366(9486):682–86.

Houskamp, B.M., Fisher, L.A., and Stuber, M.L. 2004. Spirituality in children and adolescents: Research findings and implications for clinicians and researchers. *Child Adolesc Psychiatr Clin N Am* 13(1):221–30.

Humphrey, G.M., and Zimpfer, D.G. 2008. *Counselling for Grief and Bereavement.* Los Angeles: Sage Publications.

Kagawa-Singer, M., and Blackhall, L.J. 2001. Negotiating cross-cultural issues at the end of life: "You got to go where he lives." *JAMA* 286(23):2993–3001.

Keown, D. 2005. End of life: The Buddhist view. *Lancet* 366(9489):952–55.

Klass, D., Silverman, P.R., and Nickman, S.L. 1996. *Continuing Bonds: New Understandings of Grief.* Washington, DC: Taylor & Francis.

Kobler, K., Limbo, R., and Kavanaugh, K. 2007. Meaningful moments. *MCN Am J Matern Child Nurs* 32(5):288–95; quiz 296–97.

Koenig, H.G. 2006. Annotated bibliography on religion, spirituality and medicine. *South Med J* 99(10):1189–96.

———. 2007. Physician's role in addressing spiritual needs. *South Med J* 100(9): 932–33.

Lo, B., Ruston, D., and Kates, L.W. 2002. Discussing religious and spiritual issues at the end of life: A practical guide for physicians. *JAMA* 287(6):749–54.

Markwell, H. 2005. End-of-life: A catholic view. *Lancet* 366(9491):1132–35.

Matthews, D.A. 1998. *The Faith Factor.* New York: Penguin Books. www.redlands hospital.org/pastoral_care/pastoral_care_physicians.htm.

Maugans, T.A. 1996. The SPIRITual history. *Arch Fam Med* 5(1):11–16.

Meert, K.L., Thurston, C.S., and Briller, S.H. 2005. The spiritual needs of parents at the time of their child's death in the pediatric intensive care unit and during bereavement: A qualitative study. *Pediatr Crit Care Med* 6(4):420–27.

Miller, L. 2006. Spirituality, health and medical care of children and adolescents. *South Med J* 99(10):1164–65.

Morrison, W., and Nelson, R.M. 2007. Should we talk to patients (and their families) about God? *Crit Care Med* 35(4):1208–9.

Nelson, R.M. 2005. The compassionate clinician: Attending to the spiritual needs of self and others. *Crit Care Med* 33(12):2841–42.

Puchalski, C., Ferrell, B., Virani, R., et al. 2009. Improving the quality of spiritual care as a dimension of palliative care: The report of the Consensus Conference. *J Palliat Med* 12(10):885–904.

Puchalski, C., and Romer, A.L. 2000. Taking a spiritual history allows clinicians to understand patients more fully. *J Palliat Med* 3(1):129–37.

Sachedina, A. 2005. End-of-life: The Islamic view. *Lancet* 366(9487):774–79.

Stuber, M.L., and Houskamp, B.M. 2004. Spirituality in children confronting death. *Child Adolesc Psychiatr Clin N Am* 13(1):127–36, viii.

Sulmasy, D.P. 2006. Spiritual issues in the care of dying patients: ". . . It's okay between me and god." *JAMA* 296(11):1385–92.

Worden, J.W. 2009. *Grief Counseling and Grief Therapy: A Handbook for the Mental Health Practitioner*. New York: Springer.

10

Holistic Management of Symptoms

Richard Hain, M.D., Lonnie Zeltzer, M.D.,
Melody Hellsten, M.S.N., P.N.P., Susan O. Cohen, M.A., A.D.T.R., C.C.L.S.,
Stacy F. Orloff, Ed.D., L.C.S.W., A.C.H.P.-S.W., and Dianne Gray, B.S.

TJ was a 16-year-old girl who lived with her mother and four younger sisters. She had first presented to medical attention with left arm and shoulder pain two years earlier, at which time a slow-growing tumor of the head of the left humerus was diagnosed. Unfortunately, the tumor progressed despite maximal treatment, and the oncology team felt that there were no more curative options. TJ was referred to palliative medicine.

TJ's main problem at referral was severe pain despite fentanyl by transcutaneous patch with oral morphine for breakthrough. The pain was of several types, having elements of neuropathic and musculoskel-etal pain. Exploration with TJ also disclosed sadness and concern for her family, as well as intense anger directed at both her parents. Her father had left the family home after many years of physically abusing her mother, and TJ blamed her mother for being ineffectual, failing to prevent the abuse, and allowing him to return intermittently since.

TJ's pain was brought under immediate control by rapid titration of opioids and introduction of appropriate adjuvants (nonsteroidal anti-inflammatory drugs, tricyclic antidepressants, and radiotherapy). Her opioid requirements rose quickly in the first week as titration proceeded, but then decreased by 50 percent as the adjuvants took effect over the next 2 weeks.

Because of her home situation, TJ elected to remain in the hospital over the remaining weeks of her life. During that time, she remained largely free of physical pain, and her opioid requirements remained stable with no need for further titration. Her emotional pain, however, remained, and TJ refused to allow either parent to visit her in the hospital. The palliative care team worked intensively with her to explore her anger; 2 weeks before her death, TJ relented and there was a reconciliation with both parents.

TJ's opioid requirements, having been unchanged for some weeks, then dramatically fell, and at the time of her death, TJ was peaceful and pain-free on approximately 25 percent of the opioid dose she had required at maximum.

This case illustrates the concept of "total pain," of which physical, psychosocial, and spiritual elements are all interdependent aspects. It also illustrates the value of an analytical approach in which recognizing these aspects means that they can be individually addressed. Finally, it illustrates that they are not separable in the person who experiences them, and that the therapeutic benefit of addressing spiritual issues such as anger can sometimes be measured in milligrams of morphine.

In the traditional medical model, a problem is first described, then investigated and diagnosed, and finally treated in the expectation that it will resolve. The approach is rational and analytical. Because they often rely on exogenous interventions such as medication, the treatments are sometimes described as "allopathic." As it stands, this model does not serve well the approach needed in children with life-threatening conditions. For many reasons—particularly time—there may never be resolution of many of the most important problems faced by such a child and his or her family. Furthermore, problems that are immense from the perspective of the family may not be recognized through objective assessment by a physician, particularly if there is no solution. Yet, to be compassionate, symptom control must be attained by means that maximize effectiveness and minimize adverse effects. This requires some form of rational analysis, of understanding of the evidence. Thus, it is clear that in symptom control, the traditional medical model needs to be reformed rather than simply abandoned.

Most definitions of palliative care emphasize the need for "holistic" care. In the context of symptom management, the term *holistic* requires some elaboration. Derived from the Greek word for "everything," it has acquired a number of more precise but less accurate meanings. For some, it means seeing the child in the wider context of school and family. For others, it means the antithesis of the medical model—addressing the child as a whole being, rather than as a set of problems demanding solutions. Many forms of complementary and alternative medicine (CAM) are based on such an empirical approach.

Neither of these interpretations does justice to the term. Its full breadth is perhaps best expressed in the synonym *biopsychosocial*. In its structure, this term clarifies that there are three dimensions in which all human experiences can occur. The first, physical, can refer to the physical phenomenon of a broken tibia, for example. The second, psychosocial, refers to the effect such an injury can have on the self-concept and interactive functioning of the individual. Consider the difference in importance of a broken leg to a computer operator versus a professional athlete. The third dimension, spiritual (or, perhaps better, *existential*), does not appear in the word *biopsychosocial* but is implicit. It refers to the meaning the patient ascribes to the illness or injury. It is a feature of being human to construct explanations, for not only how experiences happen, but also why. Making meaning often invokes an overtly religious framework of belief, but issues of paradigm shift, guilt, belief, and doubt are common existential concerns, irrespective of formal religious conviction.

A common error is to imagine that these dimensions are categories, and that any given symptom falls into one category or another. For example, we may imagine pain to be a physical symptom and guilt to be an existential one, while in reality both have ramifications in every dimension. All symptoms occur in all dimensions. A systematic approach may demand that we examine the three dimensions separately, but a process of reintegration is then necessary in our application of the principles to patient care.

In recent decades, there has been increasing public use of complementary and alternative medicine (CAM). The National Center for Complementary and Alternative Medicine (NCCAM) of the U.S. National Institutes of Health considers CAM as a broad range of activities and interventions that are outside standard allopathic medicine. They have become increasingly popular, often costing patients and families large sums of money.

Scientific evidence supporting CAM techniques is variable. Factors influencing individuals' choices of CAM interventions are poorly understood, but they do not rest primarily on evidence of effectiveness. Specific cultural practices and the belief systems on which they are based should therefore be fully appreciated by the professional health care team, especially in the pediatric setting. Tolerance of harmless CAM practices, encouragement of helpful practices, and knowledge of harmful practices or therapies are critical to effective patient- and family-centered care (table 10.1).

Symptom control requires a holistic synthesis of these two approaches: the analytical (allopathic), on the one hand, and the empirical, on the other. This synthesis has been termed *integrative medicine*. It would not be possible to address the whole of symptom control in a single chapter. Instead,

Table 10.1 Considering complementary and alternative medicine in palliative care for children

---

- Consider each practice separately, based on the specific situation
- Gather data on safety
- Gather data on efficacy
- Elicit patient/family beliefs and preferences
- Present recommendation to patient and family:
  - If there is sufficient evidence of unacceptable risk and efficacy data are lacking, advise against.
  - If risk is uncertain and efficacy data are lacking, advise accordingly (cannot make medical recommendation).
  - If efficacy data are sufficient, balance risk information in usual risk/benefit analysis and advise accordingly.

---

some of the more common symptoms are considered. The first section will address therapeutic approaches for individual symptoms. The second examines approaches that do not rely on analysis of cause and effect. In practice, the two have in common the recognition that symptoms do not occur in isolation, but in the context of the complex physical, psychosocial, and spiritual phenomena that make up the individual, as well as the family and community in which that individual survives and thrives.

Management of Pain and General Symptoms

Data on the prevalence of symptoms among dying children are gradually becoming available (Wolfe et al., 2000; Hain, 2005; Goldman et al., 2006; Jalmsell et al., 2006; Zebracki and Drotar, 2008). Patients present with symptom complexes related to diagnosis and stage of disease, as well as to therapeutic interventions. Symptoms change over time and in response to primary and/or palliative treatments, necessitating frequent reevaluation for effective symptom control.

PAIN

Diagnosis of Pain. A number of myths and misperceptions have traditionally been attributed to the child's experience of pain, illustrating the pitfalls of considering pain to be a single, objective, physiological phenomenon. For much of the twentieth century, it was thought that children suffered pain less intensely than adults did. The fact that a baby's response to a painful stimulus is different from that of an adult was assumed to be due to a difference in perception rather than response. One early study even concluded that "the neonate's experience of pain is equivalent to that of a deeply anesthetized adult" (McGraw, 1941).

A second observation was that the nervous system of a neonate also differs from that of an adult. The relative lack of myelination in a neonate's nervous system compared with that of an adult similarly led to the fallacious but understandable inference that demyelinated fibers transmit pain less intensely than fully mature, myelinated ones.

Recognition that a child's pain is a subjective phenomenon (World Health Organization, 1998) has led researchers to find ways to understand the child's own experience of pain, rather than relying on adult interpretation. It now appears that children experience pain at least as intensely as adults. New hypotheses to explain this unanticipated phenomenon have included the idea that many of the fibers that are unmyelinated in the neonatal period are those that inhibit pain (Anand, 2000a). Thus, neonates' experience of pain may be even more intense than adults' (Craig and Grunau, 1993). Furthermore, early experiences of pain affect childrens' subsequent perception, tolerance, and adaptation to pain (Porter, Grunau, and Anand, 1999; Anand, 2000b; Colver and Jessen, 2000; Lowery et al., 2007).

Nevertheless, there is still a tendency on the part of adults and particularly health care professionals to underestimate a child's experience of pain. Despite the availability of safe and effective anesthesia, painful procedures such as circumcision and bone marrow biopsy are still performed on conscious children without even local anesthetics or postprocedure analgesics (Hain and Campbell, 2001). Adults often judge that for children, pain is relatively trivial, while adequate analgesia is unnecessary and perhaps even dangerous. More generally, because pain is not perceived to be life threatening, it is not given sufficient priority by health care providers or funders, including third-party payers.

Pain in Pediatric Palliative Care. Until relatively recently, the study of pain control in adult palliative medicine has been essentially the study of cancer pain. Children who have cancer probably account for fewer than half of referrals to pediatric palliative care (Hain and Hughes, 2001); the remainder have a wide range of nonmalignant conditions, usually complex neurodegenerative disorders. Many of the principles of good pain control developed for adults can safely be extrapolated, but pain in children presents some unique challenges. One commonsense approach is summarized (Baker and Wong, 1987) by the acronym QUEST (table 10.2).

There are many different ways of classifying pain (table 10.3). Of these, perhaps the most helpful at diagnosis is to consider the underlying cause.

Table 10.2 QUEST acronym mnemonic summarizing aspects of pain management in children

Q—Question the child
U—Use rating tools
E—Evaluate behavior
S—Sensitize parents (and staff)
T—Take action!

Source: Adapted from Baker and Wong, 1987.

Once a management plan has been instituted, a more empirical classification based on responsiveness to opioids becomes helpful. Clearly the classification systems are linked; for example, neuropathic pain is more likely than soft tissue pain to be only partially opioid responsive. A diagnostic classification based on responsiveness to therapy emphasizes that, irrespective of the underlying cause, opioids will usually provide the most effective relief (Cherny, 2000).

Several common causative subtypes of pain are encountered in pediatric palliative care (table 10.3).

Diagnosing Pain in Nonverbal or Preverbal Children. Recognizing that a child is in pain is not always easy for the health care professional. It has been said that the normal child is always either sleeping or playing. Behavior can give a valuable clue that a child is in pain, even in the absence of verbalization. It is important always to consider pain in the differential diagnosis of altered behavior patterns, such as a child who becomes distressed when being moved. Behavioral changes that indicate pain may, however, be subtle. A child may be able to avoid pain, but only at the expense of normal social interaction, giving the child an affect resembling depression (Gauvain-Piquard et al., 1999). Because it is not always possible reliably to exclude pain in a child, a therapeutic trial of analgesia may therefore be justified; as with any therapeutic intervention, it is important that appropriate doses of the right analgesia are used during the trial period.

The longer the observation of behavior patterns in an individual child, the more reliable. Thus, the child's family and primary nurses or other consistent caregivers are more likely to accurately identify pain-related behaviors than are physicians and others with more limited contact. The treatment team, and particularly the palliative care team, should respect the assessment of those who know the child best.

In assessing whether a child is likely to experience pain as a result of an intervention, a simple technique is to ask, "Would I be in pain if it were

Table 10.3 Classifications of pain

Classification	Categories	Description
Pathophysiological	Nociceptive Physiological: Somatic, Visceral Pathological: Somatic, Visceral Neuropathic Compression: Somatic, Visceral Injury: Peripheral, Somatic, Visceral Central Sympathetic-mediated	Useful classification for understanding pathophysiology; in this way can help suggest interventions most likely to be effective. Limitation is that although it appears comprehensive, it in fact, encompasses only the physical aspects of pain and excludes behavioral components.
Causative	Soft tissue pain Bone pain: Osteopenia, Infiltration Nerve pain Central pain Muscle spasm Colic "Total pain": Emotional, Spiritual, Interpersonal	Simple, empirical clinical classification; useful as it clearly links cause for pain with interventions likely to be effective. Not all pain types fit into this classification, and there is a risk of too closely associating cause with specific intervention.
Temporal	Acute Chronic Recurrent Continuous	Important distinction to make; cause, assessment, and management are all different. Particularly important in assessment of pain in children, whose "acute" response to pain may be short-lived.
Opioid-responsiveness	Opioid responsive Partially opioid responsive Opioid resistant	Helpful pragmatic classification; emphasizes that opioids are the first line of treatment for most pain in palliative care, irrespective of underlying cause.

Source: Adapted from Twycross, 1997.

me?" If pain is likely, adequate analgesia and even anesthesia should be provided, regardless of whether or not a child is capable of verbalizing pain.

Assessment. Once pain is diagnosed, it should be measured to provide an indication of how effective treatment has been and to engage the child to provide insights into his or her perception of it. To maximize the likelihood that measurement will be accurate and used effectively, scales must be well designed so that they are practical for staff and/or families and accessible for children (Hain, 1997; Franck, Greenberg, and Stevens, 2000). Although there are numerous scales devised for children, inconsistent use or underuse is still likely, owing to weaknesses in the concept or practicality of many of the tools, or possibly the continued low priority given to pain management on many busy acute care units. Furthermore, overemphasis on the need for subjective reporting risks avoidance or underuse of valuable and innovative scales that characterize behavior in younger children (Gauvain-Piquard et al., 1999; Hunt et al., 2004; Hain, Devins, and Davies, 2008).

Quality of Life. Pain scales have a number of important roles in assessing the effectiveness of a new approach to analgesia. For example, it is important to know that an analgesic relieves pain rather than anxiety. In evaluating the effectiveness of pediatric palliative care, however, it may be that simply measuring pain is of little value. Ultimately the intention of palliative care is to improve a child's quality of life. Good pain management is an important part of this, but there is a need for reliable, accessible, and practical tools to measure more global aspects of the quality of life (Gee et al., 2000; Young et al., 2009). Currently, there are few scales relevant to palliative care, particularly for children at or near end of life.

Treatment. The WHO pain ladder (World Health Organization, 1984, 1998; Ventafridda et al., 1989) is familiar to many clinicians around the world, although perhaps not as widely in the United States (fig. 10.1). For mild pain, management starts with simple analgesics such as acetaminophen on an "as needed" basis. For more severe pain, the ladder suggests that a fixed-dose combination opioid, such as codeine plus acetaminophen, be tried. In practice, the main benefit of this step is probably simply to give the family time to adjust to the need for major opioids (step 3) such as morphine, diamorphine (not available in the United States), oxycodone, hydromorphone, and fentanyl.

Associated with this simple approach are a number of general principles:

- Medication should usually be given orally. A number of alternative routes are available, including intravenous, subcutaneous, transcutaneous, transmucosal, rectal, nasal, epidural, and intrathecal. Nevertheless, the enteral route (oral or gastrostomy) is preferred for most children, most of the time.
- The use of appropriate adjuvants should be considered at all levels of pain. Adjuvants are medications that are not usually prescribed for pain relief, but which offer analgesia in certain situations, including some

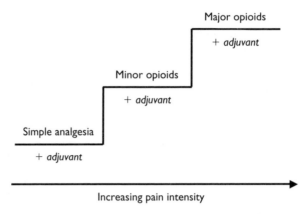

Figure 10.1. World Health Organization Pain Ladder: a straightforward approach to pain in palliative care. Some authors avoid the terms *major* and *minor* opioids, preferring instead *opioids for moderate to severe pain* and *opioids for mild to moderate pain*, respectively, to acknowledge that some opioids are intermediate. A large dose of a minor opioid is pharmacologically identical to a small dose of a major opioid; it can be argued that in children the middle step is redundant. *Source:* Adapted from WHO, 1998

anticonvulsants and antidepressants for neuropathic pain, nonsteroidal anti-inflammatory drugs (NSAIDs) for musculoskeletal pain, anticholinergics for colic, and muscle relaxants for pain caused by muscle spasm. While each of these may be effective for a particular sort of pain, opioids are usually more effective than any of them for moderate to severe pain, irrespective of the cause (Cherny, 2000).

- Opioids should be given regularly ("around the clock") to treat moderate and severe pain, with additional doses prescribed to be used as necessary for breakthrough pain.
- Nonpharmacologic methods should always be initiated in concert with medication therapy.
- Adverse drug events or side effects should be anticipated and managed expectantly.

There are three phases in initiating analgesia for pediatric patients:

1. *Selecting a Starting Dose.* The starting dose of a major opioid can be selected in one of two ways. If the child is already on a minor opioid (such as codeine), conversion can be made to the equivalent dose of oral morphine (table 10.4). Alternatively, an empiric starting dose of 1 mg/kg/day can be selected (Hewitt et al., 2008).

Table 10.4 Relative potencies of some "major" and "minor" opioids, extrapolating from adult data

Opioid	Route	Relative potency to oral morphine
Codeine	Oral	0.1
Dihydrocodeine	Oral	0.1
Tramadol	Oral	0.2
Morphine	Oral	1
Morphine SR	Oral	1
Morphine	SC	2
Morphine	CSCI	2
Diamorphine	SC	3
Diamorphine	CSCI	3
Buprenorphine	Patch	15–20
Fentanyl	Patch	150
Fentanyl	CSCI	150
Alfentanil	CSCI	30
Hydromorphone	Oral	7.5

Source: Adapted from Back, 2001.
Note: CSCI = continuous subcutaneous infusion; SC = subcutaneous.

The total daily dose should be given as six divided doses at regular 4-hour intervals. The intention of this regular dose is to keep the child from experiencing pain, and it should be given even when the child's pain is under good control. Inevitably, there will be some episodes of breakthrough pain; an additional dose of analgesia, equivalent to the regular 4-hour dose (that is to say, a sixth of the total daily dose), should be prescribed and available on an every 1- to 4-hour basis. The half-life of morphine is variable; frequency of breakthrough dosing must be tailored to the individual.

Most children will become drowsy in the first 24 to 48 hours of commencing or increasing morphine therapy. This usually resolves spontaneously, with no need to intervene or adjust the dose. Explaining this to both child and family in advance of its occurrence provides reassurance and decreases anxiety.

2. *Titrating the Dose.* The purpose of titrating the dose is to establish the individual child's opioid dose for effective relief. Good pain relief is indicated by the need for only one or two breakthrough doses per day. If more frequent breakthrough medications are needed, the regular dose should be increased by simply adding the additional

doses to the total daily dose and prescribing it, again, as six equal doses given every 4 hours. The breakthrough dose should increase proportionally, remaining a sixth of the total daily dose.

3. *Maintenance.* Once the child's opioid requirements have been established, the doses can be given in a more convenient form. For many children, slow release formulations of morphine will be appropriate. As the child's condition progresses, other approaches such as intravenous or subcutaneous infusions or transcutaneous formulations may be indicated. Whatever form regular dosing takes, it should always be accompanied by access to appropriate doses of breakthrough medications. Ideally, breakthrough medications should be complementary; for example, if using morphine or diamorphine for breakthrough to block mu1 receptors, it would be pharmacologically ideal to combine this with a mu2 receptor blocker such as fentanyl for background pain. However, for practical reasons this may not be possible, and breakthrough and background opioids are more often different formulations of the same medication (e.g., immediate and slow-release formulations of morphine).

Adverse Effects of Opioids. Constipation is almost universal among children who require major opioids. The problem is frequently exacerbated by relative dehydration and inactivity. Any prescription of major opioids for a child should therefore be accompanied by prophylactic stimulant and softening laxatives. Bulking agents are inappropriate in this setting.

Opioid-related side effects have different frequencies in adult and pediatric populations; usually nausea and vomiting occur less frequently and urinary retention and pruritus occur more often in children than adults. There is some evidence that ondansetron and oral naloxone can help (Pal, Cortiella, and Herndon, 1997); newer agents such as methylnaltrexone are also under investigation and may provide promising relief. If dose escalation results in intolerable adverse effects, consider an alternative opioid, ideally of a different type.

Special Considerations When Using Opioids in Children. Relatively little research has been published on the use of opioids in pediatric palliative care. It appears that children may clear morphine more quickly than adults and that the half-life is therefore somewhat shorter in children (Hain et al., 1999; Hunt et al., 1999; Mashayekhi et al., 2009). However, there is wide interpatient variability of morphine half-life. Scaling the adult dose of morphine down per unit weight for children does result in a similar serum concentration. Although there have been few formal studies, clinical experience indicates that the principles for use of opioids developed in adult palliative medicine can be extrapolated safely to children. If anything, children appear to be rather resistant to the toxic and beneficial effects of opioids, compared with their adult counterparts. Respiratory depression, a much-feared complication, has been reported rarely in children (Gill et al., 1996) but not in a pediatric palliative setting.

There is some pediatric research on the use of morphine and diamorphine, fentanyl, hydromorphone, and meperidine (pethidine). Of these, the incidence of seizures and its narrow therapeutic window make meperidine too toxic for use in pediatric pain relief now that experience has grown with alternatives. Proven roles for oxycodone and tramadol in pediatric palliative care have yet to be established. Methadone is particularly useful for neuropathic pain (Carpenter, Chapman, and Dickenson, 2000; Sang, 2000; Stringer et al., 2000; McDonnell, Sloan, and Hamann, 2001) and seems to be effective in children (Davies, DeVlaming, and Haines, 2008), although its use beyond the oncology population has not been robustly investigated. Diamorphine (heroin) is a highly effective opioid, which is highly soluble and therefore ideal for continuous infusion or buccal use, but unfortunately is not available in North America. Hydromorphone, which is 5–10 times more potent than morphine, but otherwise similar, is a useful alternative in the setting of fluid restriction and need for high-dose opioids. Buprenorphine and fentanyl offer the option of parenteral opioids without the need for needles, and both are sufficiently different from morphine to be appropriate for opioid substitution (Collins et al., 1999). The efficacy and safety data for fentanyl in children are considerably greater than for buprenorphine at present. (For a more specific overview of the relative potency of different opioid formulations and dosing, the reader is referred to further reviews in Drake and Hain 2006 and Friedrichsdorf and Kang 2007.)

The diagnosis of pain in children can be difficult. Some children can clearly detect and describe their pain. For others, particularly those who are non- or preverbal, a change in behavior can be the only clue. Health care professionals must respect the knowledge of usual caregivers, particularly the family. A therapeutic trial of analgesia may be the only way to distinguish pain from other causes of distress. Assessing and measuring children's pain is also difficult. Many scales are available, but most are more suitable for research than clinical applications; they work best when clinicians become familiar with a limited number of age-appropriate tools and use them consistently to best assess trends for individual patients. Beyond pain, the need remains for validated tools that assess more global aspects of quality of life, particularly for children who are terminally ill.

Although we have all been children, the memory is so far removed from our daily experience that it is difficult for most adults to draw on it. Furthermore, pediatricians rarely are experienced in recognizing and managing psychological symptoms. Comprehensive care for a child with a life-threatening condition thus requires advice and support of psychiatrists, psychologists, counselors, spiritual care providers, and other professionals outside of medicine.

A child's anxiety, like that of an adult, is based on prior experience and understanding. The child who undergoes a bone marrow aspirate while conscious may forever after find even coming into the pediatric oncology department stressful and frightening. Those working with children acknowledge the close and complex interrelationship between the attitude of children and that of their parents. It is not enough simply to explore the fears of the child; a complicated web of perception and understanding must be uncovered to reassure the whole family and help reestablish a normal family dynamic.

The mainstay of pharmacologic anxiolytic therapy in children is the benzodiazepine class; however, some young children and some who have brain injuries respond paradoxically to this class of medication. Benzodiazepines range from ultrashort acting, such as midazolam, through intermediate half-life, such as lorazepam, to longer-acting ones, such as diazepam. Midazolam is a particularly useful drug, especially for procedure-related anxiety, as it can be administered subcutaneously, by injection, by infusion, or buccally (Hussain et al., 2006). In intervening to prevent a panic spiral, in which children and parents mutually exacerbate each other's anxiety, it is clearly important to select a route with rapid onset of action.

Although benzodiazepines cause sedation as well as anxiolysis, it is important to remember that not all sedatives relieve anxiety. Chloral hydrate, for example, does little to alleviate anxiety. Nozinan (levomepromazine) is an effective soporific (Chater et al., 1998) but has an unproven role in the relief of anxiety. The distinction between soporific and anxiolytic actions should also be borne in mind when advocating the use of other medications prescribed wholly or in part for their sedative effect, such as phenobarbital.

DEPRESSION

Depression is probably under-recognized in children, and differentiating its clinical manifestations from other symptoms, such as fatigue, can be challenging. Particularly in adolescents, the syndrome closely resembles that of adults and may respond to commonly prescribed medications, such as the serotonin reuptake inhibitors. Tricyclic antidepressants, such as amitriptyline and nortriptyline, may also have a role. An advantage of these medications is that they may alleviate other symptoms. For example, they are powerful adjuvants in neuropathic pain, they may act as soporifics, and their anticholinergic activity may provide useful antiemetic effects.

AGITATION

Agitation is a difficult symptom to manage in children, as in adults. It is typically multifactorial, caused by environmental factors as much as those specific to the individual child. Multiple medications are a common cause, although children are probably more resilient than adults to the plethora of pharmaceuticals that are typically co-prescribed in the terminal phase. This underlines the need to review medications frequently, reducing the number where possible. It is also important to exclude organic causes, such as infection (particularly sepsis, respiratory or urinary tract) and undiagnosed pain, that produce, or mimic, agitation in children unable to articulate their experience. This is a particular challenge in children who are nonverbal as a result of cognitive impairment.

Where an organic cause cannot be found, neuroleptics such as haloperidol may have a role. Haloperidol is relatively nonsedating and is also a powerful antiemetic that can be combined with other medications in a single syringe (Vermeire and Remon, 1999). Benzodiazepines once again have a role. Levomepromazine, which is both neuroleptic and sedative, is often a particularly helpful medication in the terminal stages.

Phenobarbital (phenobarbitone) has been reported by clinicians to be a useful drug in the management of agitation caused by cerebral irritation, which frequently complicates an acute anoxic or septic insult to a child's brain and may be a feature of some neurodegenerative conditions. Phenobarbital can be given by mouth or by infusion. Phenobarbital is familiar to pediatricians and is an anticonvulsant, which is important because seizures commonly complicate cerebral irritation as well as metabolic disturbances and tumors.

DISORDERED SLEEP

Disordered sleep patterns are common in pediatric palliative care, particularly in patients who have a brain injury. Sleep disorder, like most other symptoms, is multifactorial. There is accordingly no single agreed-on treatment method, but the following stepwise approach is often effective:

1. Rationalize medications. Children who have disordered sleep are typically on many different medications throughout the day. Many of these are potentially sedative. As a first step, reorder medications so that all sedative ones are given at night, and readjust administration schedules as much as possible to avoid waking children who are asleep.

2. Institute or reinforce good sleep hygiene. Emphasize the distinction between day and night, including the distinction between time for sleeping and time for being awake. Thus, during the day, the child is encouraged to be active within the constraints of the condition. The curtains are open and, weather permitting, so are the windows. At night, activity and interruptions are kept to a minimum and the room is kept dark and quiet.

3. Introduce new medications. A number of medications can be useful in trying to regulate the sleep-wake cycle. Occasionally, low-dose diphenhydramine may be all that's necessary to ease a child to sleep. Melatonin is a rational choice at night because it mimics the physiology of the normal circadian rhythm (Jan, 2000; Jan et al., 2001). Short-term use of zolpidem (starting at 2.5–5 mg) can also provide relief; if no significant side effects are noted, an extended-release form is also available for children who are troubled with midsleep waking. Benzodiazepines can be useful if the child is not already receiving them. The half-life of diazepam is about 8 hours, lasting through the night. Chloral hydrate is an effective sedative but relatively irritating to the stomach. Furthermore, in the volumes required for older children it is difficult to take, and long-term use is dangerous. If the non-oral route is being considered, midazolam infusion overnight is more controllable because the drug is rapidly cleared once the infusion is discontinued in the morning.

FEEDING

The need to nurture and feed a child is a fundamental part of a parent's identity. At the first sign of flagging appetite, parents will often ask for medication to restore the child to normal food intake. Few interventions can achieve this. Reluctance to eat can, of course, be related to other gastrointestinal symptoms (see below), some of which are reversible. Where the cause is early satiety caused by gastric compression, metoclopramide, with or without steroids, may be effective. Other important organic conditions to consider and treat are oral thrush, the side effects of chemotherapy (many agents can cause metallic or other altered taste), xerostomia from radiotherapy, and untreated nausea. Steroids can produce a transient stimulation of appetite and there may be an occasional role for a short course, but prolonged use leads to disproportionate adverse effects. Megestrol acetate and cyproheptadine are commonly used, but evidence for consistent effect on quality of life is lacking, and there is probably little to be gained from considering these or other pharmacological approaches.

In fact, poor appetite is usually more of a concern to the family and professionals than it is to the child. To be forced against one's will to eat can be as unpleasant as being denied food when hungry. With this in mind, the first goal is to explore issues of feeding and appetite with the family and the child, and in particular to establish what giving or withholding feeding means to them (MacIntosh et al., 1998). This process can uncover profound differences between the family's values and understanding and those of the professional team about the child's condition and prognosis.

Even without pharmacological intervention, food can be made more attractive and palatable. A child may consider eating many small meals a day rather than a few large ones. Favorite meals, attractively presented on small plates or saucers, can often tempt the child to eat. It is important to remember that meal times are a favorite battleground for children even in the absence of life-threatening conditions; it is best to avoid food becoming an issue if at all possible.

Technical advances mean that many children are medically "fed" through nasogastric, gastrostomy, or jejunostomy tubes or with intravenous hyperalimentation. Although these modalities are often helpful and appropriate during prolonged medical illness, it may not be in the dying child's best interest for life to be artificially and unnecessarily prolonged in this way (Craig, 1996; British Medical Association, 1999; Royal College, 2004; Diekema and Botkin, 2009). Anorexia is part of the natural progression of disease, and medically provided nutrition may add to the patient's symptom burden, for example, by worsening nausea or respiratory secretions. Benefits and burdens must be assessed on a case-by-case basis; this issue is explored more fully in chapter 2.

GASTROINTESTINAL SYMPTOMS

Pain and dysfunction of the gastrointestinal (GI) tract are common in pediatric palliative care, related either to the disease process or to side effects of treatment. Assessment includes eliciting symptom intensity and symptom distress for each gastrointestinal symptom. Strategies for symptom relief depend on the presence or absence of mechanical obstruction, and potential for reversibility, if present. Inflammatory processes may be reversed if associated with infection. Noninfectious, treatment-related inflammation of the GI tract usually responds to medical therapies. Treatment of central nervous system etiologies of nausea and vomiting involves correction of the underlying process when possible (e.g., raised intracranial pressure). If obstruction is present and reversible, all attempts to promote proper motility should be undertaken. If obstruction is present and irreversible, symptoms of pain, dysphagia, nausea, vomiting, abdominal distention, and constipation must be treated aggressively. Note that opioid and other analgesics given to treat pain are likely to cause persistent bowel slowing; therefore, constipation should be anticipated and prevented.

Nausea and Vomiting. Clinicians should rationally select antiemetic agents based on the mechanism of action and an understanding of the etiology of nausea and vomiting. Centrally acting drugs can cause sedation, confusion, and extrapyramidal side effects. Newer agents that produce selective 5HT3 blockade may be more effective for chemotherapy-related nausea and vomiting. Prokinetic agents are selected when there is motility disturbance and when constipation is a concurrent problem (Peeters, 1993).

Constipation. Constipation may be relieved with dietary measures and increased fluid intake. If medications are needed, a combination of gentle stimulant laxative and stool softener is usually effective. Osmotic agents and stronger laxatives may be required. In some cases, enemas may be required to evacuate the colon and rectum before initiating an effective laxative program. Opioid antagonists can help relieve otherwise refractory opioid-induced constipation (Meissner et al., 2000; Yuan, 2007), but they must be dosed cautiously to avoid reversing the desired analgesic effects of opioids.

Irreversible Intestinal Obstruction. When intestinal obstruction is irreversible and severe nausea and vomiting accompany dysmotility of the GI tract, placement of a nasogastric tube or pharmacologic bowel paralysis is warranted. Octreotide, a long-acting analogue of somatostatin that reduces secretions, has been used to treat high-output vomiting associated with bowel obstruction in adults (Mercadante, 1994); while not yet studied in pediatric palliative care, its delivery through subcutaneous injection may limit its use.

Diarrhea. In addition to significant interference with quality of life, uncontrolled diarrhea may threaten the integrity of a patient's skin, leading to painful breakdown and increased risk of sepsis. If standard approaches are not effective in controlling diarrhea—such as eliminating offending medications, making dietary adjustments (including the addition of bulk), testing for and treating reversible causes (e.g., *Clostridium difficile* infection), and employing antispasmodic medications—anticholinergics and/or opioid derivatives can be tried. Octreotide is also helpful for high-output vomiting or diarrhea (Ripamonti, Easson, and Gerdes, 2008; Shima et al., 2008).

Oral Hygiene. Simple measures such as ice chips, wet sponges, or glycerin swabs can maintain a comfortably moist oral mucosa in the final stages of life when general dehydration naturally occurs. Pineapple chunks or ascorbic acid dissolved on the tongue can help keep the mouth feeling fresh. However, care must be taken in children whose swallowing is impaired and those who have oral or esophageal ulcerations.

Mucosal bleeding from the mouth and nose are particularly common in the setting of advanced hematopoeitic malignancy. Bleeding from the nose may originate from a single source, which can be arrested by application of a pressure dressing or by cautery. Fibrinolytic agents, such as tranexamic acid, can be effective topically (Pereira and Phan, 2004) or systemically (Dean and Tuffin, 1997). Oral agents to promote platelet aggregation may also be effective (see section on *Hemorrhage* under "Emergencies").

RESPIRATORY SYMPTOMS

Symptoms of respiratory distress (dyspnea, cough, and difficulty with secretions) are common. Clinical evaluation is directed to identify mechanical interference with breathing and structural lesions causing cough or airway irritation. Whenever possible, physical interventions to relieve mechanical interference should be considered. Simple measures such as patient positioning, better room airflow (opening a window or adding a fan), and a less physically crowded environment may relieve air hunger. Oxygen supplementation may relieve dyspnea in the setting of hypoxia, but many patients find face masks uncomfortable, as they contribute to the feeling of suffocation. Nebulized air, bronchodilators, and chest physiotherapy may be helpful. Where accumulation of cellular debris is the cause (for example, in cystic fibrosis), inhaled mucolytics such as n-acetyl cysteine can help to loosen thick secretions and make them easier to clear. Noninvasive positive pressure ventilation may be an effective means to support respiration mechanically in selected circumstances, depending on the family's goals of care and the child's comfort with the apparatus.

Systemic benzodiazepines and opioids are effective for dyspnea and cough. Nebulized morphine and fentanyl have been reported in the literature, but the results are variable (Ullrich and Mayer, 2007). Hiccup may be caused by gastric distention and is a common reversible side effect of corticosteroids. Phenothiazines may be useful for hiccup. At the end of life, noisy breathing with wet secretions (the death rattle) may be distressing to family members. Reduction of unnecessary exogenous fluids (IV, SQ, GT, etc.), as well as agents to dry secretions, such as anticholinergics (glycopyrrolate, hyoscyamine, and hyoscine), may be effective in this setting (Hain et al., 1995). Some anticholinergics are available in a transdermal patch, making them suitable for use in children.

SKIN PROBLEMS

Pruritus. Medications known to cause itching should be discontinued if possible and rashes treated with emollients, humidified air, or topical and systemic medications, as needed. In the context of individual conditions, specific interventions directed at the underlying cause may be effective. These would include the use of cholestyramine or rifampicin in pruritis associated with cholestasis, and steroids or palliative chemotherapy in the management of Hodgkin disease. Antihistamines are often used, but it is not clear whether they confer therapeutic benefit independent of their sedative effect. Less conventionally, ondansetron and oral naloxone have been tried for opioid-induced pruritus (Pal, Cortiella, and Herndon, 1997; Watterson, Denyer, and Hain, 2006). However, when opioids are the cause, it is more appropriate first to consider conversion to an alternative agent. Fentanyl may cause less pruritus than other available agents.

Pressure Sores. Pressure sores (decubitus ulcers) are usually preventable. The bedridden patient should be assessed for risk of pressure sores and predisposing factors reversed whenever possible. Excellent bed care includes skin hygiene, frequent position changes, and avoidance of hard surfaces and shearing forces on body parts. Once a bedsore is established, care is directed to promote healing of tissues and may include local dressings, debridement, and antibiotic therapy.

Malodorous Tumors. Even with excellent nursing care, tumors may progress through the skin, becoming necrotic, malodorous, and distressing to the patient and family. Good room ventilation and frequent change of room deodorizers may help. Specific charcoal- or algae-containing dressings, as well as topical and systemic antibiotics, will minimize odor and anaerobic infection. In extreme cases, short-term radiation therapy may provide relief.

OTHER SUPPORTIVE CARE CONSIDERATIONS

Family caregivers may be instructed to regularly inspect indwelling catheters for proper positioning, functioning, and signs of infection. They may also assist with catheter care and administration of medications and nutritional supplements, which may increase their personal satisfaction with caring for their child.

The patient who has impaired mobility should be assisted to be out of bed as much as is desired. Again, family members may be instructed by occupational or physical therapists in such techniques and may participate as they feel comfortable. Change of rooms and even brief trips out of doors can be beneficial to relieve patient and family boredom and feelings of entrapment.

Adequate professional support, instruction, and reassurance for family caregivers are all essential. As professionals, we are obliged to remain sensitive to family caregiver burdens and to be prepared to provide or arrange alternate hands-on care whenever needed.

Emergencies

RAISED INTRACRANIAL PRESSURE

Raised intracranial pressure is characterized by headaches, nausea, and vomiting that are typically made worse by lying down and are at their most severe first thing in the morning. Acutely elevated intracranial pressure is relatively rare, except in association with some brain tumors or shunt malfunction. A short-term solution is to give parenteral high-dose steroids, conventionally dexamethasone. Radiotherapy or surgical placement of a ventricular shunt may be needed, bearing in mind the discomfort that raised intracranial pressure can cause. In many cases, however, medical management can be effective, using a combination of acetazolamide, steroids, and appropriate pain therapy.

COMPRESSION OF THE SPINAL CORD

Compression of the spinal cord is relatively rare in childhood, in contrast with adults. It can complicate the management of cancer, in particular neuroblastoma. Even in the palliative phase, management of spinal cord compression is an emergency. Initial treatment is high-dose parenteral dexamethasone, followed by radiotherapy as the definitive treatment, depending on the family's goals of care. Surgery may be needed, if, on balance, the potential benefit to the child outweighs the burden of a possibly prolonged and painful hospital admission.

OBSTRUCTION OF THE SUPERIOR VENA CAVA

Obstruction of the superior vena cava (SVC) presents with a feeling of fullness in the head, and headaches that are worse when lying down or when the pressure is increased by Valsalva maneuvers (for example, sneezing or coughing). Findings include facial fullness and plethora, as well as dilated superficial veins over the upper thorax. The jugular vein is typically distended and nonpulsatile. Symptoms of SVC obstruction include discomfort, dyspnea, and panic. SVC syndrome commonly complicates mediastinal lymphoma, but it can also be caused by thrombosis (e.g., after long-term total parenteral nutrition through a central line). Management of the underlying cause relieves the obstruction. For tumors, treatment consists of high-dose steroids followed by radiotherapy; for clot, thrombolysis followed by anticoagulation may be indicated (Marcy et al., 2001).

INTRACTABLE SEIZURES

Children who have brain injuries, malformations, or neurodegenerative diseases often have seizures, which may increase in frequency and severity as the terminal phase nears. Often they are taking numerous anticonvulsants, but paradoxically, this profusion of medications may become epileptogenic, worsening the seizure disorder; the solution is often to simplify the regimen to one or two anticonvulsants (Richardson et al., 2004). Conversely, some children at risk for seizures toward the end of life may not be on anticonvulsants (such as children who have brain tumors); for these patients, the addition of a stable background dose of phenobarbital or phenytoin may serve to prevent distressing symptoms.

If seizures do occur, control can be secured rapidly and effectively with the use of lorazepam, phenobarbital, Tranxene, and/or midazolam. Breakthrough seizures can be managed with rectal diazepam (or paraldehyde outside of the United States). If the child is at home, these formulations allow the parents to administer the drugs rapidly as soon as the seizure begins.

It is likely that seizures are more distressing for the family than for the child him- or herself. As death draws nearer, it may not be appropriate to treat minor or short-duration seizures. It is important to be sure that the burden of the interventions we are offering the child—which will be both inconvenient and sedating—is offset by a positive impact on the child's quality of life. Parents and caregivers are often reassured when informed that seizures lasting only 5 or 10 minutes will do little harm to the child. It is always important to acknowledge, however, that even if the seizure is harmless, it may be frightening to watch.

HEMORRHAGE

Many parents greatly fear sudden catastrophic hemorrhage. In practice, it is rare; patients at highest risk are children who are dying from lymphoproliferative disorders that result in dysfunctional or deficient platelets. Some leukemias are associated with coagulopathies. These risk factors can be exacerbated by the indiscriminate use of nonsteroidal anti-inflammatory drugs, which can interfere with platelet aggregation. Once again, it is often more helpful to talk through the issue than simply to offer pharmacological solutions.

The fear of acute hemorrhage may be based on a series of much smaller bleeds, typically from the oral mucosa or from the nose. It is often possible to identify a localized bleeding point, which can be cauterized. Tranexamic acid and ethamsylate, topically or systemically, may both have a role here (Avvisati et al., 1989). Tranexamic acid is an antifibrinolytic agent that inhibits the breakdown of clots. Ethamsylate works by increasing platelet aggregation and will therefore depend on the presence of normal numbers of circulating platelets.

When severe hemorrhage is considered a likely terminal event, it may be helpful to ensure that green, black, or red towels are available at the patient's bedside. A small volume of blood can look frighteningly large when it has come from your own child, and these towels serve to reduce the visual impact of a hemorrhage. If a conscious child has a hemorrhage, sedation may be helpful; midazolam, which is both quick acting and of a short duration, is most commonly recommended (Bentley et al., 2002).

Adjunctive Therapies

CHILD-LIFE THERAPY

> The event of hospitalization seriously threatens the quality of play and the extent to which the child may engage in it. Because play is so important to the growth of the child, to impede play is to discourage normal development.
> —*Thompson and Standford*

Play has been said to be a child's work and a way for the child to make sense of the world. Having opportunities to play can help a child work through a stressful situation by gaining mastery and expressing fears and anxieties. Child-life specialists receive classroom and supervised clinical training to use medical play to facilitate a child's understanding of and comfort with medical procedures. All child-life specialists are trained in anatomy and medical terminology and have both practicum and internship experience in children's hospitals.

Parents often ask for assistance in discussing diagnosis, treatment, and prognosis with their ill child. It is important for parents to have the opportunity to meet with a child-life specialist for their concerns to be addressed, as child-life specialists are trained to communicate medical information to children in developmentally appropriate terms and can do this directly or coach parents how to do it themselves. Child-life specialists can also help parents understand the ramifications in the family system if parents withhold information from children, and they can play a significant role as an advocate for the hospitalized child and family by communicating any concerns or miscommunications to the other members of the care team.

Child-life specialists use distraction techniques to reduce procedure-related anxiety, such as bubble blowing or reading a "push the button book," providing even very young children an important sense of control and encouraging focus during uncomfortable times. An important function of child-life therapists is to provide the needed creative opportunities for ill and compromised children to express feelings and concerns (Rubin, 1992).

CREATIVE ARTS THERAPY

The creative arts therapies offer unique and novel ways to assist ill children during a time of separation and potential departure. Whether the modality is art therapy, dance/movement therapy (Mendelsohn, 1999), or music therapy, creative arts therapists help children transition from the familiar into a world that is unknown. Serious illness and dying are processes that, even in the company of others, conclude with aloneness. It is a time when sensory and bodily experiences diminish, and children turn inward toward a deep sense of ultimate quiet and stillness.

In working with children who die, the creative arts therapist attends to nuances of eye contact, body posture, images, energy level, interactive style, and verbal references, each of which may provide entry points for exploring relevant therapeutic issues. As with all caregivers, the creative arts therapist must be attuned to the family's religious and cultural beliefs to avoid imposing his or her own practices and beliefs. Through creative arts therapy, there is an acknowledgment of the completeness of the child's life, regardless of how brief. The child is empowered and reassured about potentially experiencing a wide range of emotional responses and exploring unspoken inner experiences; the creative arts therapist can provide a mechanism to delve into these important feelings. It is not possible to accompany a child fully during this intimate process if unresolved conflicts get in the way. Dealing with the vulnerabilities and personal terrors associated with loss must be addressed with a sense of dedication and commitment. The task is to be able to contain and channel one's own grief in order to allow the child fully to access his or her own (Sourkes, 1992).

Each of the following discrete developmental stages affects subsequent stages in a multifaceted manner; rigid conceptualization by age and developmental milestone thus is not helpful.

Children from birth to 3 years old chiefly express concerns such as separation anxiety and primary caregiver attachment through crying (Faulkner, 1993). The need for close and continuous physical contact is paramount. Empathic contact and stimulation can provide the basis for a secure sense of boundaries for young children when their routines are continually changing and they are exposed to aversive sensations. The dance/movement therapist may use voice, breath, touch, and movement to help young children experience various regions of the body by developing a sense of bodily organization and awareness. Use of touch and light stroking can develop a feeling of being contained within an undefined environment. It is important that stimulation across various channels (voice, breath, touch, and movement) be integrated and synchronous, facilitating greater assimilation for the young child.

General therapeutic goals include helping the young child modulate emotions and adapt to the demands of a given moment (Cohen and Walco, 1999). Dying children age 3 to 6 may have anxiety about separation, immobility, and even going to sleep. To allay some of these fears, the creative arts therapist begins where the child is and provides contact, reassurance, and gentle instruction to address the child's fears. Body movement activities provide the basis to explore a range of feelings. The dance/movement therapist may first invite the child to explore extremes in movement (e.g., strong/light, big/small, quick/slow) and then facilitate a sense of modulation and control by exploring the gradients in between. Physical contact and reassurance may provide a sense of integration on a body level, along with verbal comments that offer support and acceptance. Through art therapy, children can begin to create symbols through their drawings, depicting relevant themes and images pertaining to their experience. Their stories can be discussed and developed through the art-making process. This can enhance the child's understanding of the dying process in a less threatening manner. Creating meaningful family images and objects builds common themes and helps the whole family begin to attain a sense of closure.

For children age 6 to 12, vulnerability regarding peer rejection due to changes in physical appearance from illness and treatment may cause isolation and withdrawal. In contrast, the ability to be problem solvers and to begin to use logical thought can provide essential coping skills for children in this age group. Children begin to assimilate relational issues of isolation and separation; themes of body integrity and loss become increasingly important. Children in this phase need to have their bodies treated with careful respect, to be offered specific factual information, and to have as much control over their situation as possible.

Exploring feelings related to the dying process, both nonverbally and verbally, opens new ways of understanding challenging concerns. The creative arts therapist can offer a range of choices (e.g., choosing instruments, movement props, art materials) to facilitate a sense of control and discovery. Acknowledging the child's pace and style of expression is crucial as the therapist begins to integrate the child's thought, behavior, and emotion. Through the arts, children begin to interrelate various components about death and can integrate difficult emotional elements such as fear, anxiety, and alienation. Rituals bring in sacred elements as children attempt to attain a sense of peace when saying goodbye to loved ones.

Socially and emotionally, healthy adolescents age 12 or older are moving toward more independence and autonomy, although still dependent on parents and family members for reassurance at times. A chronically or terminally ill child is challenged in achieving these normal transitions and milestones. Personal beliefs are explored and may be influenced by symbolism in art forms and religion.

Adolescents facing the end of life are capable of speculating about the comprehensive implications and ramifications of death. They have an "adultlike" understanding about the end of their own lives, as well as the impact it has on other people and on society as a whole. Facing death may invoke anger, fear, and sorrow. Balancing a range of needs becomes an extremely delicate proposition. Professional caregivers and family members negotiate the teenager's need for privacy, closeness, and independence in just the right doses. Because their peers are such an important part of most adolescents' lives, they need opportunities to interact with friends and may also have a strong drive to document their lives in a global context.

Facing the reality of premature death can be expressed in nonverbal forms that potentially facilitate greater acceptance. Observation of the teen's body movement dynamics (e.g., gestures, postures, interactive style) can help others understand some of the issues that are otherwise difficult to communicate. Creative arts therapy provides adolescents with an important avenue in which to identify emotional material that may be difficult to access by verbal language alone. Art images and symbols, key themes in recorded music, musical improvisation, and songwriting provide teenagers with alternative, less threatening mechanisms to explore the dying process. The creation of videotapes, art objects, murals, and dances enables adolescents to say goodbye and leave a legacy.

DANCE/MOVEMENT THERAPY

Dance/movement therapy focuses on body movement as a manifestation of thoughts and feelings. It should be noted that "dance" and "movement" are each viewed in the broadest context to encompass elements of traditional dance forms, patterns of movements, gestures, postures, and more subtle aspects of nonverbal communication. A fundamental premise is that psychological processes, such as affect and cognition, are expressed consistently through nonverbal means.

ART THERAPY

Art can serve as an assessment tool to provide further information about the child's response to illness, treatment, and dying. Art therapy allows children to express their feelings by creating a visual image for their fears, anger, frustrations, and fantasies; the art therapist then communicates these feelings to the child's family and medical team. Art therapy provides tactile stimulation, distraction from pain, an opportunity for choice, and a means to achieve mastery. Art is a familiar language for all children. For children, often what cannot be said in words can be said through images.

MUSIC THERAPY

Sensitively improvised music can help a frightened child feel less threatened and can initiate the establishment of trust and rapport. Music can reduce children's isolation by including family members or medical staff in sessions, increasing opportunities for positive interactions. Improvisational music therapy is used to engage, empower, and focus children undergoing painful medical procedures and can be a useful tool for processing their experiences afterward. Active songwriting and improvisation can be used to encourage children to relate their experiences and explore their feelings within a creative structure. Various tones, musical dynamics, and rhythm are used to decrease pain, stress, and anxiety by promoting distraction, release, soothing, or comfort.

The progression of disease processes may engender a sense of lack of control. Within the music therapy experience, children can regain a sense of involvement with their own care.

Conclusion

Whatever term is used—holistic, multidimensional, person-centered—those working in pediatric palliative care recognize the need for a wide understanding of a child's experience and needs, particularly as he or she approaches death.

This chapter first examined the ways in which medical management can address some of those needs. Evidence-based, well-considered, and compassionate use of medications and other medical interventions to attenuate symptoms can dramatically improve the quality of a child's life and play an important part in palliative care for many children. This is particularly true of symptoms that have a largely physical basis, but medical management can also help address emotional and psychological dimensions of suffering.

Medical interventions alone, however, are rarely sufficient. This chapter also considered some of the nonmedical approaches that can affect the quality of a child's life and that of his or her family. While not an exhaustive list, the modalities considered here illustrate the range of therapies that can be of value. Throughout the developmental continuum, play, imagination, and creativity provide natural outlets for expression. When children want others to understand their inner experience, nonverbal communication vehicles may be essential tools.

Confronting chronic or terminal illness and end of life requires the identification of feelings as well as mechanisms to share them safely with others. Creative arts therapy brings a richness and potency to that expression. Resolving conflicts, decreasing isolation, and maximizing comfort are essential in attempting to gain ultimate peace and acceptance. For caregivers, there are unique opportunities to participate in an extremely intimate experience, as children and their families face final separation. In the words of Saint-Exupery's Little Prince, "One runs the risk of weeping a little, if one lets himself be tamed."

References

Anand, K.J. 2000a. Effects of perinatal pain and stress. *Prog Brain Res* 122:117–29.
———. 2000b. Pain, plasticity, and premature birth: A prescription for permanent suffering? *Nat Med* 6(9):971–73.
Avvisati, G., ten Cate, J.W., Büller, H.R., et al. 1989. Tranexamic acid for control of haemorrhage in acute promyelocytic leukaemia. *Lancet* 2(8655):122–24.
Back, I.N. 2001. *Palliative Medicine Handbook*. Cardiff, Wales, UK: BPM Books.
Baker, C.M., and Wong, D.L. 1987. QUEST: A process of pain assessment in children. *Orthopaedic Nursing* 6(1):11–21.
Bentley, R., Cope, J., Jenney, M., et al. 2002. Use of intranasal/oral midazolam in paediatric palliative care. *Arch Dis Child* 86(Supp 1):A76.
British Medical Association. 1999. Withholding and withdrawing life-prolonging medical treatment: Guidance for decision making. London: BMJ Publishing Group.
Carpenter, K.J., Chapman, V., and Dickenson, A.H. 2000. Neuronal inhibitory effects of methadone are predominantly opioid receptor mediated in the rat spinal cord *in vivo*. *Eur J Pain* 4:19–26.
Chater, S., Viola, R., Paterson, J., et al. 1998. Sedation for intractable distress in the dying: A survey of experts. *Palliat Med* 12(4):255–69.

Cherny, N.I. 2000. The management of cancer pain. *CA Cancer J Clin* 50(2):70–116; quiz 117–20.

Cohen, S.O., and Walco, G.A. 1999. Dance/movement therapy for children and adolescents with cancer. *Cancer Practice* 7(1):34–42.

Collins, J.J., Dunkel, I.J., Gupta, S.K., et al. 1999. Transdermal fentanyl in children with cancer pain: Feasibility, tolerability, and pharmacokinetic correlates. *J Pediatr* 134:319–23.

Colver, A., and Jessen, C. 2000. Measurement of health status and quality of life in neonatal follow-up studies. *Semin Neonatol* 5(2):149–57.

Craig, G.M. 1996. On withholding artificial hydration and nutrition from terminally ill sedated patients: The debate continues. *J Med Ethics* 22:147–53.

Craig, K.D., and Grunau, R.V.E. 1993. Neonatal pain perception and behavioral measurement. In *Pain in Neonates*, ed. K.S.J. Anand and P.J. McGrath, pp. 67–105. Vancouver: Elsevier Science.

Davies, D., DeVlaming, D., and Haines, C. 2008. Methadone analgesia for children with advanced cancer. *Pediatr Blood Cancer* 51(3):393–97.

Dean, A., and Tuffin, P. 1997. Fibrinolytic inhibitors for cancer-associated bleeding problems. *J Pain Symptom Manage* 13(1):20–24.

Diekema, D.S., Botkin, J.R., and the AAP COB. 2009. Forgoing medically-provided nutrition and hydration in children. *Pediatrics* 124(2):813–22.

Drake, R., and Hain, R.D.W. 2006. Pain: Pharmacological management. In *Oxford Textbook of Palliative Care for Children*, ed. A. Goldman, R. Hain, and S. Liben, pp. 304–41. Oxford: Oxford University Press.

Faulkner, K.W. 1993. Children's understanding of death. In *Hospice Care for Children*, ed. A. Armstrong-Dailey and S. Zarbock, pp. 9–22. New York: Oxford University Press.

Franck, L.S., Greenberg, C.S., and Stevens, B. 2000. Pain assessment in infants and children. *Pediatr Clin North Am* 47(3):487–512.

Friedrichsdorf, S.J., and Kang, T.I. 2007. The management of pain in children with life-limiting illnesses. *Pediatr Clin North Am* 54(5):645–72.

Gauvain-Piquard, A., Rodary, C., Rezvani, A., et al. 1999. The development of the DEGR(R): A scale to assess pain in young children with cancer. *Eur J Pain* 3(2): 165–76.

Gee, L., Abbott, J., Conway, S.P., et al. 2000. Development of a disease specific health related quality of life measure for adults and adolescents with cystic fibrosis. *Thorax* 55(11):946–54.

Gill, A.M., Cousins, A., Nunn, A.J., et al. 1996. Opiate-induced respiratory depression in pediatric patients. *Ann Pharmacother* 30:125–29.

Goldman, A., Hewitt, M., Collins, G.S., et al. 2006. Symptoms in children/young people with progressive malignant disease: United Kingdom Children's Cancer Study Group/Paediatric Oncology Nurses Forum survey. *Pediatrics* 117(6): e1179–86.

Hain, R., Devins, M., and Davies, R. 2008. Douleur enfant Gustave Roussey scale in an English-speaking population: Correlation with visual analogue scale. *Arch Dis Ch* 93(Suppl 1):A64.

Hain, R.D., and Campbell, C. 2001. Invasive procedures carried out in conscious children: Contrast between North American and European paediatric oncology centres. *Arch Dis Child* 85(1):12–15.

Hain, R.D., Hardcastle, A., Pinkerton, C.R., and Aherne, G.W. 1999. Morphine and morphine-6-glucuronide in the plasma and cerebrospinal fluid of children. *Br J Clin Pharmacol* 48(1):37–42.

Hain, R.D.W. 1997. Pain scales in children: A review. *Palliat Med* 11:341–50.

———. 2005. Palliative care in children in Wales: A study of provision and need. *Palliat Med* 19:137–42.

Hain, R.D.W., and Hughes, E. 2001. Children referred for specialist palliative care: First 25 patients. *Arch Dis Child* 85:12–15.

Hain, R.D.W., Patel, N., Crabtree, S., et al. 1995. Respiratory symptoms in children dying from malignant disease. *Palliat Med* 206:203–8.

Hewitt, M., Goldman, A., Collins, G.S., et al. 2008. Opioid use in palliative care of children and young people with cancer. *J Pediatr* 152:39–44.

Hunt, A., Goldman, A., Seers, K., et al. 2004. Clinical validation of the paediatric pain profile. *Dev Med Child Neurol* 46:9–18.

Hunt, A., Joel, S., Dick, G., and Goldman, A. 1999. Population pharmacokinetics of oral morphine and its glucuronides in children receiving morphine as immediate-release liquid or sustained-release tablets for cancer pain. *J Pediatr* 135(1):47–55.

Hussain, N., Regan, E., Gosalakkal, J., et al. 2006. Use of buccal midazolam in children. *Arch Dis Child* 91(12):1041–42.

Jalmsell, L., Kreicbergs, U., Onelov, E., et al. 2006. Symptoms affecting children with malignancies during the last month of life: A nationwide follow-up. *Pediatrics* 117(4):1314–20.

Jan, J.E., Tai, J., Hahn, G., et al. 2001. Melatonin replacement therapy in a child with a pineal tumor. *J Child Neurol* 16(2):139–40.

Jan, M.M. 2000. Melatonin for the treatment of handicapped children with severe sleep disorders. *Pediatr Neurol* 23(3):229–32.

Lowery, C.L., Hardman, M.P., Manning, N., et al. 2007. Neurodevelopmental changes of fetal pain. *Semin Perinatol* 31(5):275–82.

MacIntosh, N., Alderson, P., Bates, P., et al., eds. 1998. *Withholding or Withdrawing Life Saving Treatment in Children: A Framework for Practice*. London: Royal College of Paediatrics and Child Health.

Marcy, P.Y., Magne, N., Bentolila, F., et al. 2001. Superior vena cava obstruction: Is stenting necessary? *Support Care Cancer* 9(2):103–7.

Mashayekhi, S.O., Ghandforoush-Sattari, M., Routledge, P.A., et al. 2009. Pharmacokinetic and pharmacodynamic study of morphine and morphine 6-glucuronide after oral and intravenous administration of morphine in children with cancer. *Biopharm Drug Dispos* 30(3):99–106.

McDonnell, F.J., Sloan, J.W., and Hamann, S.R. 2001. Advances in cancer pain management. *Curr Pain Headache Rep* 5(3):265–71.

McGraw, M. 1941. Neural maturation as exemplified in the changing reactions of the infant to pin prick. *Child Dev* 12(1):31–42.

Meissner, W., et al. 2000. Oral naloxone reverses opioid-induced constipation. *Pain* 84:105–9.

Mendelsohn, J. 1999. Dance/movement therapy with hospitalized children. *Am J Dance Therapy* 21(2):65–80.

Mercadante, S. 1994. The role of octreotide in palliative care. *J Pain Symptom Manage* 9(6):406–11.

Pal, S.K., Cortiella, J., and Herndon, D. 1997. Adjunctive methods of pain control in burns. *Burns* 23(5):404–12.

Peeters, T.L. 1993. Erythromycin and other macrolides as prokinetic agents. *Gastroenterology* 105:1886–99.

Pereira, J., and Phan, T. 2004. Management of bleeding in patients with advanced cancer. *Oncologist* 9(5):561–70.

Porter, F.L., Grunau, R.E., and Anand, K.J. 1999. Long-term effects of pain in infants. *J Dev Behav Pediatr* 20(4):253–61.

Richardson, S.P., Farias, S.T., Lima, A.R., et al. 2004. Improvement in seizure control and quality of life in medically refractory epilepsy patients converted from polypharmacy to monotherapy. *Epilepsy Behav* 5(3):343–47.

Ripamonti, C.I., Easson, A.M., and Gerdes, H. 2008. Management of malignant bowel obstruction. *Eur J Cancer* 44(8):1105–15.

Royal College for Paediatrics and Child Health. 2004. *Withholding or Withdrawing Life Sustaining Treatment in Children: A Framework for Practice*, 2nd ed. London: Royal College of Paediatrics and Child Health.

Rubin, S. 1992. What's in a name? Child life and the play lady legacy. *Children's Healthcare* 21(1):4.

Sang, C.N. 2000. NMDA-receptor antagonists in neuropathic pain: Experimental methods to clinical trials. *J Pain Symptom Manage* 19(1 Suppl):S21–25.

Shima, Y., Ohtsu, A., Shirao, K., et al. 2008. Clinical efficacy and safety of octreotide (SMS201–995) in terminally ill Japanese cancer patients with malignant bowel obstruction. *Jpn J Clin Oncol* 38(5):354–59.

Sourkes, B.M. 1992. The child with a life-threatening illness. In *Countertransference in Psychotherapy with Children and Adolescence*, ed. J. Brandell. New York: Aronson Press.

Stringer, M., Makin, M.K., Miles, J., et al. 2000. d-morphine, but not l-morphine, has low micromolar affinity for the non-competitive N-methyl-D-aspartate site in rat forebrain: Possible clinical implications for the management of neuropathic pain. *Neurosci Lett* 295(1–2):21–24.

Thompson, R.H., and Standford, G. 1981. *Child Life in Hospitals: Theory and Practice.* Springfield, IL: Charles C. Thomas.

Twycross, R. 1997. *Symptom Management in Advanced Cancer.* Oxford: Radcliffe Medical Press.

Ullrich, C.K., and Mayer, O.H. 2007. Assessment and management of fatigue and dyspnea in pediatric palliative care. *Pediatr Clin North Am* 54(5):735–56.

Ventafridda, V., Tamburini, M., Caraceni, A., et al. 1989. A validation study of the WHO method for cancer pain relief. *Cancer* 59:850–56.

Vermeire, A., and Remon, J.P. 1999. Compatibility and stability of ternary admixtures of morphine with haloperidol or midazolam and dexamethasone or methylprednisolone. *Int J Pharm* 177(1):53–67.

Watterson, G., Denyer, J., and Hain, R.D.W. 2006. Skin symptoms. In *Oxford Textbook of Palliative Care in Children*, ed. A. Goldman, R. Hain, and S. Liben, pp. 448–59. Oxford: Oxford University Press.

Wolfe, J., Grier, H.E., Klar, N., et al. 2000. Symptoms and suffering at the end of life in children with cancer [see comments]. *N Engl J Med* 342(5):326–33.

World Health Organization. 1984. *Cancer as a Global Problem*. Geneva: WHO.

———. 1998. Guidelines for analgesic drug therapy. In *Cancer Pain Relief and Palliative Care in Children*, pp. 24–28. Geneva: WHO/IASP.

Young, N.L., Varni, J.W., Snider, L., et al. 2009. The Internet is valid and reliable for child-report: An example using the Activities Scale for Kids (ASK) and the Pediatric Quality of Life Inventory (PedsQL). *J Clin Epidemiol* 62(3):314–20.

Yuan, C.S. 2007. Methylnaltrexone mechanisms of action and effects on opioid bowel dysfunction and other opioid adverse effects. *Ann Pharmacother* 41(6):984–93.

Zebracki, K., and Drotar, D. 2008. Pain and activity limitations in children with Duchenne or Becker muscular dystrophy. *Dev Med Child Neurol* 50(7):546–52.

Bereavement

Stacy F. Orloff, Ed.D., L.C.S.W., A.C.H.P.-S.W., Suzanne S. Toce, M.D., Lizabeth Sumner, R.N., B.S.N., and Lee Ann Grimes

Nine months after her child's death, a mother shares that it wasn't until 2 months ago that she could acknowledge that she wasn't bringing him home.

A father whose son died of cancer despite valiant efforts becomes angry when he remembers his son's ordeal. He has never cried since his son died 3 years ago, admitting that he lives behind a hard, protective shell that only his wife and daughter can penetrate.

The death of one's child can be among the most difficult losses to grieve. This is especially true when the child is underage and depends on the parent for life-sustaining activities. One goal of hospice and palliative care programs is to assist the family in being "prepared" for the death. Many hospice/palliative care professionals also speak about a "good" death. However, for family members facing the death of a child, no death is good and no one in the family is ever truly ready or prepared. The best that health care professionals can do is to assist the family in finding a way for the death to occur in a manner that reflects their goals, values, cultural practices, and religious and spiritual beliefs.

Health care professionals know much more about the experience of bereavement than in years past:

- A commonality in loss exists for all bereaved families.
- There may be particular nuances and unique features of the grief process for families whose child dies suddenly or with an uncertain prognosis.

- A perinatal loss often entails unique meanings and is experienced differently from an older child's death.

This chapter will address the common bereavement experience as well as some unique features associated with perinatal, sudden, or uncertain death.

Health care providers understand that they are not the experts in showing families how to grieve. Just as the goals of care for the living child are mutually derived by the patient, family, and clinicians, the bereavement plan of care is directed by the surviving family members. The hospice/palliative care team serves as a guide and fellow traveler on this uncharted journey, providing support if the family feels they are losing their way.

For families, the death of a child symbolizes the loss of a future—the dream that this child will continue the family's legacy. The effect of this death may reverberate through the family in untold ways. Heartfelt grief is also noted by the larger community that surrounded the child, such as the child's peers and classmates, teachers, members of the family's faith community, and the health care professionals involved in the child's care. According to a recent study, regardless of the number of years that have passed, memories of the child's life and death remain fresh (Arnold and Gemma, 2008). Families and individual family members are forever changed by this experience. Parents must learn to integrate their grief in such a way that they can focus on their loss in a controlled manner while restoring their capacity for daily functioning (Barrera et al., 2007). Parents, siblings, grandparents, and all others who were a part of the child's life need the informed support of health care professionals as they grieve.

When a child dies, a large void is left, both physically and figuratively. There is an empty bed, toys no longer played with, perhaps an empty kitchen chair. These reminders are present day in and day out for all members of the family. For some, these are painful reminders, while for others tangible objects such as a favorite doll or sweatshirt provide great comfort.

Common Themes

Some generalities about parental grief are universal. A study found two factors to decrease parental grief: the parents' ability to say goodbye to their child (this could have been said at or before the time of death or could have been completed through a symbolic ritual at a later date) and the decision to have their child laid out at home (Wijngaards-De Meij et al., 2008).

Many factors may influence how the family grieves the death of the child.

In trying to effectively assist them, health care professionals need to note such things as

- how the family has coped with prior losses;
- whether or not the family has experienced the death of any other children;
- how effective the family's support system is; and
- whether or not the family has a spiritual grounding or religious faith.

It is important to monitor for withdrawn behaviors, comments indicating that an individual is contemplating self-harm, and inability to carry out day-to-day functioning.

Guilt plagues most bereaved parents. Clinicians can frequently address parents' doubts about having made the right treatment decisions for the child by honoring requests to review the medical events of the child's illness and death with different members of the medical health care team. Parents may question medical decisions they made, concerned they have hastened their child's death or altered the treatment outcome. In a study assessing parental grief patterns (Barrera et al., 2007), one mother stated, "I still feel guilty. As being a mother. I think I, I did everything I could for her but, ah . . . maybe I, I should, I could do, I could cuddle her much longer, if I knew she's not going to make it. . . . I just can't stop thinking maybe I did something wrong during my pregnancy."

Guilt may arise from questions of having made the right treatment decisions for the child, the decision to pursue palliative rather than life-prolonging treatment, or even having conceived or given birth to a child who developed a terminal illness or "genetically infecting" the child with the disease. Guilt may also result from breaking the perceived cultural injunction to protect one's child against harm or from either behaviorally or emotionally abandoning other children or family members while caring for the deceased child.

Bereaved parents sometimes feel a need to blame someone for the death of their child. Such a need is strong when the child died in an accident, by suicide, or by homicide, but the same can hold true for the child who dies of natural causes. Sometimes the need to blame is targeted toward a marriage partner or other family member, placing stress on the whole family system. It is also possible for parents to treat a family member, such as a child, as a scapegoat after a death. Clinicians need to be aware of these dynamics and help families find the appropriate ways to deal with anger and blame.

Long after the acute pain of the death has subsided, graduations, marriages, births, children playing, and other life events remind the bereaved of what might have been if the child had survived. These events bring about renewed pain. One grieving mother said, "All I know is that this will go on for a long time but I look forward to the day when the pain will not be so intense. I know that life will never be the same as if my child had survived, but I hope one day to make some sense of all of this and perhaps even find some meaning for what we are going through." By addressing the pain, seeking to feel understood and not judged, negotiating painful events, and perhaps discovering some meaning in the loss, grieving parents may find that life can return to normal—not the normal as it was or would have been, but a new normal.

Many family members struggle with a central task of mourning: accepting the reality of the child's death (Worden, 2002). In a study (Arnold and Gemma, 2008), 64 parents were asked to describe what acceptance meant for them when thinking about their deceased child. Most parents offered that the death must be accepted because it could not be changed, and acceptance was not possible because the loss was not tolerable. They may appear to understand and accept the death, but emotionally they are not ready. It is common for family friends and health care professionals, out of their own discomfort with death, to encourage the bereaved family to reconnect socially with others, return to work, and clean out the child's room and belongings. It is more comforting to reassure parents that they will know when they are ready to take care of cleaning the room or resuming regular activities.

Expression of feelings is another task of mourning and is influenced by personality, ego strength, and cultural and religious values. Expression of feelings is an important goal of bereavement counseling. Rituals and other nonverbal means (e.g., keeping a journal, art activities, a balloon release or tree planting) to commemorate special dates are useful ways to express feelings. Children are especially comforted by rituals.

Grieving is a social phenomenon. For grief to progress and the tasks of mourning to be accomplished, grieving persons need an opportunity to share their grief and experiences with others. Such sharing includes talking about the events leading up to the death, including the diagnosis, treatment, and interactions with others and with the deceased. Some people feel uncomfortable around bereaved parents and may cut off such conversations. A thematic analysis of parental grief showed that for parents, sharing keeps memories vivid and parents are happy to talk about their child's life and death and memories. Bereaved parents desire to share their grief, but few ask or are willing to listen (Arnold and Gemma, 2008). Support groups for bereaved parents can be a safe haven to share their thoughts and feelings with others who have also lost a child.

Meert et al. (2007) conducted a study in which they asked parents to determine how they felt regarding the desirability, content, and conditions of a physician-parent conference after the death of their child in the pediatric intensive care unit (PICU). What parents most desired to gain from the meeting was more information. Second, they wanted to provide feedback to the physician regarding their PICU experience. To a lesser extent, they expressed a need for emotional support. Other informational topics parents mentioned included chronology of events leading to PICU admission and death, cause of death, treatment, autopsy, genetic risk, medical documents, discontinuation of life support, ways to help others, bereavement support, and what to tell other family members. When asked to rank the importance of predefined topics, they gave the order of importance as information about treatment, autopsy, cause of death, medical records, and bereavement support.

Prevalent in the medical community is the notion that the family's experience of the death of a child results in a higher divorce rate for the parents of that child. It is felt that the child's death places stressors on the marriage that can cause the marriage to dissolve. A review of the literature on this subject showed that the death of a child is likely to affect the marital relationship; however, these effects can be negative or positive. In fact, evidence suggests that a greater number of couples remain married and that the marriage may be strengthened as a result of their experiences (Reiko, 1998).

PARENTAL GRIEF

There is some evidence to suggest that mothers and fathers grieve the loss of their child differently. Several studies have shown that bereaved mothers grieve more intensely and are more distressed than bereaved fathers (Lang and Gottlieb, 1993; Moriarty, Carroll, and Cotroneo, 1996; Murphy et al., 1998). However, other studies have found that the intensity of fathers' grief is equal to that of mothers but fathers' ways of grieving can be incongruent; that is, parents do not grieve in the same ways or over the same period of time (Hunfeld et al., 1993; Aho et al., 2006; Lannen et al., 2008). Also these perceived gender differences depend on which measures are used as indicators of grief (Vance et al., 1995a). If only measures of anxiety and depression are used, it appears that women are considerably more disturbed than men by the loss of their child. However, when measures of alcohol use are included as a reaction to stress, the difference in responses between men and women becomes much smaller or even nonexistent.

Some explain the difference between mothers' and fathers' ways of grieving by looking at the nature of the relationship between the parent and the child (Lang and Gottlieb, 1993; Gamino, 1999). This is particularly relevant when newborns die. Gamino (1999), whose infant son died a few hours after birth, reported that his grief differed from his wife's grief because each was attached differently to the baby. For him, the relationship was more abstract, while for his wife, Marla, it was more physiologic. Because of the fetus's small size, Gamino felt his son move only a couple of times while in utero. Marla, however, often felt the baby kick her internal organs and had a stronger sense of his aliveness, which, at times, gave her comfort in her grief, while her husband was more often sad. Others have also studied pregnancy loss and found similar findings (Samuelsson, Radestad, and Segesten, 2001; McCreight, 2004).

MOTHERS' GRIEF

In most families, the mother is the primary caregiver. It is therefore not unexpected that mothers can become consumed in grief after the loss of their child. A study that looked at parental grief patterns after the loss of a child found that only mothers experienced overwhelming grief (Barrera et al., 2007). These mothers had difficulty finding a way to reframe their loss in a positive way, and some were unable to accept the death of their child.

Mothers of disabled children also struggle with long-term care needs and bereavement. In a study interviewing mothers after the deaths of their developmentally disabled children, mothers reported that parenting a child with a disability and then losing that child had transformed many aspects of their life—sense of identity, world view, relationships, spirituality, and priorities—and they viewed the experience as a blessing (Milo, 1997).

FATHERS' GRIEF

Although the death of a child greatly affects the entire family, the mother-child dyad commonly receives the most attention from the health care team. This attention first begins with concern for the mother's health during pregnancy and continues with a focus on the mother-child relationship. This emphasis is reflected both within clinical practice and in the literature, as studies of mothers and children are by far more common than studies of fathers. It is, therefore, not surprising that this emphasis is also found with bereavement research, in which studies of mothers' grief are in abundance in comparison with studies of fathers' grief.

Fathers may not be allowed to sense and express their own emotions, because they are expected to be "strong" for the sake of their wife and other family members. One father asked, "When is it my turn to cry?" He offered his own answer: "I'm not sure society or my upbringing will ever allow me a time to really cry, because of the reaction and repercussion that might follow. I must be strong for my wife because I am a man. I must be the cornerstone of our family because society says so, my family says so, and, until I can reverse my learned nature, I say so" (DeFrain et al., 1991, p. 112). This father's statement illustrates society's perspective of fathers' grief and raises the question of how this perception of fathers' experiences affects clinicians as they care for bereaved fathers.

Clinicians and researchers specializing in men's grief agree that men's emotional life consists of the tension between the need for expressing unhappy feelings and fear of the consequences of doing so. Pollack (1998) claims that historical, cultural, and economic forces have affected parenting styles in such a way that men experience a premature psychic separation from both maternal and paternal caregivers. This may later become problematic for men as they unconsciously try to protect themselves from further loss by blocking expression of all strong emotions except anger. Consequently, their ability to grieve and mourn is impaired, as they have an inability to tolerate feelings of vulnerability or to express and bear sadness. Moreover, men often find themselves in a dilemma stemming from the societal expectation that men should comfort their wives and from the cultural notion that healthy grieving requires the sharing of feelings. A female bias in conceptualization and measurement of grief and in bereavement interventions makes fathers' grief invisible to both clinicians and researchers.

Before their child's death, many fathers experienced anticipatory grief, which often began when the father learned that his child was seriously ill and/or the prognosis was poor. Anticipatory grief was shown to inhibit subsequent grieving owing to the long-term stress that it had caused. One father stated, "I was stressed and nervous already a long time before the death of our child. . . . The stress caused by the death and worrying about my wife and child probably added to my grief" (Aho et al., 2006).

Fathers also experienced despair and hope. The illness at times could be so burdensome that fathers felt they had lost control over their lives and experienced mental exhaustion. Feelings of conflict were not uncommon. Often, on watching their children suffer, fathers wished for their child's death, yet if aggressive therapy was forgone, emotions ranged from relief to agony to anger. Fathers felt guilty that they could not prevent their child from dying and worried that their flawed genes or actions contributed to their child's death. Not all emotions were negative. Gratitude, joy, and relief after the child's death occurred when fathers felt that their children were no longer experiencing pain and suffering; however, these feelings often spurred feelings of guilt later (Aho et al., 2006).

Fathers were not immune to physical reactions. Fathers described "shivering," "a strong feeling of pressure," "migraine," "arrhythmia," "physical pain," and "tiredness" as physical manifestations immediately after their child's death. They also acknowledged causing themselves pain and feelings of agony after the deaths. As one father stated, "Last spring I got a tattoo, it was Peter's [dead son] handprint . . . getting the tattoo was so hard, well there was a physical side to it and pain. . . . It was also like living again those days, and now I have it [tattoo], every morning and evening . . . when I see it, I kind of jump to those feelings again" (Aho et al., 2006).

Socially, fathers suffered as well. Fathers withdrew from relationships, were less motivated for work, and had difficulty concentrating. Some turned to alcohol. To cope, physical activity was a frequent theme, with fathers describing weeping, shouting, expressing rage, and physical work and activity as helpful coping activities (Aho et al., 2006).

However, men seem to work hard at their "grief work." Their coping strategies commonly emphasize suppressing and blocking of thoughts about the death, controlling upsetting emotions in order not to hurt others, and earnest attempts to deal with their wives' need for their husbands' expressiveness. Bereaved fathers exert considerable effort at managing their emotions, despite seeming to be less affected by the loss when assessed through various measures (Cook, 1988). Instead of expressing their grief, men are more likely to be active and to keep themselves busy by working long hours and/or physically exhausting themselves through participation in sports (Worden, 1996; Wood and Milo, 2001). Nevertheless, there is room for individual differences in the response to the loss of a child. Some fathers are silent and stoic, not liking to openly express emotions; other fathers need to talk about and express their emotions to facilitate their own healing. Two fathers grieving the loss of their sons to cancer illustrate the range of fathers' grief reactions (Davies et al., 2004).

Mike's 12-year-old son Alex died of brain cancer despite several treatments, including treatment in another state. Mike had a win/lose perspective of his family's battle with cancer. He became angry when the cancer relapsed, "chewing the cancer out" at his son's deathbed.

In the 3 years since Alex's death, Mike has never cried; his strongest emotion is anger. He is less tolerant of other people's struggles and admits that he has a hard, protective shell around him. The only people who can penetrate it are his wife and surviving daughter. From the beginning, Mike felt the need to be strong for his family. Although he has wanted to cry, as soon as he feels tears approaching, he unconsciously "shuts it off" by changing his thoughts, talking through it, or going somewhere else. When asked how and when he had learned to prevent himself from crying, he said, "I guess we were brought up that guys never cry," while at the same time admitting that his wife and daughter believe crying would help him in his grief. Mike even sought bereavement therapy for 18 months, but he was still unable to cry. He is aware of his restricted emotional repertoire. Although he believes that it would be better for him to express his hidden emotions, he is not ready for that.

Andrew lost his 15-year-old son Daniel to leukemia. Andrew initially believed that he needed to be strong, resourceful, and confident for his family. However, he also realized that this experience might destroy his family and discovered that he needed and wanted to talk about it. Moreover, his wife needed him to show his fears, worries, and sadness as they lived through this challenging time, and as he says, "I learned to get over my sort of rock of Gibraltar routine." Andrew's way of dealing with his newfound need to talk honestly about how he felt was to tell anyone who asked exactly what was troubling him, instead of saying that he was doing fine if he wasn't.

Andrew also finds comfort in his faith and spirituality. He describes himself as having an "ecumenical or postdenominational outlook on religion," but he found that his life experience brought him in touch with his own spirituality on a much deeper level than before his son's illness. He learned to pray anew, and as he sat on his son's deathbed, holding his hand and reading aloud from "The Tibetan Book of the Dead," he realized that his son was not just his child, but "a soul in his own destiny." Andrew's spirituality continues to nurture him 2 years after Daniel's death. He views life as bittersweet without Daniel but says that he still has loving to give and receive. He believes that celebrating life honors the memory of his son.

There is much to learn from these two fathers. Mike fits the stereotype of a man who has a difficult time expressing his emotions. Andrew discovered that it helped him and his family to open up and to learn to express his emotions characteristic of "women's ways" of coping with sorrow.

It is important to emphasize that no one way of grieving is better than another. However, clinicians need to be aware of and open to the many ways in which men express their grief. By accepting differences among men, clinicians will better support bereaved fathers as they uniquely grieve for their child.

Clinicians might help fathers by acknowledging the particular way each father is grieving. For example, fathers who are trying to be strong for the sake of their family need to be complimented for their endeavor. It may also be important for other family members, such as the mother, to understand that her husband's limited emotional expression may represent his inherent need to protect his family.

Mike saw his inability to cry as a deficit. Acknowledging that he may not be the kind of person who cries when faced with a tragedy and talking about the strong feelings he has, namely, his anger and frustration, and how they affect his life may be more therapeutic. Andrew's spirituality was helpful to him. Helping fathers evaluate their strengths and use them to heal is an important way to help.

Attendance at support groups is often recommended to the newly bereaved, but many fathers do not find them helpful, and if they go, they frequently go only to support their wives (Worden and Monahan, 2000). This behavior may emanate from their gender socialization and their common need to be more private about their grief (Cook, 1988; Murphy et al., 1998). As we learn more about the unique ways in which fathers live with the loss of a beloved child, we will be better able to offer care that is attuned to the special needs of fathers and thereby provide optimal care to all members of the family.

SIBLINGS' GRIEF

Siblings are often forgotten or, at the very least, poorly informed and rarely included during the time their brother or sister is ill, and this often continues after the death. Surviving siblings report that they often were not well informed about their sibling's illness and would have welcomed the opportunity to discuss the implications of the disease (Nolbris and Hellström, 2005). These siblings also felt they would have benefited from meeting individuals in a similar situation, both before and after their sibling's death, as loneliness was a prevalent feeling for them (Nolbris and Hellström, 2005).

Surviving children may attempt to take over the role(s) of their deceased sibling, such as the "good" child, the athlete, or the "funny" child. It is important to assure bereaved siblings that they are loved for being themselves (Davies, 1999). Assisting families in finding ways to memorialize the deceased child will increase family members' understanding that the dead child cannot be replaced. Bereaved siblings often hold on to private memories and special objects that represent their deceased sibling to them (Nolbris and Hellström, 2005).

Siblings frequently misunderstand the cause of death, often attributing partial responsibility to themselves (Davies, 1999). Concrete and developmentally appropriate information can do much to allay siblings' fears and concerns. Parents will be needed to help gather and share such information with their children. Expressive arts (music, art, and play) are especially helpful in reaching siblings. Siblings may exhibit expressions of sadness or may change their behavior with parents, with caregivers, and at school. As potential sources of comfort and reassurance, caregivers and school personnel should be kept informed of the death so that they are not ill prepared to offer support.

Despite a growing body of literature regarding the needs of bereaved siblings, they continue to be an underserved and vulnerable group. The healthy brother or sister who has lived with the uncertainty of an illness carries the often silent scars of that experience. Bereavement support for such children and adolescents is highly important. Research suggests that sibling bereavement camps or programs for siblings who have shared common experiences can be highly beneficial (Packman et al., 2005).

INTERVENTION

Bereavement intervention begins before the death of the child. One role of palliative care teams in the inpatient setting may be to provide or coordinate family support. Bereavement is an example of such a support service (Knapp and Contro, 2009). The bereavement plan of care should be tailored to specific goals, depending on the age of the child, the illness, the family, and the type of care setting and program. These goals include the following (Worden and Monahan, 2000):

1. *Help the family stay connected with their child until death.* While relatively easy for some, many families who see their child declining find it too painful and may have trouble staying connected with the child until the end. One mother whose son was born with major congenital defects found living with him during his 6 years to be demanding and difficult to manage. During his final hospitalization, his mother was not there with him; she developed serious clinical depression related to guilt feelings because of "abandoning" him. It

took considerable therapy to help her work through her feelings (Worden and Monahan, 2000).

2. *Facilitate communication.* This involves communication not only between the family and the caregiving staff, but also among family members themselves. Being sensitive to what a parent, patient, or sibling wants to know or does not want to know is important. Helping parents say to their child what they need to say before the child dies may prevent regrets after the death. A study by Kreicbergs et al. (2004) found that parents whose children were imminently dying did not regret talking to their child about death. The study also found that 27 percent of parents who did not talk to their imminently dying child about death regretted that decision.

3. *Help the family develop memories that they can cherish long after the death.* Pictures and videotapes of the child and other family members are concrete memorials that the family will cherish and replay over the years (Worden and Monahan, 2000).

4. *Help parents negotiate the medical system.* Some parents are well skilled in this and do not need help. Others are more intimidated by the system and are hesitant to ask questions or to assert their preferences. Helping parents develop these skills through role-playing and providing them encouragement to do what they need can be an important part of pre-bereavement counseling (Worden and Monahan, 2000).

5. *Provide respite care.* The demands of caring for a sick child are many. They often fall on the mother's shoulders. Hospice volunteers are typically good resources for this type of respite care, allowing the parents to take a break from their caregiving responsibilities. However, the closer to death the child is, the more the family may want to be with the child (Worden and Monahan, 2000).

6. *Help parents with the concept of "appropriate death."* An appropriate death, according to Worden (2000), is a death consonant with the goals, values, and lifestyle of the individual. Although used more with adults, it can be a useful concept with children, particularly adolescents.

7. *Help parents talk about choices for the funeral or memorial service in advance, if they choose to do this.* While difficult, it allows them to plan a service reflecting the uniqueness of their child. Including family members, particularly siblings, in this activity can be very

valuable. For some parents, this activity may be difficult or contrary to long-standing cultural and/or religious/spiritual beliefs (Worden and Monahan, 2000).

What do bereaved parents feel would be helpful to adjust effectively to the death of a child? D'Agostino, Berlin-Romalis, and Barrera (2008) met with a focus group of seven parents to ascertain what services were, or would have been, helpful during early bereavement. They found that parents wished to do the following:

1. Have formal bereavement services offered by their deceased child's treatment center shortly after the loss. Parents expressed a need to stay connected with their child's health care professionals to prevent secondary losses and feelings of abandonment.
2. Have good communication with health care professionals before and after the loss.
3. Have flexibility of bereavement services. Some parents wanted telephone follow-up, others wanted one-on-one sessions, and still others preferred group therapy.
4. Have their treating center act as a conduit for social networking, allowing them to meet with other parents and share their experiences.
5. Have palliative care support and anticipatory grief services during the period before their child died. Parents would have appreciated specific information packages they could review at their own pace.

PRACTICAL IMPLICATIONS

After a child's death, the child is gone, but not forgotten. Keeping an updated list of supportive and varied community resources for families is helpful. Provide one or two small booklets or printed handouts of relevant information and a list of appropriate books and booklets for when family members feel ready to read them. Finally, give the family the name of one person at the hospice, grief center, or other related agency they can phone if they wish to ask a question or follow up on some advice that has been given. Families often feel a special bond with the professionals who cared for their child at the end of his or her life; this bond needs to be withdrawn gently to avoid the family's feeling abandoned and isolated. In the words of a support group known as Mothers in Sympathy and Support (MISS), "It is our hope that you discover the enormity and depth of the love you have for your child; a love that transcends time and distance, heaven and earth, life and death."

Uncertain Prognosis

Living with an uncertain prognosis is a demanding task that forces all involved to walk a precarious line, wavering between periods of hope and times of despair. In pediatric palliative care an uncertain diagnosis means moving between two worlds, understanding on some level that the outcome of the illness will most likely be death while simultaneously maintaining hope for a cure or a miracle. Rando (1988) describes both the opportunity and difficulty of witnessing the progression of an illness and the impact on later bereavement. Families can use the time during the illness to make sure they have said and done the important things that they may not have actualized before the illness. However, she states that the mourning starts well before death with the loss of the healthy child, and all that will be lost in the future. The challenge is to stay connected to the child in spite of the impending loss.

The relentless uncertainty coupled with caring for an ill child creates a persistent strain on the family, often leaving them lacking resources physically, emotionally, and for some financially as well. Families readjust their routines to cope with the illness of a child. Siblings are parceled out to friends and family, one parent often spends large amounts of time away from home at the hospital, and out of necessity roles are divided up, sometimes stressing relationships. Siblings experience a myriad of feelings: anger that this has happened to their family, jealousy at the attention given to the ill sibling, and of course sadness over the loss of a healthy sibling and guilt because they feel they are somehow a causative factor. The child facing an uncertain prognosis straddles identities between that of a "sick" child and a "healthy" one, attempting to master normal developmental tasks.

The child, like other family members, experiences grief around the loss of usual activities, friends, and normal routines, such as attending school. Anticipatory grief involves rehearsing a variety of future scenarios and, depending on the age of the child, can include feelings of loss and sadness associated with the realization that life is ending coupled with associated fears and concerns about leaving family, friends, pets, and all that is familiar. Each member of the family goes through similar experiences tailored by their unique beliefs and personalities.

Daniel, a tall, lanky 16-year-old, was diagnosed with a brain tumor at age 14. His initial prognosis, as he and his parents understood it, was uncertain. His parents, Cammy and Luke, were intelligent, resourceful, and adept advocates for their son. However, their disagreement over discussing the possibility that Daniel might die led their oncologist to refer them to a social worker for counseling. Their daughter, Caitlin, was 7 years old and often stayed with a neighbor while Cammy cared for Daniel in the hospital and Luke worked long hours as an executive.

Even when Daniel's treatment options became few, his parents continued to disagree about whether or not to discuss the possibility of his death between themselves, with Daniel, or even with his physician. Luke felt to do so would mean to give up hope, and he feared that such talk would affect Daniel's willingness "to fight" his disease. Consequently, he dove into researching all possible treatment options, contacting experts across the country and spending hours on the Internet looking for help. Cammy believed she needed to talk about all possible outcomes of treatment to prepare herself for whatever might come. She contacted a social worker from the palliative care team and set up weekly appointments. A therapeutic relationship was established quickly between Cammy and the social worker, but Luke resisted invitations to talk, stating that he didn't want to be "judged or forced to talk about things." Daniel's sister, Caitlin, was invited to meet with the social worker, who then referred her to a child-life specialist. Eventually, Luke came to a meeting but clearly indicated that he would not entertain the possibility that Daniel would not make it. He continued researching experimental treatments and always emphasized the positive comments made by Daniel's physician while rebuffing any talk of a poor prognosis. The social worker met with both parents periodically, with Cammy individually on a weekly basis, and with Daniel on a regular basis during his clinic visits. Daniel stated that he did not want to hear news from his physician and gave instructions to have all medical information filtered through his parents.

After exhausting all treatment options, 4 years after diagnosis, Daniel was sent home on hospice care and died 3 months later with his family at his bedside. The family wanted to care for Daniel at home but was angry because they felt their hospital family had abandoned them at such a difficult time. Surprisingly, during his time at home, Daniel talked with teenage peers about dying and even distributed his favorite belongings ahead of time. However, he continued to protect his family from such discussions. He extracted a promise from the social worker that she would continue to work with his family after his death because he said, "they are going to need a lot of help, especially my dad."

Although Cammy talked openly to friends and family about Daniel dying, Luke never did. However, he openly grieved and took an active role in memorializing Daniel. Years later he stated, "If anyone had told me Daniel wasn't going to make it, I would have fired them on the spot. That's just not the way I wanted to approach the whole thing."

The social worker was able to continue to work with the family through their bereavement, at first intensely and later as needed. Each member has grieved Daniel's loss in their own way. Luke continues to be task oriented and not inclined to discuss Daniel's loss but instead raises funds for brain tumor research and various activities Daniel had been involved in. Cammy continues to express her sadness openly and has found a variety of ways to commemorate Daniel's life. Caitlin remains quiet and pensive and has used art to express herself but continues to worry about her parents and is fearful of burdening them in any way. The family now tells their story when invited to educational forums, illustrating their different perspectives, coping styles, and needs throughout the process. Luke always jokingly adds that without the ongoing support of the social worker, they would have surely been divorced by now. "She gave Cammy the opportunity to express the things that I couldn't tolerate thinking about."

This vignette illustrates the unique perspective of each family member in the way he or she approached the illness, death, and bereavement. Families who have lived with an uncertain prognosis have potentially had time to prepare for death, but certainly not everyone is willing or able to do so. Bereavement is a highly individual process. As in this family, mothers and fathers may find themselves "out of sync" with each other, and the grief of siblings can sometimes be forgotten or ignored in the face of the turbulence that follows a death. Families like Daniel's have already experienced many losses and hardships prior to the actual death, such as losing the ability to lead a "normal" life, for parents to be actively present with siblings, and hopes and dreams for the future. At the time of death, this accumulation of hardships has already taken its toll on the family.

Pediatric palliative care includes psychological intervention and support services from the time of diagnosis through treatment, death, and bereavement. The efficacy of these services depends on a carefully formulated assessment that is comprehensive and fluid over time, mirroring the progression of the family. The assessment must include a variety of key features: the family composition, cultural and spiritual perspectives, experience with prior loss/

trauma, the mental health history of the family members, stability of familial relationships prior to the illness, drug/alcohol use, support systems, and the individual strengths of each family member. A history of prior psychiatric problems, suicidal behavior or thoughts, or multiple prior losses or traumas may complicate the bereavement process, and a safety net may need to be put in place.

For this family as well as many others, the ongoing connection to the hospital "family" was critical after the death of the child. They expressed outright despair over the loss of those relationships. There is a growing body of literature that underscores the importance of continuity of care after the death of child, particularly with a long-term illness (deCinque et al., 2006; D'Agostino, Berlin-Romalis, and Barrera, 2008).

Families highly value a continued relationship with key members from the care team through bereavement. Many families report compounded distress when faced with the loss of a child and their hospital family concurrently. In an interview conducted as part of a bereavement needs assessment at a children's hospital, one nurse in the oncology clinic tearfully described comments made to her by a recently bereaved mother: "She was so angry at me. She sat in the clinic waiting room for an hour and finally came up to me at the end of the afternoon. She questioned me intensely, 'How come I haven't heard from you? None of my friends know what I'm going through. They don't understand. It's only my hospital family that can really know what I have been through. How could you abandon me right when Jonathan died?'" (Contro and Sourkes, 2009).

As noted above, families often rely heavily on their care team and the comfort of the clinical setting where people know them and understand their experiences. Consequently, it becomes even more important to keep these lifelines intact after the child dies. One study identified insufficient contact with the child's health care team as the second-most-common stressful event for parents after the loss of a child (Kreicbergs et al., 2004). Families often find themselves exhausted and unable to tell their story to new people. Families also report benefit from connecting with other families who have had like experiences, and consequently peer-based interventions can be useful (D'Agostino, Berlin-Romalis, and Barrera, 2008).

Sudden Death

Although the majority of children in palliative care programs will die of an illness diagnosed sometime in the past, palliative care programs must also address the grief and bereavement needs of families who have a child die suddenly. Consider the following:

- A 5-year-old boy is running across the street after his T-ball game. He's wearing his new baseball shoes with cleats, which cause him to slip in the street. An oncoming car doesn't see him in time.
- An 18-year-old boy was the valedictorian of his high school class. Now he's a freshman at a large state university. His first-quarter grades include one B. He's so distraught he jumps out the eighteenth-floor dormitory window.
- A young couple wakes up one morning well rested after their first full night's sleep only to find their 4-month-old daughter lying lifeless on the Winnie the Pooh sheets in her crib.
- A 10-year-old girl was thought to have the flu, only to be brought to the ER in full arrest due to viral myocarditis.

Scores of children who have equally gut-wrenching stories arrive at emergency departments (EDs) daily. Traumatic injury is the main cause of death in children age 1–19: 42.4 percent of all deaths were caused by accidents, and 10.9 percent were caused by assault. In children less than 1 year of age, sudden infant death syndrome (7.4%) is the third-leading cause of death, and accidents (~4%) are the sixth-leading cause of death (Martin et al., 2008). Although these families interface with the health care system for only a brief time, palliative care principles can be applied in the care of these children to improve the long-term outcomes of the surviving family members.

In sudden death, parents, who normally function as their child's protector, enter the ED with feelings of helplessness, loss, and perhaps guilt depending on the circumstances. According to policy (Knapp et al., 2005), providers in the ED must be sensitive to the family's beliefs and cultural backgrounds. Translators should be available to help avoid barriers to communication. This sensitivity spans being aware of the family's methods for decision making, how they would like the body to be cared for after death, and how grief is expressed in their culture. It is recommended that a representative of the health care team be assigned to the family throughout the attempt at resuscitation. He or she should answer questions, explain procedures, and/or prepare the family and bring them to the resuscitation area. The emergency physician is responsible for notifying the family of the patient's death. He should explain to them the circumstances of the death and should also notify the family if there are concerns regarding maltreatment that will require reporting and investigation (Truog et al., 2006).

ED care does not stop after the child's death. After death, the family should be encouraged to be with their child. Families may choose to hold their child or bathe their child. Some authors have emphasized that this is a critical part of bereavement. The creation of handprints, or the collection of a lock of hair, has been found to be useful to families during the bereavement process. Support staff such as a chaplain, social worker, child-life therapist, and/or psychologist should be at the family's disposal during this time (Cook, White, and Ross-Russell, 2002; Stack, 2003; Knapp et al., 2005; Truog et al., 2006).

Although in medicine we often can give a tentative prediction regarding the likely cause of death and the trajectory of a patient's illness, sometimes the patient does not die according to an anticipated timetable, or does not die in the expected way. If the parents are given a particular illness trajectory, they may not be mentally prepared for a death that occurs earlier than predicted. The parents may respond in a similar manner to parents whose child dies of an accidental or intentional injury. If a child is expected to die as a result of a specific complication, such as aspiration pneumonia, but instead dies of a different complication, such as diarrhea and dehydration, the parents may react with shock and disbelief. Parents of a child with a known terminal condition may function with some degree of denial and react like parents of a child who died suddenly. They may even react to their child's expected death with shock, disbelief, or hysteria.

Some parents secretly harbor the belief, or fantasy, that their child will be different, that somehow their child will make it, even when they know at an intellectual level that this cannot happen. The death of the child assaults the parents' protector role and is one of the major stressors when a child dies. Regardless of the cause of a child's death, parents lament, "How could I have not prevented this from happening?"

Perinatal Loss

> Those things were not supposed to happen to us. Those things happen to other families.
>
> —*A mother (RTS, 2007)*

Loss in the perinatal period is unique in that it occurs in a setting where parents are expecting the welcomed birth of a normal healthy baby. Mourning replaces celebration. Perinatal death is not the normal order of things.

The scope of these deaths is so broad and diverse that terminology does not exist to describe in a single word all types of deaths that occur in pregnancy and the newborn period. How does the loss of the fetus or newborn affect these families, and how can we as health care providers influence the experience of the families and support them through the difficult times ahead? Consider the following situation:

> Miranda is a 23-year-old woman who was weeping inconsolably at work. It was the 1-year anniversary of the death of her baby James, who had died at 5 days of age of prenatally diagnosed congenital heart disease. Although Miranda was given bereavement support group literature, she attended no meetings. She rarely speaks about James and had thought she was "over it." While she used to find solace in prayer, she finds that she can no longer pray. She is 22 weeks pregnant and has sought no prenatal care. She is fearful that her current baby has heart disease and will die.

THE SCOPE OF THE PROBLEM

Each year there are nearly 19,000 neonatal deaths: about 1 per 200 neonates less than 28 days old (Ventura, Abma, and Mosher, 2004; Kung et al., 2008). Lethal congenital anomalies are a major cause of perinatal loss. This underestimates the scope of perinatal loss, as there are over a million spontaneous fetal losses each year (~20% of all pregnancies end in a miscarriage or stillbirth; Ventura, Abma, and Mosher, 2004). Before the late 1960s, these losses were considered inconsequential in society's view (Hoeldtke and Calhoun, 2001) and were rarely discussed, even between the mother and father. Siblings and grandparents were forgotten mourners, and fathers' grief was underrecognized. Since the 1970s, there has been an increasing awareness of the grief associated with perinatal loss and the need for strategies to aid families to cope with and validate the loss. What was once spoken of in private between mother and daughter is now recognized among women friends as far more common. These losses do not have any age or socioeconomic boundaries. In almost any group gathering, professional or social, one can ask who has had a perinatal or pregnancy loss and someone will raise a hand.

IMPACT ON THE FAMILY

> She wasn't just alive for eleven days. She was alive for nine months and eleven days.
> —A father (RTS, 2007)

As many parents are young, they likely have had limited experience with loss. Parental attachment clearly precedes the birth of an infant, making even an early miscarriage a significant loss for many parents (Weiss, Frischer, and Richman, 1989).

Recognition of the loss is reinforced by the burgeoning technology available to "connect with one's baby" with ultrasound, headphones to hear the heartbeat, and even 3-D imaging. Many parents are learning of a potentially lethal condition long before delivery. In an instant, the parents begin saying goodbye even before a chance to say hello. These parents not only experience the pain of loss but also may need to make difficult decisions (Weiss, Frischer, and Richman, 1989). Among a variety of reports, as few as 10 percent and as many as 75 percent of parents who receive a lethal diagnosis for their unborn fetus may elect to continue the pregnancy (Schechtman et al., 2002; D'Almeida et al., 2006; Breeze et al., 2007).

Although early pregnancy losses may produce less intense grief than stillbirth or neonatal loss, grief intensity and complications are highly personal responses, not related to birth weight, gestational age, parental age, or participation in decisions to discontinue support. The intensity of grief over a perinatal loss can be as great as losing a spouse or close relative and may persist for years. In the early months after the death, frequent emotional and somatic signs of distress of grieving parents include aching arms, feeling the presence of the baby, hearing baby sounds, and hallucinations of the dead baby.

Parental emotions after perinatal loss may encompass shock, denial, anger, depression, and acceptance, similar to other grief responses (Murray et al., 2000). Depression and anxiety are more common in the first 6–8 months (Vance et al., 1995b) but may persist in a less intense form 12–16 months after the pregnancy loss. Although mood levels improve over time, there is significant interpersonal variability. Parents may benefit from understanding the range of anticipated emotional responses. Not only do the parents experience loss of the wished-for baby, but also they may experience loss of self-esteem, loss of their role as parent, and loss of confidence in their ability to produce a healthy child (Weiss, Frischer, and Richman, 1989). They also lose the commonality of what others go through in the experience of pregnancy: planning, celebrating, showers, the social element of sharing the anticipated child, as well as the secondary losses of losing the future they had hoped for their child, the experiences and milestones, rites of passages as parents they too will miss in the future. In many cases after hospital discharge the parents face a home, family, and community readied for a new baby. Some families adapt well and find ways to integrate the child's short life into the fabric of the family; others never speak of the baby again; still others mourn for a long time.

Guilt may arise as a result of genetic issues or because of a maternal sense of being responsible for the death. With stillbirths, the fetus literally dies inside her. Grieving mothers must also contend with some real physical pain or discomfort and the lingering effects of the pregnancy. Despite the absence of their baby, they may experience engorged breasts, healing wounds, hormonal influences, and physical exhaustion. Mothers' grief seems to be more intense and longer in duration than their partners', but the studies are inconsistent (Callister, 2006). Women are generally more willing to talk about their emotions and participate in support groups.

Society's expectations of men as being strong supports for their partners may conflict with the strong grief responses of men. Men and women do seem to grieve differently, but the intensity of men's grief relative to their partners' is variable (Hunfeld et al., 1996). Men tend to be less verbally expressive concerning the loss and participate less in support groups.

Siblings who may be anticipating being a big brother or sister are faced with loss of that role, a disrupted family life, loss of their sense of invulnerability, and parents who are stressed and poorly able to care for them. They are sad, may not understand death, and are unable to overcome their parents' sadness. For those siblings who may have resented the future sibling's arrival in the family, guilt over their perceived role in causing the death by feelings they had can be frightening (Orloff, 2005).

COMPLICATED GRIEF

One-fifth to one-third of parents experience pathologic grief at 1–2 years after perinatal loss (Rowe et al., 1978). Pathologic grief is a continued inability to work through the sense of loss, with resultant continued feelings of self-hatred and deflation of self-esteem, extreme isolation, inability to return to work or previous activities of daily living, severe depression, and suicidal ideation. Diagnostic clues include the intensity, duration, or rigidity of the grief symptoms. When one of a set of multiples dies, it presents a challenge for parents who have a constant reminder of their loss. Decision making appears to be similar to that when singletons are involved (Pector, 2004). When all of a set of multiples dies, the loss can be compounded. Other factors predisposing to complicated grief include crises or ambivalence during pregnancy; lack of spousal, social, or family support; and a history of prior mental health problems (Rowe et al., 1978; Murray et al., 2000).

The impact of foreknowledge of the fetal or neonatal likelihood of death on the intensity of grief is unknown. Grief can be adversely affected by the behavior of family, friends, and health care providers. Although well intended, the common verbal blunders of friends and relatives can worsen the pain and isolation in the grieving parents, who may feel that no one really does understand. The reality is that our society does not teach us how to support one another in these difficult times. Some health care professionals also lack the discretion and sometimes the sensitivity to recognize the impact, often lasting, of their words (Gold, 2007).

DISENFRANCHISED GRIEF

Stillbirth: "a nonevent in which there is guilt and shame with no tangible person to mourn."

—*Bourne (1968, p. 110)*

Mothers who have experienced stillbirth may feel disenfranchised as there are few societal rituals recognizing the loss of stillbirth. Fetuses have not traditionally been viewed as members of the family and community and may be unnamed. States have just recently begun to allow burial of stillborns. When the fetus dies before it is born, parents may be left to grieve in an isolated, misunderstood way.

The grief response of parents electing termination can be as intense as parents experiencing stillbirth or neonatal loss (Weiss, Frischer, and Richman, 1989; Hoeldtke and Calhoun, 2001), yet often this grief is not acknowledged by the woman, the partner, or medical professionals. The need for support can be just as great, however. Perinatal loss support programs and/or group facilitators need to decide how and if they will include these "elective" losses in the general perinatal loss support group model and to anticipate the differences in circumstances in advance.

HOW TO HELP FAMILIES WHO ARE
EXPERIENCING PERINATAL LOSS

Scales such as the Perinatal Grief Scale (Toedter, Lasker, and Alhadeff, 1988; Hunfeld et al., 1993, 1996) have been used to assess grief and coping after a perinatal loss. It is unclear how useful they are in clinical practice. During a telephone or in-person follow-up, the health care provider should assess the impact of the loss, parental grief response and coping mechanisms, and available family and community support. The depression and suicide risks should be evaluated.

Attitudes and actions of health care providers are powerful factors, which may impede or facilitate future grief work (Weiss, Frischer, and Richman, 1989). Health care providers and other sources of support can validate the loss and validate the grief. Placing a card with a recognized picture or symbol signifying perinatal loss outside the door to the mother's room ensures that all staff that enter the room are aware of the loss. The physician can review the baby's problems, diagnoses, cause of death, and autopsy results, if available. Referral for genetic counseling may be recommended depending on the circumstance. Psychosocial and spiritual support of the family is critical, regardless of the timing of the loss.

During antenatal or postnatal discussions, health care providers can inform parents of the issues and needs of siblings and provide strategies to support grieving. Having a trusted adult present for the siblings during and after the delivery is especially important. Attention should also be placed on the needs of the siblings when returning home or to school. Teachers can be important in supporting bereaved siblings and encouraging peers to recognize their grief. Consultation by a child-life specialist may be beneficial.

After the delivery of a stillborn, it is unclear whether or not holding the baby is traumatizing and promotes depression and posttraumatic stress disorder (Hughs et al., 2002) or supports adaptation with less anxiety and depression (Cacciatore, Rådestad, and Frederik Frøen, 2008). It is important to empower parents to make decisions based on their own values.

Photographs, crib cards, locks of hair, baby blankets, hand and foot prints and casts, and other mementos are treasured by grieving parents. When one or more multiples die, parents may value pictures and mementos of all the babies together.

For babies dying in the hospital, some centers provide a bereavement packet and/or memory box including a disposable camera, baby clothes and a blanket, a baby book to record memories, and information about bereavement, including contact information for community-based support groups. Tangible items of the baby's life as keepsakes may bring comfort to parents long after they leave the hospital, even if they choose not to access them for some time. These are also worth considering for siblings as well. Walking the family to their car with a bereavement packet or stuffed animal to fill their empty arms aids the transition out of the NICU (or ED) for the last time (Catlin and Carter, 2002). In some locations, laws allow parents to transport their infant's body to the funeral home themselves. Staff should support the parents' choices that are consistent with their values, religion, and/or culture.

While few rituals pertain to perinatal death, rituals can help provide meaning, document transitions, and connect the people who participate (Kobler, Limbo, and Kavanaugh, 2007). Bathing and clothing the dead baby is a ritual that appears in many cultures. Many families develop their own rituals if given support to think of what might comfort them or given suggestions on what has helped other parents.

We celebrated because she was one week old. We made cards for Valentine's Day.
—a sister (RTS, 2007)

Models of standardized grief follow-up or in-hospital procedures to follow at time of death are available and serve as good training guides for staff. Bereaved parents are excellent resources as policies are reviewed that address care of the newborn and support of the family. For complicated or prolonged grief, referral to a mental health care professional who has expertise with bereaved parents may be indicated in some cases when peer support or community bereavement support groups are not adequate.

Hospital-based health care providers are wise to inventory and update annually the local follow-up supports available and investigate what services are available through local hospice programs. This offers an excellent opportunity to collaborate, to extend limited resources further, and to avoid duplication of groups or efforts.

The subsequent pregnancy poses unique challenges and concerns. A pregnancy less than 5–6 months after the loss may cut short the mourning process and cause mental health problems (Rowe et al., 1978). The next pregnancy may be fraught with mental, emotional, and physical challenges (Armstrong, 2007). Failure to mourn may have dire consequences for mothering a subsequent child. There may be overprotective and replacement feelings with the next child. The family may feel disloyalty toward the dead child. The new child is perceived as having more health and behavior problems. Problems are especially acute if the birthday is near the anniversary of the death of the earlier baby, if grief is not resolved, if the mother is anxious, or if there is poor social support. On the other hand, if the parents have been able to grieve in a healthy manner and are trying to work through the loss issues, the perceptions and rationale for another baby may be positive in the context of the individual family. Conceiving again and the subsequent birth may lessen grief, bring the couple closer, be positive to a sibling, and integrate the memory of the dead child into the family experience. Interconceptual counseling might be indicated to answer remaining questions about the cause of death, rule out recurrent pregnancy risks, and allow informed decisions regarding future pregnancies. The health care provider can support the mother during pregnancy, relieve anxiety, validate the normal progression of pregnancy, and reinforce the health of the new baby (Weiss, Frischer, and Richman, 1989).

Depending on the individual needs of the mother and father, support groups may help the couple find meaning in the loss of their newborn and find ways to deal positively with their emotions and relationships. Hospital medical professionals should be familiar with community resources for grief follow-up. To aid in seamless consistent care, bereavement counselors can be introduced to the family during antenatal visits or in the NICU or nursery and continue providing counseling through death and as long as the family needs support (Harvey, Snowdon, and Elbourne, 2008). Being familiar with what local hospices offer for bereavement support is also important. It may create an opportunity for collaboration and better coordination for a continuum of support before, during, and after the death. Some bereavement support groups are professionally facilitated, and some may be facilitated by others who have experienced these deaths themselves. Parents may need to try a few options to find what best meets their needs and styles.

Parent bereavement support groups such as Share Pregnancy & Infant Loss Support Organization, Inc. (SHARE) and Resolve Through Sharing (RTS) are important resources for families experiencing perinatal loss, especially fetal loss. Bereavement support groups offer families an environment in which they can comfortably speak openly about their dead child (Brosig et al., 2007). Support programs are effective in increasing the understanding of autopsy findings and burial options, increasing confidence in a future pregnancy, and improving parent satisfaction and paternal involvement (Murray et al., 2000). Psychological and spiritual support, either professional or from a peer support group, can decrease anger and hostility, physical symptoms, depression, and intensity of grief, particularly in the first 6 months after the loss (Murray et al., 2000). This support is particularly important in the absence of family and social support. The higher the parent's risk, the greater is the benefit of the support and the satisfaction with the support program.

PRACTICAL IMPLICATIONS

There is a role for health care providers in the management of grief and loss. Silence is not golden. There are many specific ways to be supportive in anticipation of a neonatal death or delivery of a stillborn infant (Weiss, Frischer, and Richman, 1989; Brosig et al., 2007; Carter, 2007; Fitzsimons and Seyda, 2007; Gold, 2007; Marron-Corwin and Corwin, 2008; Williams et al., 2008). The two tables in this chapter help explain many "dos and don'ts" when caring for families experiencing loss.

Health care providers can compassionately affirm the death and validate the loss. Consider the following:

Jessica and Mark eagerly awaited the birth of their quadruplets even though they understood the significant risks of death or complications. Jessica spent many weeks in the hospital to optimize their chances. Jason (Quad C) died in utero 24 hours before the preterm birth of the rest of the babies. When the neonatologist who had provided antenatal counseling to the family saw that the incubators were labeled A, B, and C, she made sure that they were relabeled A, B, and D and gently corrected those who talked about the "triplets."

Health care providers can educate the family about the grieving process, make sure each individual family member's needs are expressed and met, and ensure that the family makes a seamless connection to bereavement follow-up care. Caregivers can be sympathetic listeners and sensitive informants. They can make sure that the death of the newborn doesn't fall into a medical void with neither the obstetrician nor the pediatrician assuming responsibility for counseling the family and providing follow-up. As nearly one-third of parents choose a different physician after the death of a child, satisfaction with care is an important issue. Parents' satisfaction with health care positively correlates with the providers being available, bearing witness, giving them honest appropriate medical information, and supporting empowered decision making. Other aspects of care include allowing them to grieve and adapt, including a supportive physical environment, faith/trust in nursing care, emotional support for them, information about grieving, and support from other hospital care providers such as chaplains, social workers, the palliative care team, and child-life specialists (Weiss, Frischer, and Richman, 1989; Harper and Wisian, 1994; Brosig et al., 2007; Carter, 2007; Williams et al., 2008). Interestingly, the involvement of hospice/palliative care does not affect grief or adaptation scores (Brosig et al., 2007). On the other hand, avoidance, poor communication between staff members, actions that diminish the loss or minimize grief, isolation, insensitive communications, perception of unequal treatment because of finances, and lack of emotional support are associated with parental dissatisfaction (Gold, 2007). To help care providers assess their performance, there is a recently developed tool for assessing quality of neonatal end-of-life care. While parents are generally satisfied with the process of discontinuation of support, their needs are not consistently met with regard to in-hospital and follow-up

Table 11.1 Dos and don'ts when caring for grieving families

Do

Allow your own human caring and concern to show through; take the initiative to contact them.

Recognize that families are systems, and that a child's death affects everyone, not just the parents.

Acknowledge the depth of family members' loss; reassure the parents they did everything they could have; allow parents to express their grief over time.

Recognize the dead baby/child/adolescent as a person; refer to the child by name.

Encourage collection of memories, mementos, and keepsakes.

Educate parents and other family members about the range of grief responses over time.

Pay attention to individual differences among family members, taking into account cultural, religious, personality, and other differences.

Give practical help.

Repeat information as needed, realizing that the stress of the situation may preclude parents and others from grasping facts the first time.

Be available to listen and follow up. Attend the funeral or memorial service or send sympathy cards. Give attention to the surviving siblings.

Refer the parents to other bereavement resources.

Develop a plan to help the school/community cope with the death of a child or adolescent.

Pay attention to your own needs for emotional support.

Don't

Minimize the loss ("At least you have your other children [your big brother]" or "You can always have another child").

Judge parents' grief reactions or minimize their grief.

Say, "It has been _____ months, aren't you over it yet?"

Expect expression of grief to fit a protocol or be uniform.

Interfere with the father's demonstrations of grief by reinforcing the male stereotype of strength.

Tell them what they "should" feel or do.

Offer platitudes or artificial consolation.

Avoid them because you feel helpless or uncomfortable.

bereavement support (Williams et al., 2009). After discharge with or without the baby, there should be follow-up contact, referral to support groups, and continuity of care, if possible, with the next pregnancy.

Doctors, nurses, and other staff members who have been intimately involved in the care of the mother and newborn may also experience intense grief over the loss of the newborn and the loss of the relationship with the family. Their needs are addressed in chapter 12. As noted there, staff at hos-

Table 11.2 Dos and don'ts when helping with perinatal loss

Do

Refer to the baby by name.

Encourage access by parents, siblings, and significant support people in a private setting.

Offer holding, touching, skin-to-skin contact.

Acknowledge parents' loss and their grief.

Give honest answers to questions.

Involve parents in decision making and support them in their decisions.

Provide anticipatory guidance and logistical planning, including potential home hospice/palliative care if the baby lives to discharge.

Provide a supportive environment in the mother's room, NICU, contiguous room, or home.

Be accessible, flexible, genuine, and compassionate.

Be present. Listen and be quiet; be receptive to their emotions.

Choose words carefully. They matter.

Ask about siblings and sources of support.

Explore spiritual, religious, and cultural issues.

Encourage closure and support the meaning of this life through rituals.

Ensure consistent team communication.

Keep in contact; send cards, attend funerals and memorials, etc.

Provide anticipatory guidance about normal and abnormal grief.

Don't

Minimize the loss or grief, or assume that a mother who has an early miscarriage is not grieving.

Avoid, abandon, or isolate the parents.

Give inaccurate information.

Confuse the sex or name of the baby.

Deny access by limiting visiting hours, preventing holding, etc.

Use terms like "incompatible with life," "lethal," etc. Parents are focusing on the life of their child, however short.

Assume that the father grieves less.

Think that your relationship ends with death or discharge.

Presume that you know how they feel.

Assume that their value system or worldview is the same as yours.

Assume that bonding with the baby in utero or knowing of in-utero diagnosis of life-limiting condition will cause more pain.

Be insensitive as a result of lack of awareness of death.

pitals inexperienced in perinatal loss may need consultation and support from the tertiary center if a baby with a condition incompatible with prolonged life is delivered and is cared for in the community.

While each family member copes in his or her own way, the health care team can offer strategies to optimize outcomes. With interdisciplinary collaboration, support of the family experiencing perinatal loss can lead to an intact family finding meaning in the brief life and death of their hoped-for newborn and adapting to life after the loss.

Conclusion

The death of a fetus, infant, or child has a profound and lifelong impact on parents, siblings, grandparents, and sometimes the larger community. Each person has an individual way of expressing grief. Protective factors enabling successful bereavement are presented, including adequate information and prebereavement counseling. Suggestions for an effective prenatal program are provided. However, our society frequently ignores the grieving and bereavement needs of those who are most profoundly affected. Parents of unborn children who die; families of children who die of sudden causes; and fathers, siblings, and grandparents bereaved of infants and children need informed attention to their concerns. They need affirmation and support through direction to resources, continued contact with a designated health care professional, peer groups, professional counseling, or companioning. Tables 11.1 and 11.2 present practical lists of "dos and don'ts" for all caregivers. In summary, while it may be difficult to provide ideally for all the needs of a bereaved family, simple measures that depend on only one individual can make the experience significantly better for the majority of families.

References

Aho, A.L.,Tarkka, M.T., Astedt-Kurki, P., et al. 2006. Father's grief after the death of a child. *Issues Ment Health Nurs* 27(6):647–63.

Armstrong, D. 2007. Perinatal loss and parental distress after the birth of a healthy infant. *Advanc Neonat Care* 7:200–206.

Arnold, J., and Gemma, P.B. 2008. The continuing process of parental grief. *Death Studies* 32:658–73.

Barrera, M., D'Agostino, N.M., Schneiderman, G., et al. 2007. Patterns of parental bereavement following the loss of a child and related factors. *OMEGA* 55(2): 145–67.

Bourne, S. 1968. The psychological effects of stillbirths on women and their doctors. *J Royal Coll Gen Practitioners* 16:103–12.

Breeze, A., Lees, C., Kumar, A., et al. 2007. Palliative care for prenatally diagnosed lethal fetal abnormality. *Arch Dis Child Fetal Neonatal Ed* 92:F56–58.

Brosig, C., Peirucci, R., Kupst, M., et al. 2007. Infant end of life care: The parents' perspective. *J Perinatol* 27:510–16.

Cacciatore, J, Rådestad, I., and Frederik Frøen, J. 2008. Effects of contact with still-born babies on maternal anxiety and depression. *Birth* 4:313–20.

Callister, L.C. 2006. Perinatal loss: A family perspective. *J Perinat Neonat Nurs* 20: 227–34.

Carter, B. 2007. Neonatal and infant death: What bereaved parents can teach us. *J Perinatol* 27:467–68.

Catlin, A., and Carter, B. 2002. Creation of a neonatal end-of-life palliative care protocol. *J Perinatol* 22:184–95.

Contro, N., and Sourkes, B. 2009, Bereavement services at a children's hospital: A needs assessment. Unpublished manuscript. Stanford University Medical Center, Palo Alto, CA.

Cook, J. A. 1988. Dad's double binds. Rethinking fathers' bereavement from a men's studies perspective. *J Contemp Ethnography* 17:285–308.

Cook, P., White, D.K., and Ross-Russell, R.I. 2002. Bereavement support following sudden and unexpected death: Guidelines for care. *Arch Dis Child* 87:36–38.

D'Agostino, N.M., Berlin-Romalis, D., and Barrera, M. 2008. Bereaved parents' perspectives on their needs. *Palliat Support Care* 6:33–41.

D'Almeida, M., Hume, R.F., Lathrop, A., et al. 2006. Perinatal hospice: Family-centered care of the fetus with a lethal condition. *J Am Phys Surg* 11:52–55.

Davies, B. 1999. *Shadows in the Sun*. Philadelphia: Brunner/Mazel.

Davies, B., Gudmundsdottir, M., Worden, B., et al. 2004. Living in the dragon's shadow: Fathers' experiences of a child's life limiting illness. *Death Studies* 28:111–35.

deCinque, N., Monterosso, L., Dadd, G., et al. 2006. Bereavement support for families following the death of a child from cancer: Experience of bereaved parents. *J Psychosoc Oncol* 24(2):65–83.

DeFrain, J., Ernst, L., Jakub, D., et al. 1991. *Sudden Infant Death: Enduring the Loss.* Lexington, MA: Lexington Books.

Fitzsimons, A., and Seyda, B. 2007. A "primer" on perinatal loss and infant death: Statistics/definition, parents' needs, and suggestions for family care. NHPCO, *ChiPPS Pediatric Palliative Care Newsletter* 7:2–6.

Gamino, L.A. 1999. A father's experience of neonatal loss. *The Forum* 3:14–15.

Gold, K. 2007. Navigating care after a baby dies: A systematic review of parent experiences with health providers. *J Perinatol* 27:230–37.

Harper, M.B., and Wisian, N.B. 1994. Care of bereaved parents: A study of patient satisfaction. *J Reprod Med* 39:80–86.

Harvey, S., Snowdon, C., and Elbourne, D. 2008. Effectiveness of bereavement interventions in neonatal intensive care: A review of the evidence. *Sem Fetal/Neonat Med* 13:341–56.

Hoeldtke, N., and Calhoun, B. 2001. Perinatal hospice. *Am J Obstet Gynecol* 185: 525–29.

Hughs, P., Turton, P., Hopper, E., et al. 2002. Assessment of guidelines for good practice in psychosocial care of mothers after stillbirth: A cohort study. *Lancet* 360:114–18.

Hunfeld, J.A., Wladimiroff, J.W., Passchier, J., et al. 1993. Reliability and validity of the perinatal grief scale for women who experienced late pregnancy loss. *Br J Med Psychol* 66:295–98.

Hunfeld, J.A.M., Mourik, M.M., Tibboel, D., et al. 1996. Parental grieving after infant death [Letter to the editor]. *J Fam Practice* 42:622–23.

Knapp, C.A., and Contro, N. 2009. Family support services in pediatric palliative care. *Am J Hosp Palliat Med* 26(6):476–82.

Knapp, J., Mulligan-Smith, D., and the Committee on Pediatric Emergency Medicine of the American Academy of Pediatrics. 2005. Death of a child in the emergency department. *Pediatrics* 115(5):1432–37.

Kobler, K., Limbo, R., and Kavanaugh, K. 2007. Meaningful moments: The use of ritual in perinatal and pediatric death. *MCN* 32:288–95.

Kreicbergs, U., Valdimarsdóttir, U., Onelöv, E., et al. 2004. Talking about death with children who have severe malignant disease. *N Engl J Med* 351(12):1175–86.

Kung, H., Hoyert, D., Xu, J., et al. 2008. Deaths: Final data for 2005. *National Vital Statistics Report* 56:95–102.

Lang, A., and Gottlieb, L. 1993. Parental grief reactions and marital intimacy following infant death. *Death Studies* 17:233–55.

Lannen, P.K., Wolfe, J., Prigerson, H.G., et al. 2008. Unresolved grief in a national sample of bereaved parents: Impaired mental and physical health 4–9 years later. *J Clin Oncol* 26 (36):5870–76.

Marron-Corwin, M.J., and Corwin, A. 2008. When tenderness should replace technology: The role of perinatal hospice. *NeoReviews* 9:e348–52.

Martin, J.A., Kung, H., Mathews, T. J., et al. 2008. Annual summary of vital statistics, 2006. *Pediatrics* 121:788–801.

McCreight, B.S. 2004. A grief ignored: Narratives of pregnancy loss from a male perspective. *Sociol Health Illness* 26(3):326–50.

Meert, K.L., Eggly, S., Pollack, M., et al. 2007. Parents' perspectives regarding a physician-parent conference after their child's death in the pediatric intensive care unit. *J Pediatr* 151(1):50–55.

Milo, E.M. 1997. Maternal responses to the life and death of a child with a developmental disability: A story of hope. *Death Studies* 21:443–76.

Moriarty, H.J., Carroll, R., and Cotroneo, M. 1996. Differences in bereavement reactions within couples following death of a child. *Res Nurs Health* 19:461–69.

Murphy, S.A., Johnson, C., Cain, K.C., et al. 1998. Broad-spectrum group treatment for parents bereaved by the violent deaths of their 12-to-28 year-old children: A randomized controlled trial. *Death Studies* 22:209–35.

Murray, J.A., Terry, D.J., Vance, J.C., et al. 2000. Effects of a program of intervention on parental distress following infant death. *Death Studies* 24:275–305.

Nolbris, M., and Hellström, A. 2005. Siblings' needs and issues when a brother or sister dies of cancer. *J Pediatr Oncol Nurs* 22(4):227–33.

Orloff, S. 2005. Bereaved siblings. NHPCO, ChiPPS Newsletter August. www.nhpco .org/i4a/pages/Index.cfm?pageID=4664 (accessed April 30, 2010).

Packman, W., Greenhalgh, J., Chesterman, B., et al. 2005. Siblings of pediatric cancer patients: The quantitative and qualitative nature of quality of life. *J Psychosoc Oncol* 23(1):87–108.

Pector, E. 2004. Views of bereaved multiple-birth parents on life support decisions, the dying process, and discussions surrounding death. *J Perinatol* 24:4–10.

Pollack, W. S. 1998. Mourning, melancholia, and masculinity: Recognizing and treating depression in men. In *New Psychotherapy for Men*, ed. W. S. Pollack, pp. 147–66. New York: John Wiley & Sons.

Rando, T. 1988. *How to Go On Living When Someone You Love Dies*. Lexington, MA: Lexington Books.

Reiko, S. 1998. A child's death and divorce: Dispelling the myth. *Death Studies* 22(5): 445–68.

Rowe, J., Clyman, R., Green, C., et al. 1978. Follow-up of families who experience a perinatal death. *Pediatrics* 62:166–70.

RTS. 2007. Waiting for birth and death: Knowing your baby will not survive. Bereavement Services the RTS People. Gundersen Lutheran Medical Foundation, Inc., LaCrosse, WI.

Samuelsson, M., Radestad, I., and Segesten, K. 2001. A waste of life: Fathers' experience of losing a child before birth. *Birth* 28:124–30.

Schechtman, K., Gray, D., Bary, J., et al. 2002. Decision-making for termination of pregnancies with fetal anomalies: Analysis of 53,000 pregnancies. *Obstet Gynecol* 99:216–22.

Stack, C.G. 2003. Bereavement in paediatric intensive care. *Paediatr Anaesth* 13: 651–54.

Toedter, L.J., Lasker, J.N., and Alhadeff, J.M. 1988. The perinatal grief scale: Development and initial validation. *Am J Orthopsychiatry* 58:435–49.

Truog, R.D., Christ, G., Browning, D.M., et al. 2006. Sudden traumatic death in children: "We did everything, but your child didn't survive." *JAMA* 295(22): 2645–54.

Vance, J.C., Boyle, F.M., Najman, J.M., et al. 1995a. Gender differences in parental psychological distress following perinatal death or sudden infant death syndrome. *Br J Psychiatry* 167:806–11.

Vance, J.C., Najman, J.M., Thearle, M.J., et al. 1995b. Psychological changes in parents eight months after the loss of an infant from stillbirth, neonatal death, or sudden infant death syndrome: A longitudinal study. *Pediatrics* 96:933–38.

Ventura, S., Abma, J., and Mosher, W. 2004. Estimated pregnancy rates for the United States, 1990–2000: An update. *National Vital Statistics Report* 52:1–12.

Weiss, L., Frischer, D., and Richman, J. 1989. Parental adjustment to intrapartum and delivery room loss: The role of a hospital-based support program. *Clin Perinatol* 16:1009–19.

Wijngaards-De Meij, L., Stroebe, M., Stroebe, W., et al. 2008. The impact of circumstances surrounding the death of a child on parents' grief. *Death Studies* 32:237–52.

Williams, C., Cairnie, J., Fines, V., et al. 2009. Construction of a parent-derived questionnaire to measure end-of-life care after withdrawal of life-sustaining treatment in the neonatal intensive care unit. *Pediatrics* 123:e87–95.

Williams, C., Munson, D., Zupancic, J., et al. 2008. Supporting bereaved parents: Practical steps in providing compassionate perinatal and neonatal end-of-life care— a North American perspective. *Semin Fetal Neonat Med* 13:335–40.

Wood, J.D., and Milo, E. 2001. Fathers' grief when a disabled child dies. *Death Studies* 25:635–61.

Worden, J.W. 1996. *Children and Grief: When a Parent Dies.* New York: Guilford.
———. 2000. Towards an appropriate death. In *Clinical Dimensions of Anticipatory Mourning,* ed. T. Rando, pp. 267–80. Champaign, IL: Research Press.
———. 2002. *Grief Counseling and Grief Therapy.* New York: Springer.
Worden, J.W., and Monahan, J. 2009. Caring for bereaved parents. In *Hospice Care for Children,* 3rd ed., ed. A. Armstrong-Dailey and S. Zarbock. New York: Oxford University Press.

Perinatal Loss Resources (all accessed April 30, 2010)

Forgotten Grief: www.forgottengrief.com
Hygeia: www.hygeiafoundation.org/homeqm.htm
Now I Lay Me Down to Sleep: www.nowilaymedowntosleep.org
Share Pregnancy and Infant Loss, Inc.: www.nationalshareoffice.com
Wisconsin Association for Perinatal Care: www.perinatalweb.org/index.php?option =content&task=view&id=123

12

The Other Side of Caring: Caregiver Suffering

Cynda H. Rushton, Ph.D., R.N., and M. Karen Ballard, M.C.M., B.C.C.

Caring for children with life-threatening conditions and their families can be a source of profound satisfaction, renewal, and affirmation. Sharing the journey with sick and dying children and their families is a privilege that only a few experience. For these caregivers, suffering for and with is an integral dimension of caring.

By definition, to care is to suffer with, to share solidarity. Suffering for and with another person ignites our innate capacities for compassionate action. Caring for others signifies concern or interest in them as persons and in their well-being. It involves creating and sustaining relationships, emotional involvement, and a commitment to act on behalf of another; it connotes a strong sense of responsibility to attend to the holistic needs of another and, in the case of health care professionals, to provide needed services. Being with suffering can be transformative: the impetus for personal growth and social change (Halifax, 2008) and a source for the remarkable resiliency of the human spirit (Stamm, 2002).

The act of caring for seriously ill and dying children demands empathy, sympathy, and compassion, three closely related responses. *Empathy*, the ability to feel and relate to the suffering of the other, invites mutual vulnerability and connection. It is the ability to perceive the experience of the other, to understand and convey one's validation and understanding of the other's experience without judgment (Sabo, 2006). In contrast, *sympathy* refers to a genuine feeling of concern for another's welfare or situation, conveying recognition or understanding of the circumstances or feelings ("I'm sorry for your loss"). Oriented toward the other rather than the self, sympathy may be impersonal or personal and invoke feelings of pity, sorrow, or anguish (Eisenberg, 2004). Although empathy and *compassion* are closely related, "compassion is the ability to be present to all levels of suffering, to experience it, and aspire or act to transform it without attachment to outcome or being overwhelmed by emotions or circumstances" (Rushton et al., 2009, p. 408). Compassion invites a quality of presence that conveys stability and resilience with a balanced concern and heartfelt connection but is not depleting or overwhelming to either person. It reflects the individual's character through a virtuous concern for the welfare of others and conveys an "inherent regard and respect" for another who shares a common human destiny (Sabo, 2006, p. 137). For the caregiver, each response has the potential to create meaning, satisfaction, and renewal. But there is another side of care and caring that must also be acknowledged: the potential cost of caring so much.

Professionals who listen to and witness the pain and suffering of children and their families may themselves experience pain and suffering (Cadge and Catlin, 2006). Health care professionals may experience frustration and anguish as they observe children struggling against formidable odds and parents grappling with some of the most difficult decisions a family can ever confront. Children bear the consequences of disease, injury, and medical interventions in an often hectic health care environment. Professionals face demands that are at times unrelenting, accomplishing their tasks under high personal and professional tension. Ethical dilemmas grow as some children's lives end before their potential is reached, while other children's lives continue in time but not in quality.

Caring for children and their families requires specialized knowledge and skill, sustained relationships, and courageous advocacy. In sum, it calls on tremendous physical, emotional, and spiritual energies from health care professionals. When demands exceed energies, integrity and self-worth can be threatened. Caregivers may begin to question the threshold of suffering they should be expected to endure. Clearly, when suffering becomes so great that it threatens the professional's sense of identity and integrity, it can no longer be justified (Rushton, 1992). Imbalanced sympathy and hypersensitivity to the emotions or suffering of others can lead to depletion and suffering (Cadge and Catlin, 2006; Halifax, 2008) and undermine compassionate action. Health care professionals are not expected to be martyrs or to sacrifice their own well-being to carry out their caregiving roles. Nor can they be expected to deliver good-quality care when their integrity is shattered. Family caregivers experience these same dynamics; the difference, of course, is that they are not in caregiving situations by choice and usually cannot, or would not, want to walk away.

On a positive note, however, clinicians and family members embrace caregiving relationships because of the tremendous joy and satisfaction inherent in the role. As mentioned above, suffering and witnessing suffering can be transformative. Various descriptions of this process are available in the literature—posttraumatic growth, vicarious posttraumatic growth, healing connections (Boston and Mount, 2006; Kearney et al., 2009)—and are explored further in this chapter. When systems and processes are designed and maintained with proactive attention to boundaries and preservation of integrity, caregiving provides unparalleled opportunities to bear witness to suffering and assist in the transformation of that experience into sustained meaning for professionals and family members alike.

This chapter opens by relating two contrasting clinical scenarios that raise very different issues for caregivers. We then define caregiver suffering and its sources, evaluate those sources, and examine responses and behaviors associated with suffering. In a final section, we offer strategies that may help health care professionals and family caregivers address their own suffering—and, by doing so, provide better care for their patients and their families. At present, little evidence-based information exists surrounding issues of caregiver suffering for children with life-threatening conditions and their families. As the field of pediatric palliative care continues to grow and salient research is conducted, the theories and practices delineated in this chapter may take on more or less relevance for our population; currently, however, we offer helpful perspectives for families and health care professionals to develop awareness.

> Mark, a 16-year-old high school junior, has a 4-year history of osteogenic sarcoma of the leg, which has recurred in several other locations. He is an attractive, gregarious adolescent who excels in everything he attempts. Each recurrence of the cancer has been treated with extensive surgical resection and multiple chemotherapeutic regimens. Most recently, the tumor recurred in his spine. It was surgically debulked; stabilization rods and radiation implants were inserted. After the initial treatment, he was referred for an autologous bone marrow transplant as the best option for possible cure. During the preparation phase, the tumor continued to enlarge, causing spinal cord compression that required aggressive surgical intervention. After Mark recovered from surgery, the bone marrow transplant was performed. Recurrent infections, medically managed kidney failure, and wound dehiscence have complicated the post-transplant period. Mark has become bedridden because of the weakness, the large back wound that requires frequent debridement, and constant diarrhea. He is often in pain, although he is receiving patient-controlled analgesia.

Mark has always prided himself on his independence, meticulous appearance, and self-sufficiency. His new dependence on the nurses and his family for basic human needs is devastating for him. He often apologizes for needing to be cleaned up. The nurses caring for him empathize with his suffering and respond with compassion to the indignity of the disease and the assault of treatment on his self-image. They treat him with the utmost respect, physically and emotionally. They make every possible effort to restore his dignity by maintaining his privacy, allowing him choices, and honoring the coping mechanisms he uses to deal with the treatment and disease. They consistently advocate for better management of his pain and spend time with him, listening to his concerns while keeping silent to honor him.

Anna, an 8-month-old infant who has human immunodeficiency virus (HIV), has been hospitalized repeatedly with a variety of HIV-related health problems, including opportunistic infections, recurrent fever and sepsis, thrombocytopenia, impaired myocardial function, chronic diarrhea, encephalopathy, failure to thrive, and developmental delay. Six weeks ago, she was admitted to the hospital with respiratory distress, poor oxygenation, and failure to thrive. Her respiratory compromise worsened, and she was electively intubated and mechanically ventilated. Her liver and spleen were greatly enlarged, and she had severely diminished myocardial function. Over the next week, she received maximal ventilatory support, but her lungs did not improve and she was unable to be weaned from the ventilator. She also had pain due to muscle aches, mouth sores, Candidiasis, hepatosplenomegaly, and frequent procedures.

When Anna was 5 months old, her 19-year-old mother died of AIDS-related complications. Anna had been placed in foster care as a newborn because of her mother's age, history of drug abuse, and a positive drug screen at birth. Anna's grandmother was unable to care for her because of her own history of schizophrenia and child neglect. No other relatives were available to assume Anna's care, so she was placed in the care of a specially trained foster mother. As Anna's condition worsened, however, she needed to be admitted to a chronic care facility for children.

As Anna's condition deteriorates, controversy regarding the goals of her treatment emerges among the health care team. Upon her admission to the ICU, invasive measures are used to treat the respiratory and multisystem organ failure. Multiple therapies are instituted, some not proven to be effective in the treatment of AIDS-related syndromes in children. Some members of the health care team believe that, because the trajectory of AIDS in children is evolving, it is imperative that the goal of care be to prolong life. Other caregivers for Anna, especially her bedside nurses, are increasingly concerned about her level of pain and the number of painful interventions she is undergoing. Despite the efforts to date, they believe that Anna is still undermedicated for pain. They believe that Anna is dying and that the interventions are prolonging her suffering.

The situation is further complicated because Anna's legal guardian is the state, which must be involved in any decisions to initiate or forgo medical intervention. Decision making is compromised by the bureaucratic process and by the fact that her primary health care team has assumed a major role in advocating for Anna in the absence of an invested and available decision maker. As long as there is controversy within her care team, the state is unlikely to decide to withhold or discontinue medical intervention (adapted from Rushton et al., 1993).

Issues

Shared human encounters give rise to an empathetic identification by the health care professional with the patient's suffering and invite compassion to arise. In the words of Arthur Frank, "One of our most difficult duties as human beings is to listen to the voices of those who suffer" (Frank, 1995, p. 25). In Mark's case, clinicians are able to intimately enter his world and remain grounded in themselves and their professional roles with unencumbered hearts and minds. While cases such as Mark's invoke myriad emotional, spiritual, and moral questions among patients, families, and clinicians, his caregivers are able to honor him as a person and believe that their actions are congruent with their professional values and ideals. In contrast, Anna's story is characterized by moral tension and distress among the care team, whose members disagree about what will best serve the patient. Some of Anna's caregivers feel as if they are expected to act against their moral beliefs, thereby diminishing their integrity. In the absence of a designated advocate, moral tension is heightened by conflicts among those acting as surrogates for Anna and attempting to define her interests. Certainly, the goal is for each clinical situation to result in outcomes similar to Mark's case, yet this is often difficult to achieve.

Several factors influence caregivers' experiences, particularly those involving children with life-threatening conditions. First, the context for providing palliative and end-of-life care is fraught with the ambiguities that accompany such conditions. Decisions regarding treatment for these children inevitably must be made under conditions of uncertainty. Determining the child's best interests can be particularly difficult when the diagnosis, prognosis, or disease trajectory is unclear. In such cases, assessing the benefits or burdens that will result from disease-directed and/or purely palliative goals of care is exceptionally difficult, often challenging core values and igniting conflict.

The unpredictability of a child's response to disease-directed therapy may motivate caregivers or parents to try to reduce uncertainty by pursuing additional diagnostic studies and innovative therapies. This creates ambiguity and controversy about whether the child's condition is reversible or is the terminal phase of the disease. Depending on how uncertainty is viewed, as either threat or opportunity, caregivers or parents may be willing in some instances to accept a greater degree of burden to give the child an opportunity for a longer life and the possibility of future beneficial treatments (Mishel, 1988). At times, however, the quest for certainty may result in disproportionate burden for the patient. In cases like Anna's, health care professionals may experience frustration and ridicule if they question the plan, suggest that the burden of treatment has exceeded the benefit of sustaining life, or voice concerns that the desire to innovate or scientific curiosity has supplanted the patient's best interests.

Second, technologic achievements in pediatric care have created unanticipated dilemmas as powerful diagnostic techniques, sophisticated surgical procedures, effective drugs, and expedient therapeutic interventions have interrupted the usual course of illness and disability. Problems have become magnified because life can be sustained for a significant period if the patient or family has accepted dependence on a specific procedure, device, or machine. The uncertainties and ambiguities that result from disease, injury, and the use of technology often force health care professionals to demand a path that they believe will effect a "cure," in the absence of otherwise compelling evidence that the child will inevitably die of the condition.

Even in providing routine care, health care professionals must balance competing obligations, to their institution, their coworkers, and themselves as individuals. Situations can and do arise in which the safety and quality of care are jeopardized as a result of institutional policies, lack of administrative support, inter- and intraprofessional conflicts, poor communication, or legal constraints. Cases like Mark's and Anna's, in which patient acuity and the intensity of interventions are high, carry increased risk of provider errors (Institute of Medicine, 2000). Institutional decisions to admit every critically ill patient despite limited resources exacerbate such risks and create intense moral distress among health care professionals. The end result—despite care-givers' efforts to put on a professional face and appear "strong"—is all too often a downward spiral of mistakes, guilt, diminished self-esteem, and sub-optimal patient care. Provision of care that is incongruent with their core values threatens health care professionals' self-image and integrity (Solomon et al., 2005).

In addition to highlighting conflicts within health care itself, Anna's case illustrates the convergence of societal ills in one troubled inner-city family, beset by poverty, drug and alcohol abuse, illness, violence, and grief. In the face of these overpowering misfortunes, Anna's caregivers struggle to make a difference in her life and to protect her interests. No small task, this requires that they balance their values as individuals and professionals with the reali-ties of Anna's condition, while only the state has the legal authority to decide on her behalf. They must also acknowledge that the medical model is inad-equate to address social problems such as those facing Anna and find some way to accommodate the tensions that result from this fact.

Suffering

DEFINITION

Suffering and loss are intrinsic and inevitable dimensions of caring for chil-dren with life-threatening conditions. According to Reich, suffering is "an anguish experienced as a threat to our composure, our integrity, the fulfill-ment of our intentions, and more deeply as a frustration to the concrete meaning that we have found in our personal experience. It is the anguish over the injury or threat to the injury to the self and thus the meaning of the self that is at the core of suffering" (Reich, 1989, p. 85). Eric Cassell describes suffering, "the state of severe distress associated with events that threaten the intactness of person," as happening to the whole person who ascribes to it his or her personal meaning (Cassell, 1991, p. 33). When mean-ing and purpose in life are threatened, suffering occurs at a spiritual or existential level. This construct clarifies why professionals caring for criti-cally ill children feel threatened if they "get too close" and allow themselves to experience grief. At the most profound level, they fear that this level of intimacy will threaten their ability to continue to function in their profes-sional roles (Cassell, 1991; Barnard, 1995).

In such instances, caregivers struggle to retain integrity in their relation-ships so that they do not suffer for and with others to the point of their own ineffectiveness or withdrawal. To avoid becoming overwhelmed with the suffering of the other, the boundaries of intimacy with patients and families require a balance between overempathizing and cultivating a stance of equanimity through embodying a healing presence (Peter and Liaschenko, 2004; Halifax, Dossey, and Rushton, 2006; Halifax, 2008). As they fulfill their obligations and expectations as professionals, caregivers may encounter threats to their ideal of their profession and professional goals, self-image, moral character, and personal identity. They may judge themselves harshly if the outcomes they pursue do not occur, if they are treated with disrespect or punished by other health care professionals or the institution where they practice, or if they fail to act because they lack skills or courage. The assault on caregivers' basic values—their understanding of life, death, disability, and relationships—may compromise how they perceive the meaning of their work. Disruptions of self may emerge as changes in the health care professional's autonomy, moral well-being, character, or self-esteem and may manifest themselves in many ways, described below, in the care the professional provides.

Whether real or perceived, powerlessness—the inability to cause or prevent change—contributes to caregiver suffering and undermines moral agency. A health care professional's perceived inability to minimize or eliminate tragic outcomes brings on feelings of powerlessness and helplessness. These feelings are magnified when professionals feel that they have no control over their practice, no input into the treatment plan, or no recourse in carrying out a plan they find morally objectionable (Penticuff and Waldren 2000; Corley et al., 2005), such as participating in unduly burdensome interventions with dying patients. In short, if caregivers believe that they receive little, if any, validation by other members of their health care team or the institution, their moral agency is threatened. Enforcing rules or imposing policies that limit or discount the legitimate role of any health care professional in the decision-making process renders them powerless, suppresses their values, and ultimately undermines their capacity for compassion (Rushton, 1995; Halifax, Dossey, and Rushton, 2006).

Understanding these threats is the key to understanding professional caregiver suffering. Underlying them all is a threat to the individual's integrity, that internal state of wholeness in all dimensions of a person's being—physical, emotional, and spiritual. Integrity relies on balance and harmony among the various dimensions of human existence. Because we are whole beings, suffering occurs at the level of the whole being (Singh, 1998). Threats to bodily integrity, for instance, can become evident as disease, injury, or illness. For caregivers, the occurrence of physical symptoms may reflect their own suffering within their professional roles (specific examples are discussed later in the chapter). Similarly, psychological integrity may be undermined by psychopathology or threats to personhood, potentially culminating in disintegration of the self. The self-image of health care professionals can be undermined by various threats: unrealistic expectations, suppressed feelings that mute the authentic self, maladaptive coping, dysfunctional relationships, and absent or ineffective communication. Because spiritual integrity involves integration of moral character, adherence to moral norms, and coherent and consistent behavior within a set of principles or commitments, it too is vulnerable to disruptions. For caregivers, treatment decisions may threaten their understanding of justified and unjustified burdens, obscure or extinguish the meaning of their work, or even lead to a crisis of faith. Consider the two cases described earlier in this chapter: in Mark's case, integrity was promoted; in Anna's case, it was fractured.

Threats to the integrity of health care professionals may be caused by arbitrary or capricious decisions that are made and acted on. Such actions may alienate them from their convictions and cause them to neglect what matters most—in many cases their sense of being a "good" physician, nurse, social worker, or other professional (Cadge and Catlin, 2006). When caregivers act in a way they believe to be wrong, their loss of integrity results in suffering. Physicians, nurses, child-life specialists, social workers, chaplains, family caregivers, and others may struggle to determine whether they did all they could to help a child or whether they missed any signs or symptoms that could have altered the outcome, were inaccurate in diagnosis, or did not fulfill their professional obligations or moral code. Their expectations and desire to alleviate or improve the patient's condition often frame their sense of what is required in their role. They may believe that if they "try hard enough" or are "smart enough," they can accomplish the outcomes they desire. When death is the outcome, their self-image may be altered, their integrity compromised because the outcome is incongruent with the ideals of their profession (Rushton, 1995; Catlin et al., 2008a; Kearney et al., 2009).

The caregiver's sense of doing the right thing may also be challenged, particularly in the face of significant ambiguity and uncertainty. Consider some questions that may arise:

- Am I helping this child or harming her by the treatments we are providing?
- Can I live with the image of myself as a doctor, nurse, chaplain, social worker, parent, etc., if I carry out a particular action?
- Can I live with the choices that I have made on behalf of this patient?
- Can I live with my participation in implementing the choices made by others (health care professional, parents, and administration)?

Each of these questions reflects a concern about acting in a way that undermines personal integrity. Commonly, when integrity is threatened or compromised, a "moral remainder or residue" persists (Webster and Baylis, 2000). Similarly, one's attunement to the moral dimensions of clinical practice reflects the development of moral sensitivity and may have both positive and negative effects on the individual (Wilkinson, 1987; Tiedje, 2000).

An environment in which these questions can be deliberated openly and intentionally among the care team is essential for the well-being of each of the team members and the prevention of moral distress. Doctors in training will especially benefit from such open inquiry as a model for collaboration and support in the midst of difficult situations and decisions. Chaplains, social workers, and psychologists can be instrumental in initiating conversations about the suffering and distress that accompanies difficult decisions made in the best interest of the child, even as all involved had been hoping for a different outcome. All caregivers need the emotional support from the entire team for those times when there is no medicine to offer but the need to be present as a caring human being still exists and, in fact, intensifies.

Suffering can arise intermittently or be sustained over long periods. In Mark's case, the intensity of the suffering increased when caregivers were asked to perform procedures that caused him to lose bodily, psychological, and/or spiritual integrity. Through their responses, Mark's nurses transformed his suffering into compassionate action and healed their own threatened integrity. By contrast, Anna's caregivers were unable to transform their suffering into compassionate action. The repeated threats to their integrity resulted in a sense of alienation from their self-identity, the goals of treatment, and the integrity of their work—in short, a climate of moral distress.

Tattlebaum differentiates suffering from painful feelings; suffering is the "persistence of painful feelings long after they were provoked" (Tattlebaum, 1989, p. 3). In other words, suffering leaves an indelible imprint on the psyche of the person experiencing it. We are hard-wired, it seems, to remember our suffering. The details of our suffering are integrated into both conscious and unconscious parts of our psyche. Often caregivers can recount the events surrounding a situation that caused them suffering many years later, with more vivid detail than they can give for an event occurring only a few days previously (Cadge and Catlin, 2006). When a suffering experience is unprocessed or unresolved and remains in the unconscious, the response to it will likely reappear whenever similar experiences of suffering or grief occur; it may also appear as inappropriate or disproportionate responses to other situations.

The experience of suffering often leaves the person feeling exposed and vulnerable. At its root is the sense of having no control over one's destiny, of submitting to or being forced to endure some particular set of circumstances (Hauerwas, 1986). This view of suffering as a passive process tends to leave the person feeling victimized and powerless; it is often reinforced by a view of suffering as an inevitable part of certain experiences, diseases, or roles. Some believe that suffering has redemptive value and "builds character," while others hold that it does not build character, but rather reveals it. Regardless of the meaning assigned to the experience, suffering carries immense spiritual and religious connotations, and both positive and negative consequences are possible.

Culture, personal experiences, and belief systems all influence the impact of suffering. Chaplains are trained and chaplaincy programs designed to attend to suffering and the search for meaning in life as these experiences challenge patients, families, and professional caregivers. Through ritual, worship, remembrance services, debriefing, or one-on-one encounters, chaplains and others often provide a caring presence to hear the personal narrative of the suffering person and to assist him or her in expressing and integrating the experience of suffering.

RELATED CONCEPTS

Several concepts—burnout, compassion fatigue syndrome, and moral distress—are related to the concept of caregiver suffering (Sundin-Huard and Fahy, 1999). The terms *burnout* and *compassion fatigue syndrome* describe the sense of being disconnected from oneself that characterizes caregiver suffering. Burnout is "a state of physical, emotional, mental exhaustion caused by long-term involvement in emotionally demanding situations" (Pines and Aronson, 1988, p. 9). It emerges gradually and is a result of emotional exhaustion and job stress. In contrast, compassion fatigue is characterized by a sense of helplessness, confusion, and isolation and can have a more rapid onset and resolution than burnout (Figley, 1995; Najjar et al., 2009). Despite the increasing use of the term, compassion fatigue may more accurately reflect what Figley later called "secondary traumatic stress" that results from helping or desiring to help a suffering person. With this definition, it is not compassion that causes fatigue but rather the inability to relieve the suffering or relate to it in ways that are not draining or exhausting because of repeated exposure or reexposure to suffering and trauma (Figley, 1995). Methods to differentiate these concepts are still lacking (Najjar et al., 2009).

The third term, *moral distress*, is "the pain or anguish affecting the mind, body or relationships in response to a situation in which the person is aware of a moral problem, acknowledges moral responsibility, and makes a moral judgment about the correct action; yet, as a result of real or perceived constraints, participates in perceived moral wrongdoing" (ANA, 2002). Acting in a manner contrary to personal or professional values undermines the individual's sense of integrity (Jameton, 1993). When health care professionals cannot live up to their personal values by acting in an ethical manner or when their conscience is violated, they experience moral distress in response to their own suffering (Solomon et al., 2005; Hamric et al., 2007). Initially, caregivers may experience feelings of frustration, anger, and anxiety in response to obstacles and conflicts with others about important values. Once recognized as a situation in which action is needed, they then respond to a real or perceived inability to act on their initial moral distress. This process involves an appraisal of how the situation and the actions taken—or not taken—promote or undermine integrity and/or result in participation in actions that are viewed as wrong (Jameton, 1993).

At the core of each concept is the sense of loss—of integrity, self-image, relationships, and hopes for the future—and of grief in the face of loss. For health care professionals, this includes threats to their integrity when they cannot resolve core issues. They may feel unable to honor their core commitments to their patients, for example, or incapable of seeing dignified deaths as a healing act.

As shown in table 12.1, many interrelated factors may undermine the integrity of health care professionals, cause moral distress, and ultimately result in caregiver suffering. Many of the factors listed here have also been associated with burnout and compassion fatigue syndrome. For instance, institutional policies and politics may lead to a sense of powerlessness; in

Table 12.1 Factors that may threaten integrity

Internal	*External*
Powerlessness	Lack of leadership
Competing obligations	Institutional policies, priorities, values
Values conflicts	Lack of administrative support
Religious/spiritual belief conflicts	Inter- and intraprofessional conflicts
Inability to articulate the ethical problem or source of suffering	Interpersonal disrespect
Conscience violations	Disintegrated models of care delivery
Lack of knowledge, skill	Communication failures
Lack of confidence	Legal, regulatory, or financial constraints
Lack of awareness	Politics of "being in the middle"
Misplaced guilt, blame, shame	Responsibility without authority
Uncertainty	

like manner, other external causes of moral distress work their way through to internal manifestations. This dynamic may exist among internal and external factors that may threaten integrity; for example, a lack of confidence might result in inter- and intraprofessional conflicts (Janvier et al., 2007).

THE EXPERIENCE

By nature subjective and unique to the person experiencing it, suffering is intensely personal and private. With the potential to destroy, suffering can erode a person's sense of integrity and undermine physical, emotional, and spiritual health. However, suffering can also transform, serving as the catalyst for self-understanding and growth. Suffering can signify a sense of endurance, perseverance, and courage rather than disintegration and degradation. The cause of suffering, according to Tattlebaum (1989), is not the situation or its consequences, but the way the individual views and responds to the situation.

A compassionate response to suffering invites empathy and connection rather than alienation or isolation. Health care professionals witness the suffering that accompanies illness or injury beyond the obvious physical and emotional suffering of the child in the situation—the indignities and the damage to the patient's self-image, the depletion of financial and human resources, the stress of parents who desperately hope for their child's recovery, and the anxiety born of the sense of powerlessness in a situation beyond their control. Health care professionals suffer because they understand and identify with the sufferings of the patient and family.

Nurses in particular experience this suffering in an intimate way. In their roles, they have the most sustained proximity to the patient and directly carry out the treatment plan. They witness the impact of their ministrations on the child and family and sometimes struggle to make sense of interventions they may view as harmful or senseless (Jameton, 1987; Peter and Liaschenko, 2004; Ferrell, 2006). This intimate connection gives nurses the opportunity to confront their own mortality and losses. Nurses and other health care professionals who are parents confront the fragility of their own children's lives and their helplessness to protect them from disease or injury. Caring deeply and genuinely for patients as individuals involves identifying with their experiences while acknowledging their independent existences and experiences. Nurses demonstrate compassion by "being there," staying attuned to the patient, and taking actions to relieve the patient's physical, emotional, or spiritual distress (Rushton 2005; Rushton, Halifax, and Dossey, 2007; Rushton et al., 2009).

Parents and health care professionals experience an unspeakable sense of grief and failure when a child is dying. Often this leads them to try to extinguish any uncertainty surrounding treatment. When interventions do not yield the desired outcomes, health care professionals question whether they have done "everything" to help the child (Keene-Reder and Serwint, 2009). They may compartmentalize the child's care into organ systems and examine the evidence for any suggestion of progress; they may consider interventions and approaches that have not been proven useful in a particular population. If health care professionals view death as a failure, then "doing everything" becomes the modus operandi to forestall the inevitable threat to their integrity. In such instances, efforts to avoid "failure" may contribute to clinical interventions or practices that result in premature declarations of futility or, alternately, burdensome overtreatment.

Feelings of guilt have many dimensions. For parents (Miller and Ober, 1999), feelings may manifest themselves as the guilt of helplessness, survivorship, and ambivalence; perceived misdeeds; shame; or codependence. While some of these are particular to parental grief, Miller's data suggest that professional caregivers may manifest similar forms of grief, although clearly of a lesser magnitude. For example, professionals may experience feelings of guilt at their helplessness to prevent the child's death. This guilt often results in blaming themselves or others for the failure of medical interventions or in expressions of regret and remorse. Health care professionals may also feel the guilt of ambivalence about their interactions with the child and family, their advocacy efforts (or lack thereof), or their level of attentiveness to the child or family. In some cases, this guilt leads to shameful feelings and loss of self-esteem. For most caregivers, the most profound form is causal guilt, guilt that accompanies an unspoken suspicion that in some way they caused the child's death—either by contributing to, failing to prevent, or figuratively causing the death, through acts of omission or commission. At its core, this is the guilt of perceived responsibility for the child's death.

FAMILY CAREGIVERS

Most of the concepts discussed here are applicable, and perhaps even more salient, when the caregiver is a parent or family member. Over the past few decades, the survival of children with life-threatening conditions and special health care needs has increased substantially. Concurrently, health care has shifted to ambulatory and community-based settings, which translates into increased demands on family members; at the same time, families have become smaller in size. The result is that fewer family members are taking on more and more caregiving responsibilities. Family caregivers differ from health care professionals in several obvious but important ways. Their psychoemotional relationships with their "patients" (biological children, foster/adopted children, siblings, nieces/nephews, grandchildren, etc.) are multilayered—based in love and best interest, yet complicated with guilt, stress, and other exhausting emotions. Their roles as caregivers are mostly unexpected; family caregivers don't usually choose or plan to raise a child with a complex, chronic, and/or life-threatening condition. Preparation and training usually occur "on the job," and the consequences of "trial-and-error" learning are laden with stress and fear (Aneshensel et al., 1995).

Informal caregivers also lack the advantages that usually accompany a formal career as a caregiver, whether practical (salary and benefits) or integrity based (societal worth and status). While there appear to be stages in the formal development of the role—preparation, acquisition, enactment, and eventual disengagement (Blacher, 1984)—progression along the "career" pathway is driven more by the child's trajectory of decline and dependence than by ambition or desire to pursue higher knowledge. Mostly, of course, the role is not one that can usually be started and stopped when convenient or desired (Raina et al., 2005).

Research on the particular suffering of family caregivers for children who have palliative care needs remains to be done. Literature from some distinct family caregiving paradigms (cerebral palsy, developmental disability, cancer) has begun to shed light on the unique journey undertaken by family caregivers, as well as their responses and helpful strategies. Until more is known, and for the purposes of this chapter, we include family caregivers in the remainder of the discussion about addressing suffering in the caregiver without specific differentiation. Suffice it to say, however, that the cost of unrecognized and untreated suffering in family caregivers is extremely high. Compassion fatigue or burnout obviously has broad-reaching impact on the family itself, the community, the child's health care system, and even society, if the suffering caregiver develops compromised health or becomes lost as a productive member of the workforce. Apart from all these issues, however, is the most important point: children with life-threatening conditions need and want their family caregivers, and for this reason if for no other, family caregiver suffering must be addressed proactively and successfully.

RESPONSES

Caregiver suffering may present itself through a wide array of symptoms, as shown in table 12.2. These symptoms or responses are derived from concepts related to suffering and cluster in four main categories: physical, emotional, behavioral, and spiritual. Individual caregivers manifest varying patterns of responses to suffering. Some individuals may find themselves seeking a

Table 12.2 Common responses to suffering

Physical	Emotional	Behavioral	Spiritual
Fatigue	Anger	Addictive or compulsive behavior	Loss of meaning
Exhaustion	Fear	Controlling behaviors	Crisis of faith
Lethargy	Guilt	Shaming others	Loss of control
Hyperactivity	Resentment	Offender behavior	Hopelessness
Weight gain	Sorrow	Victim behaviors	Loss of self-worth
Weight loss	Depression	Depersonalization	Disrupted religious practices
Persistent physical ailments	Grief	Apathy	Disconnection with people, work, community
Headaches	Anxiety	Indifference	
GI disturbances	Confusion	Avoidance	
Impaired sleep	Sarcasm	Boundary violations / overidentification	
Impaired mental processes (judgment, concentration, etc.)	Emotional outbursts	Erosion of relationships	
	Emotional shutdown	Mistrust	
	Feeling overwhelmed	Splitting	
Susceptibility to illness	Cynicism	Isolation from others	
	Feeling ineffective	Passive-aggressive behavior	
	Rigidity	Perfectionism	
		Omnipotence (others not capable of handling situation)	

Source: Adapted from Figley, 1995; Collins and Long, 2003; Rourke, 2007; Sinclair and Hamill, 2007; Kearney et al., 2009.

physician's help with persistent gastrointestinal (GI) problems, for example, while ignoring their underlying suffering. Others may find anger "easier" than showing vulnerability or admitting to suspect behaviors. Distinctions among the categories are not always clear. For example, fatigue and depression may be closely linked. Distinctions between emotional and behavioral responses are even more difficult to draw. Sarcasm may be considered a distancing behavior, and resentment an avoidance response. It may be helpful to identify emotional responses as "feelings," internal in nature, and behavioral responses as "actions," or external manifestations of suffering.

Professionals who feel constrained from taking the moral actions they believe to be right may respond with resentment. Others may experience guilt because they believe they lacked the courage to do what they knew was right. In cases like Anna's, caregivers experience guilt when they believe they inflict unjustified pain and suffering on their patient. In extreme instances, health care professionals experience emotional shutdown and become so disconnected with themselves that they walk around as "a shell of a person," no longer capable of compassion or engagement with others (Kearney, 1996; Hefferman and Heilig, 1999).

Like physical and emotional symptoms, behavioral responses take many different forms. Avoidance behaviors are common among caregivers who feel victimized and powerless. These include avoiding contact with the patient or family, developing a pattern of absenteeism, making frequent job changes, and so on. Addictive behaviors range from self-medication with drugs or alcohol to gambling or other less overtly destructive activities, such as compulsive shopping or "workaholism" (Kearney et al., 2009).

Another category of behavioral responses involves shaming or victimizing others. For example, some individuals adopt attitudes of arrogance or superiority based on their credentials, expertise, or roles; they may go so far as to use their status to disrespect, discount, or minimize the expertise or contributions of others. Some adopt "offended" behaviors to protect themselves at the expense of others, making themselves essentially impenetrable to human dimensions and situations. Some professionals resort to focusing on the behaviors of others rather than taking responsibility for their own behavior or participation; this may contribute to a failure to engage in moral discourse with others, undermining community integrity. Beyond these, there may be a pervasive expression of indifference and cynicism. Each of these behaviors can result in destructive relationships of every level and type (Stanley et al., 2007).

Behavioral responses can also include boundary violations, either constricted or diffuse. Health care professionals may employ constrictive controlling behaviors to create a sense of safety from the uncertain and unpredictable events inherent in caring for children with life-threatening conditions. Their rigidity may manifest itself in lack of flexibility in their own actions and thought, or as criticism of others who do not practice in the same way or share their beliefs and values.

Rigidity often presents with distancing behaviors, such as emotional withdrawal, physical isolation, and superficial and cool interactions with patients, families, and colleagues. Other distancing behaviors include rage, hostility, or distraction in a flurry of activity (i.e., staying busy as a means to avoid having to deal with feelings). For caregivers who believe that death represents failure, distancing behaviors may be an attempt to avoid situations that arouse feelings of guilt, sorrow, or grief.

Diffuse boundary violations are also indicative of caregiver suffering. They include patterns of "overinvolvement" to meet personal needs and behaviors that have been labeled as codependent (Holder and Schenthal, 2007). Inappropriate disclosures and interactions, including breaches of confidentiality, are also symptoms of diffuse boundary violations. Whether diffuse or constricted, boundary violations can undermine relationships in every sphere—personal, professional, and community.

Threats to spiritual integrity may manifest as feelings of loss of meaning in one's role or work, relationships, or life generally. Health care professionals who experience cumulative suffering may search for meaning in their work in the face of pain and suffering. Some individuals may experience a crisis of their faith in God or higher being. Questions about how and why the suffering of children is permitted may arise. Loss of spiritual integrity can also result in a disruption in religious practices and disconnection with relationships, work, or community. Feelings of hopelessness, loss of control, and erosions in self-worth pervade threats to spiritual integrity. Grief, both acute and cumulative, may affect the spiritual energy of the caregiver. Grief is inevitable as the professional understands and responds to the suffering of patients and families. Rashotte referred to health care professionals as "disenfranchised grievers" because their grief is not recognized by society or by the work environment. This becomes a liability for the clinician who strives to demonstrate deep and caring relationships with patients. Such caring can be enhanced if clinicians are encouraged to name and attend to their feelings of grief (Rashotte, 2005).

When suffering becomes severe and unacknowledged, the result can be described as soul pain: "the experience of an individual who has become disconnected and alienated from the deepest and most fundamental aspects of himself or herself" (Kearney, 1996, p. 60). The intense distress inherent in soul pain creates an overwhelming need to do something to alleviate painful feelings. This need may manifest itself in the symptoms and behaviors discussed earlier. When soul pain and its manifestations lead to loss of confidence, erosion of self-esteem, and loss of integrity, individuals may compensate by constantly seeking approval of others or compartmentalizing themselves.

The physical symptoms arising from underlying suffering may intensify and fail to respond to usual treatments. Behavioral responses, at least initially, tend to be characterized by denial. Because it is too threatening to accept that some children will not benefit from our efforts, health care professionals may deny that the treatment they are providing may be overly burdensome or compromise important values. Instead, they narrowly focus on the functioning of individual body systems of the patient rather than on integrating efforts to address the holistic needs of the patient and family. The temporary reassurance this gives ultimately results in alienation and disconnection as the evidence of impending death escalates. Denial of the possibility of death and the impact of the death on the caregiver can give way to feelings of emptiness, hopelessness, numbness, and meaninglessness. Unable to experience feelings fully, such caregivers can no longer respond to the suffering of others and of themselves. In essence, they deny—or, more precisely, try to deny—the existence of suffering. Paradoxically and tragically, this pattern can lead to just what the clinician wants most to prevent: causing increased suffering for children and their families.

Strategies to Address Caregiver Suffering

The suffering of health care professionals within their caregiving roles is real. Despite the potential downsides and dangers, however, the opportunity to participate so intimately in the lives of children and families facing life-threatening conditions can instead be positive, growth inspiring, and extremely satisfying. In short, "compassion fatigue" can be transformed into "compassion satisfaction" (Stamm, 2002; Kearney et al., 2009).

For caregivers of children with life-threatening conditions, the framework of integrity provides a road map to address suffering. If integrity is the goal, health care professionals and the institutions where they practice must share a vision of the behaviors and character traits they value. In such an environment, persons of integrity consistently exhibit the virtue of integrity, honoring the integrity of self and others. They understand that integrity encompasses autonomy but is not synonymous with self-determining actions or exerting their will on others. As persons of integrity, they are willing to subject their views to scrutiny and criticism. They engage in a process of assessing good and bad reasons for making concessions in situations where values conflict. They are committed to revising or reassessing principles based on an open process of analysis that leads to justifiable moral modifications. Persons of integrity cultivate trust through their trustworthy behaviors, relationships, and commitments; they honor the boundaries and limits of relationships (Pellegrino, 1990; Reina, Reina, and Rushton 2007).

Creating an environment that allows caregivers to practice with integrity is no simple task. Strategies to promote the integrity of the person being cared for, the family, the health care professional, the institution, and the community require multipronged efforts. Only through commitment to a shared vision can health care professionals and institutions successfully modulate the experience of suffering and its effect on the quality of patient care.

The process of addressing this important issue involves much more than individual interventions. Initially, single-discipline sessions may help to create trust and illuminate and explore the issues. To evolve to a place where interdisciplinary sharing and problem solving are possible, the entire care team needs to participate in interdisciplinary forums where suffering can be discussed and coping strategies defined. Table 12.3 provides selected strategies for addressing suffering.

Table 12.3 Strategies for addressing suffering

Name it

Discuss, reflect

Create a respectful environment

Foster respectful communication

Create a mechanism to process grief and loss

Transform suffering by creating meaning, compassion, satisfaction, healing connections

Celebrate the caregiving role

Develop self-care practices

Seek skilled mentorship

Cultivate healthy boundaries

Address violations of integrity

ACKNOWLEDGE AND NAME THE SOURCES OF
AND EXPERIENCE OF SUFFERING

To accept and understand the suffering of others, health care professionals must first acknowledge its existence and relate to their own suffering and emotions with compassion, tenderness, and forgiveness (Halifax, Dossey, and Rushton, 2006; Rushton et al., 2009). Identifying the sources of and responses to suffering can ease the process of transforming suffering into meaning. Although sharing suffering makes it bearable, it also involves participating in the entire process, not in an isolated moment of pain. This entails recognizing the suffering of others and being willing to enter into a dynamic process with them to help give meaning to the experience. For health care professionals, making sense out of situations that undermine their integrity requires an environment of trust where they are able to say what they *really* think and feel, not censor their comments and obscure who they really are.

The Latin root of the word *suffering* means "to allow" or "to experience," yet our natural inclination is to try to relieve ourselves of feelings of sadness, anguish, and despair. The most healing approach may be to simply "be with" and experience the full pain of our loss and suffering (Rushton, 2005; Rushton, Halifax, and Dossey, 2007). Although professionals are often unable to extinguish their own suffering or the suffering of others, bearing witness allows them to lend their nonjudgmental presence to others, to acknowledge their own suffering, and to acknowledge suffering as an integral dimension of their practice—a reality that many may wish to deny (Rushton et al., 2009). The practice of *exquisite empathy* or *bidirectionality* has also been shown to enhance professional satisfaction for caregivers; this involves developing the self-awareness necessary to be fully engaged and highly present with patients and families while remaining "well boundaried" (Katz, 2006; Harrison and Westwood, 2009). Similarly, reframing suffering as "compassion satisfaction," and celebrating that pleasure derived from the work of helping others, can counterbalance compassion fatigue (Stamm, 2002).

DEVELOP FORUMS FOR DISCUSSION,
REFLECTION, AND SHARED UNDERSTANDING

Forums can help give voice to suffering. Small inter- and unidisciplinary groups can be an important strategy to build community and openness (Austin et al., 2005). Facilitated discussions in these forums can provide the freedom and the safety health care professionals need to discuss moral issues and the intense feelings associated with the experience of suffering. Creating a safe place for sharing disappointments, fears, and concerns about patient situations can help caregivers as they struggle to identify sources of suffering, responses, and ways of creating meaning. Telling their own and listening to coworkers' stories can help them negotiate meaning and make sense of incomprehensible and confusing situations (Raines, 2000).

Stories help because the meaning an individual assigns to a particular situation is unique, derived from a unique set of personal, social, cultural, familial, religious, and political values. Understanding this context gives insight into how meaning is derived, and the search for meaning can lead to understanding (Coles, 1989). This understanding does not simply mean "knowing" certain facts or concepts, but requires integrating information into one's values, beliefs, and commitments. Meaning making is a way for caregivers to make sense of what is happening to patients, families, and themselves.

Reich (1989) suggests four questions to guide professionals as they struggle to make sense of their own suffering and the suffering they witness and inflict on patients under their care:

1. How can I see myself as a healer in the face of death and profound suffering?
2. What gives meaning to me personally?
3. What gives meaning to my work?
4. How have I grown personally and/or professionally as a result of this experience?

Facilitators of groups aimed at addressing caregiver suffering must be respectful, skillful, and trustworthy to hold emotions and responses of others' suffering and grief. For this reason, it is desirable to have a person with specialized expertise who is not a direct member of the health care team but whom the team trusts to facilitate these discussions (Rushton et al., 2006). Chaplains or psychologists may be ideally suited for this role.

CREATE AN ENVIRONMENT OF RESPECT FOR PATIENTS, FAMILIES, AND CAREGIVERS

Although health care professionals and organizations hold respect to be a core value, disrespect is often pervasive in the health care environment and can be a major contributor to erosion of integrity and caregiver suffering. Disrespect can occur during interactions with patients and families, other health care professionals, and administrators. When people are not treated with respect, it is less likely that they will treat others or themselves with respect.

Creating an environment of respect requires a robust understanding of what is required of individuals and the institutions where they practice (Penticuff and Waldren, 2000; Corley et al., 2005). Respect is an intentional act of acknowledging another person. It involves valuing the knowledge, skill, and diversity of each person. Respect invites us to see beyond a person's characteristics, personality, role, title, or discipline to appreciate the essence of who he or she is. An environment of respect creates norms of behavior that breed trust and integrity (Reina, Reina, and Rushton, 2007; Rushton, 2007). Respect does not imply that everyone agrees on every decision, value, or behavior. Rather, it is demonstrated in the ways in which conflict and diversity are handled. Respect cannot be demanded; it must be earned through trustworthy actions. Respect relies on members of an organization to respect themselves, because without self-respect, externally imposed norms or structures are unlikely to create respect in the workplace.

FOSTER RESPECTFUL COMMUNICATION, DECISION MAKING, AND CONFLICT RESOLUTION

Creating norms of communication and decision making based on respect and integrity provides the foundation for addressing suffering. Caregivers are more likely to experience the negative dimensions of suffering when they perceive that they are marginalized from the process of decision making. The same is true when the goals of care are communicated unclearly or left unsaid, and when there is no mechanism for resolving conflicting goals and values within the team in a respectful manner.

One "safe" way to foster dialogue and discussions about palliative and end-of-life care and caregiver suffering is to establish regular interdisciplinary care rounds (Rushton et al., 2006). Medical and nursing leadership can play an important role in establishing, and making routine, ongoing discussions of this type. Palliative care and ethics rounds or educational events using a case-based format can focus on the sources of suffering, responses, and ways of creating meaning. They can also provide forums in which health care professionals can discuss challenging patient care situations and engage in problem solving and care planning to address potential threats to integrity in a proactive manner. In addition, integrating quality indicators of palliative care into morbidity and mortality conferences can help diminish the intensity and frequency of situations that threaten the integrity of health care professionals. When particular cases instigate caregiver suffering and moral distress, patient care conferences and institutional mechanisms for examining and resolving conflict, such as ethics consultations, can provide supportive structures and processes for caregivers (Rushton, 2006). Whenever conflict arises, efforts to create more inquiry, dialogue, and understanding are needed (Rushton, 2009; Rushton and Adams, 2009).

CREATE MECHANISMS FOR ACKNOWLEDGING AND PROCESSING GRIEF AND LOSS

Responses to patient deaths affect health care professionals both personally and professionally in terms of caregiver suffering and responses to grief. Papadatou (2001) identified special considerations for health care professionals facing the death of pediatric patients. These include the level of investment in the relationship with the patient and family, expectations of the health care professional's identity and roles, and personal/social constructs. Each death can affect one or more levels of loss:

- Loss of the relationship with the patient
- Loss due to identifying with the pain of the patient's family
- Loss of unmet goals and expectations of professional self-image
- Loss of beliefs and assumptions about self, life, and death
- Past unresolved or future anticipated losses
- The inevitable death of oneself

Interventions to address health care professionals' needs to acknowledge and process their own grief and loss will be necessary to promote healthy grieving and restore integrity. Such interventions should be aimed at several tasks (Sanders and Valente, 1994; Papadatou, 2001):

- Managing emotional responses to the death in personally meaningful ways
- Restoring or maintaining professional integrity
- Finding meaning in the death
- Transcending the present suffering in order to reinvest in life

As the health care team experiences multiple deaths, sadness can become the overwhelming response from all team members. The sadness should be honored and staff supported by allowing them time to complete duties and then have a brief respite to grieve and refocus before being assigned to another patient. In a study at Children's Hospital of Wisconsin, staff in the pediatric ICU reported that they welcomed the sadness because they saw it as a sign of their humanity and their ability to be emotionally available to the patient and family. Physicians reported the same feeling of sadness, although it was accompanied by feelings of helplessness and frustration in not being able to help the patient get better (Lee and Dupree, 2008). Surgeons, although often considered emotionally detached, are actually at high risk for caregiver grief owing to factors that connect them on an emotional level to their patients. Hinshaw denotes these factors as (1) the "high-stakes" nature of surgical interventions that may result in death or significant long-term suffering or disability, (2) the intimate nature of interventions that invade the "privacy" of the patient, (3) the juxtaposition of the experience of great joy when the intervention is successful with the fear of things not going well, and (4) the tradition of emotional detachment. The inherent danger is that the grief will be masked and therefore unresolved, resulting in burnout and uncertainty about the value of one's work (Hinshaw, 2005).

Approaches that are aimed at providing information, clinical reviews, emotional support, and meaning making can help to address clinician grief. Group activities, such as debriefing sessions after a child dies, can help create a space for grief and provide caregivers with opportunities to reflect on the events leading to a child's death, the meaning of the child's life and death, personal responses, and self-care strategies (Rushton et al., 2006). Debriefing sessions also provide health care professionals an opportunity to identify things that went well and opportunities for future changes in practices and structures (Keene et al., 2010). Activities and interventions that address anticipatory grief and bereavement are of particular import for family caregivers, especially as unaddressed grief may begin to interfere with appropriate decision making for children who have palliative care needs (Wada and Park, 2009).

TRANSFORM SUFFERING BY CREATING MEANING

Within the search for meaning, the critical task is to transform suffering into an act of healing. Healing is facilitated when individuals find within themselves the resources to nurture their own healing or to bring wholeness into that which has been broken. Some clinicians will seek and find solace in the doctrines, practices, and rituals of their personal faith traditions; others will benefit from the support of spiritual caregivers in their own institutions to find ways of grounding themselves in the inner wellsprings that give them peace and hope (Catlin et al., 2001, 2008b; Ecklund et al., 2007). Spiritual renewal and creating ritual can help a person remain a witness to and not so much a victim of suffering. This transformation requires nurturing compassion rather than yielding to the negative and destructive dimensions of suffering (Rushton, 2005; Rushton, Halifax, and Dossey, 2007). Accomplishing this depends in large part on recognizing that compassion can affect the experience of suffering.

The search for meaning requires addressing physical, emotional, psycho-social, and spiritual needs. Individuals will often need additional support and encouragement to move beyond denial of their suffering to become willing to engage in activities that will assist them in their own process. Reframing the relationship between health care professional and patient as establishing "healing connections" gives caregivers an enhanced sense of being part of something greater than themselves and helps to deepen integrity and whole-ness (Boston and Mount, 2006). Resources such as employee assistance pro-grams, personal coaches, and mental health and spiritual care professionals should be made available.

For family caregivers, the opportunity to see the growth or the good that can emerge from suffering is essential. Despite the stress and overwhelming responsibility, parents caring for children at home on ventilators in one small study reported "deep enrichments and rewarding experiences that they could not imagine living without" (Carnevale et al., 2006, p. e49). Children and families in these and other palliative care situations are often in unfair situ-ations that create moral dilemmas for them and their health care providers, and yet they are able to synthesize their experiences as a duality of "daily living with distress and enrichment" (Carnevale et al., 2006).

Beyond this lies an opportunity for "depth" work to achieve an experi-ence of soul. Meditation, bodywork, imagework, dreamwork, creative arts, journaling, or music can help to "reconnect" the soul with significant and meaningful aspects of living (Kearney et al., 2009). Creating ritual that will help to affirm the sacred in the midst of the profane can also be instrumen-tal in transforming suffering. Through ritual, a caregiver can take a creative and perhaps even a playful stance in facing the suffering (Duvall and Chris-tie, 2009). Robert Johnson suggests using rituals that set in motion changes "at deep levels where attitudes and values originate" (Duvall and Christie, 2009, p. 6). Mindfulness meditation programs for health care professionals or programs that focus on restoring meaning to professional work can be particularly helpful (Kabat-Zinn, 2003; Cohen-Katz et al., 2004; Connelly, 2005; Kearney et al., 2009). Moreover, clinicians find contemplative and reflective practices to be meaningful, useful, and valuable tools for support-ing their own well-being (Rushton et al., 2009).

Meaning making can also be supported through memorial rituals, be it a formal service or a butterfly garden. Healing gardens or reflective spaces now exist in many health care institutions, giving staff and families a quiet, safe place to go to contemplate or process emotional responses. Many institu-tions have annual tribute services to honor and remember the children who have died in their care. Similarly, some institutions are developing regular memorial services and rituals for staff to acknowledge the children they care for and to create opportunities for closure, especially when it is not possible to attend the funeral or family memorial service (Allen, 2003; Kane, 2007; Tiak, 2007).

Caregiver support can also be accomplished informally. In one large pediatric palliative care program, the chaplain engages direct caregivers one on one in the midst of busy units to pause and remember the children who recently died, and performs a personal healing of the hands if desired by the caregiver. Most hospice and palliative care interdisciplinary team rounds usually begin with bereavement updates and moments of reflection to acknowledge the transitions of children in their care. Following this model, encouraging managers to begin staff meetings with a "memorial moment" in which the children who have recently died are called by name is an effective way to allow staff to pause and remember the significance of those lives and of the meaningful care they provided for those children. This is a nonthreatening way to engage staff members who avoid formal services or debriefings. Closure can also be facilitated by providing the opportunity for the care team to participate in bereavement follow-up.

One concrete method to transform suffering is simply to celebrate the caregiving role. For all of the potential negative consequences and downsides, the blessings and advantages of the role—whether as a health care professional or a family caregiver—are innumerable and worth revisiting regularly. For example, clear benefits to family caregiving, such as promotion of patient autonomy and dignity, may need to be named, especially during times when stress or overwhelming responsibility appears to cloud perception. Health care professionals can do this for the families with whom they work, as well as for each other (Rabow, Hauser, and Adams, 2004).

DEVELOP SELF-CARE PRACTICES

Health care professionals need to develop self-care practices for themselves and their colleagues (Rushton, Halifax, and Dossey, 2007). Practices as simple as regular exercise, leisure activities with friends and family, solitary time for reflection and renewal, memorializing a child by planting a flower or lighting a candle, or reaching out to other professionals with a kind word and compassionate query have great value. All too often, professionals look to their own needs last. They must remember that they have certain duties to themselves, duties that must be given moral weight within the boundaries of professional responsibility. The Code for Nurses (ANA, 2001) specifies these and should help nurses as they work to lessen caregiver suffering within their profession.

Institutions must also begin to invest in the health and well-being of their employees. This includes intentional attention to aspects of the work environment that may exacerbate the suffering of health care professionals (Ewing and Carter, 2004; American Association of Critical Care Nurses, 2005). Attention to workload, reward systems, decision-making authority, and the organizational ethics culture is essential to create an environment that promotes integrity. So too are measures that contribute to the development of personal self-care practices, including allowing employees time for self-care in the workplace or time away to attend patient funerals. For example, a critical care unit engaged a massage therapist to give weekly seated-chair massages to the staff. As mentioned above, spiritual support staff such as chaplains can provide support for clinicians and families alike.

For family caregivers, self-care practices may be broadly interpreted to include family functioning. Multiple studies have demonstrated that important predictors of family caregiver physical and psychological health include child behavior, caregiver demands, and family function (Raina et al., 2005; Laurvick et al., 2006). To address these issues, preventive cognitive and behavioral strategies to manage child behavior problems along with stress management techniques have been shown to contribute directly to psychological and physical health in caregivers (Raina et al., 2005). Additionally, direct caregiving assistance (such as respite), support to maintain other roles, financial assistance, sibling support, and interpersonal and marital support are all family "self-care" practices that improve caregiver function. In short, clinical interventions that support holistic, family-centered care management, instead of short-term, child-focused strategies, are most helpful for families.

CULTIVATE HEALTHY BOUNDARIES

Health care professionals caring for children with life-threatening conditions are particularly vulnerable to boundary violations. Developing processes to monitor personal and team involvement and responses to patient care situations can help them protect their integrity while allowing them to connect with others and say "no" when appropriate. These efforts require the development and use of support systems to assess involvement and responses. Although it is possible to exercise advocacy without compassion, the act of caring necessitates a measure of sacrifice and suffering within appropriate boundaries. For health care professionals, this means setting proper limits for compassion and self-sacrifice for their patients and their families—and for themselves.

ADDRESS VIOLATIONS OF INTEGRITY

Health care professionals cannot ignore violations of their integrity. Although they must make compromises, they must make them conscientiously, assessing which are moral and which are not. Acting in opposition to moral principle involves self-betrayal. Integrity demands that professionals, on occasion, raise a conscientious voice and make a conscientious refusal (Catlin et al., 2008a). In some instances, they may need to employ responsible whistleblowing or make a principled exit.

Fortunately, such circumstances are relatively rare. Jameton (1993) suggests the following important questions that caregivers must ask themselves when confronted with an issue that threatens their integrity:

- What is possible for me to do?
- What is the extent of my responsibility?
- When others are not meeting their responsibilities, what is the extent of my responsibility to compensate for their omissions?
- What personal risks are health care professionals obligated to take for patients? For their profession? For themselves?
- When I assist others who are making decisions, and the decisions prove harmful to patients, to what extent do I share the blame?

Asking these questions can clarify issues and roles in situations that threaten professional integrity. Answering them can guide caregivers in their choice of actions and support them in knowing their consciences as professionals and their own hearts as individuals. Health care professionals must also weigh ethical responsibilities, professional standards, and legal statutes (May and Aulisio, 2009).

Conclusion

Caring for sick and dying children and their families is a privilege that carries profound responsibilities and offers great rewards but also requires understanding and accepting suffering. Caregivers need to find a balance in voicing their concerns, striving to learn and understand the reasons behind others' perspectives, learning how to manage stress in effective and healthy ways, determining when they have exceeded their limits of stress, and choosing a course of action in line with their moral compass.

Our capacity to feel grief and to identify with the misfortune of others is the basis of our humanity. The ability to recognize their own suffering empowers caregivers to adopt strategies to protect their patients and families and to preserve their own professional integrity. Without the recognition of suffering, there can be no compassion for children with life-threatening conditions and their families or for their caregivers.

References

Allen, K.Z. 2003. Ritual for a premature Jewish baby whose death is imminent. *Chaplaincy Today* 19(2):31–34.

American Association of Critical Care Nurses. 2005. AACN standards for establishing and sustaining healthy work environments, ed. C. Barden. Aliso Viejo: American Association of Critical Care Nurses.

American Nurses Association (ANA). 2001. Code of ethics for nurses with interpretive statements. Washington, DC: ANA.

———. 2002. Moral distress among nurses.

Aneshensel, C.S., Pearlin, L.I., Mullin, J.T., et al. 1995. *Profiles in Caregiving: The Unexpected Career.* San Diego: Academic Press.

Austin, W., Lemermeyer, G., Goldberg, L., et al. 2005. Moral distress in healthcare practice: The situation of nurses. *HEC Forum* 17(1):33–48.

Barnard, D. 1995. The promise of intimacy and the fear of our own undoing. *J Palliat Care* 11(4):22–26.

Blacher, J. 1984. Sequential stages of parental adjustment to the birth of a child with handicaps: Fact or artifact? *Ment Retard* 22:55–68.

Boston, P.H., and Mount, B.M. 2006. The caregiver's perspective on existential and spiritual distress in palliative care. *J Pain Symptom Manage* 32(1):13–26.

Cadge, W., and Catlin, E.A. 2006. Making sense of suffering and death: How health care providers construct meanings in a neonatal intensive care unit. *J Religion and Health* 45(2):248–63.

Carnevale, F.A., Alexander, E., Davis, M., et al. 2006. Daily living with distress and enrichment: The moral experience of families with ventilator-assisted children at home. *Pediatrics* 117(1):348–60.

Cassell, E. 1991. *The Nature of Suffering and the Goals of Medicine.* New York: Oxford University Press.

Catlin, A., Volat, D., Hadley, M.A., et al. 2008a. Conscientious objection: A potential neonatal nursing response to care orders that cause suffering at the end of life? Study of a concept. *Neo Network* 27(2):101–8.

Catlin, E.A., Cadge, W., Ecklund, E.H., et al. 2008b. The spiritual and religious identities, beliefs and practices of academic pediatricians in the U.S. *Acad Med* 83(12):1118–52.

Catlin, E.A., Guillemin, J.H., Thiel, M.M., et al. 2001. Spiritual and religious components of patient care in the NICU. *J Perinatol* 21(7):426–30.

Cohen-Katz, J., Wiley, S. D., Capuano, T., et al. 2004. The effects of mindfulness-based stress reduction on nurse stress and burnout. *Holistic Nurs Prac* 18(6): 302–8.

Coles, R. 1989. *The Call of Stories: Teaching and the Moral Imagination.* Boston: Houghton Mifflin.

Collins, S., and Long, A. 2003. Working with psychological effects of trauma: Consequences for mental health professionals: A literature review. *J Psychiatr Mental Health Nurs* 10:417–24.

Connelly, J. 2005. Narrative possibilities: Using mindfulness in clinical practice. *Perspect Biol and Med* 48:84–94.

Corley, M.C., Minick, P., Elswick, R.K., et al. 2005. Nurse moral distress and ethical work environment. *Nurs Ethics* 12(4):381–90.

Duvall, R., and Christie, C. 2009. In the strong current of emotion. *Healing Spirit* 4(1):4–7.

Ecklund, E.H., et al. 2007. The religious and spiritual beliefs and practices of academic pediatric oncologists in the U.S. *J Pediatr Hematol Oncol* 29(11):733–35.

Eisenberg, N. 2004. Empathy and sympathy. In *Handbook of Emotions*, 2nd ed., ed. M. Lewis and J.M. Haviland-Jones, pp. 677–88. New York: Guilford Press.

Ewing, A.C., and Carter, B.S. 2004. Once again, Vanderbilt NICU in Nashville leads the way in nurses' emotional support. *Pediatr Nurs* 30(6):471–72.

Ferrell, B.R. 2006. Understanding the moral distress of nurses witnessing medically futile care. *Oncol Nurs Forum* 33(5):922–29.

Figley, C.R. 1995. Compassion fatigue as secondary traumatic stress disorder: An overview. In *Compassion Fatigue: Coping with Secondary Traumatic Stress Disorder*, ed. C.R. Figley, pp. 1–20. New York: Brunner/Mazel.

Frank, A. 1995. *The Wounded Storytellers: Body, Illness, and Ethics.* Chicago: University of Chicago Press.

Halifax, J. 2008. *Being with Dying: Cultivating Compassion and Fearlessness in the Presence of Death.* Boston: Shambhala.

Halifax, J., Dossey, B., and Rushton, C. 2006. *Compassionate Care of the Dying: An Integral Approach.* Santa Fe: Prajna Mountain Publishers.

Hamric, A.B., et al. 2007. Nurse-physician perspectives on the care of dying patients in intensive care units. *Crit Care Med* 35(2):422–29.

Harrison, R.L., and Westwood, M.J. 2009. Preventing vicarious traumatization of mental health therapists: Identifying protective practices. *Psychotherapy: Theory, Research, Practice Training* 46(2):203–19.

Hauerwas, S. 1986. *Suffering Presence: Theological Reflections on Medicine, the Mentally Handicapped and the Church.* Notre Dame, IN: University of Notre Dame Press.

Hefferman, P., and Heilig, S. 1999. Giving "moral distress" a voice: Ethical concerns among neonatal intensive care unit personnel. *Camb Q Healthc Ethics* 8:173–78.

Hinshaw, D. 2005. Spiritual issues in surgical palliative care. *Surg Clin N Amer* 85: 257–72.

Holder, K., and Schenthal, S. 2007. Watch your step: Nursing and professional boundaries. *Nurs Manage* 38(2):24–29.

Institute of Medicine. 2000. *To Err Is Human.* Washington, DC: National Academy Press.

Jameton, A. 1987. Duties to self: Professional nursing in the critical care unit. In *Ethics at the Bedside*, ed. M.D. Fowler and J. Levin-Arliff, pp. 115–35. Philadelphia: Lippincott.

———. 1993. Dilemmas of moral distress: Moral responsibility and nursing practice. *AWHONN'S Clinical Issues Perinatal Women's Health Nursing* 4(4):542–51.

Janvier, A., Nadeau, S., Deschenes, M., et al. 2007. Moral distress in the neonatal intensive care unit: Caregivers' experience. *J Perinatol* 27(4):203–8.

Kabat-Zinn, J. 2003. Mindfulness-based interventions in context: Past, present, and future. *Clin Psychol* 10(2):144–56.

Kane, G.C. 2007. A dying art? The doctor's letter of condolence. *Chest* 131:1245–47.

Katz, R. 2006. When our personal selves influence our professional work: An introduction to emotions and countertransference in end of life care. In *When Professionals Weep: Emotional and Countertransference Responses in End-of-Life Care*, ed. R.S. Katz and T.A. Johnson, pp. 3–12. New York: Routledge.

Kearney, M. 1996. *Mortally Wounded.* New York: Scribner.

Kearney, M.K., Weininger, R.B., Vachon, M.L., et al. 2009. Self-care of physicians caring for patients at the end of life: Being connected . . . a key to my survival. *JAMA* 301(11):1155–64, E1.

Keene, E., Hutton, N., Hall, B., et al. 2010. Bereavement debriefing sessions: An intervention to support health care professionals in managing their grief after the death of a patient. *Pediatr Nurs* 36(4):185–90.

Keene-Reder, E.A., and Serwint, J. 2009. Until the last breath: Exploring the concept of hope for parents and health care professionals during a child's serious illness. *Arch Pediatr Adolesc Med* 163(7):653–57.

Laurvick, C.L., Msall, M.E., Silburn, S., et al. 2006. Physical and mental health of mothers caring for a child with Rett syndrome. *Pediatrics* 118(4):e1152–64.

Lee, K.J., and Dupree, C.Y. 2008. Staff experiences with end-of-life care in the pediatric intensive care unit. *J Pall Med* 11(7):986–90.

May, T., and Aulisio, M.P. 2009. Personal morality and professional obligations: Rights of conscience and informed consent. *Perspectives Biol Med* 52(1):30–38.

Miller, S., and Ober, D. 1999. *Finding Hope When a Child Dies: What Other Cultures Can Teach Us.* New York: Simon & Schuster.

Mishel, M.H. 1988. Uncertainty in illness. *Image J Nurs Sch* 20(4):225–32.

Najjar, N., Davis, L.W., Beck-Coon, K., et al. 2009. Compassion fatigue: A review of the research to date and relevance to cancer-care providers. *J Health Psychol* 14(2): 267–77.

Papadatou, D. 2001. Caring for dying children: A comparative study of nurses' experiences in Greece and Hong Kong. *Cancer Nurs* 24(5):402–12.

Pellegrino, E. 1990. The relationship of autonomy and integrity in medical ethics. *Bull Pan Am Health Organ* 24(4):361–71.

Penticuff, J.H., and Waldren, M. 2000. Influence of practice environment and nurse characteristics on perinatal nurses' responses to ethical dilemmas. *Nurs Res* 49(2): 64–72.

Peter, E., and Liaschenko, J. 2004. Perils of proximity: A spatiotemporal analysis of moral distress and ambiguity. *Nurs Inquiry* 11(4):218–25.

Pines, A.M., and Aronson, E. 1988. *Career Burnout: Causes and Cures.* New York: Free Press.

Rabow, M.W., Hauser, J.M., and Adams, J. 2004. Supporting family caregivers at the end of life: "They don't know what they don't know." *JAMA* 291(4):483–91, e1.

Raina, P., O'Donnell, M., Rosenbaum, P., et al. 2005. The health and well-being of caregivers of children with cerebral palsy. *Pediatrics* 115(6):e626–36.

Raines, M.L. 2000. Ethical decision making in nurses: Relationships among moral reasoning, coping style, and ethics stress. *JONA's Healthcare Law, Ethics and Regulation* 2(1):29–41.

Rashotte, J. 2005. Dwelling with stories that haunt us: Building a meaningful nursing practice. *Nurs Inq* 12(1):34–42.

Reich, W.T. 1989. Speaking of suffering: A moral account of compassion. *Soundings* 72:83–108.

Reina, M.L., Reina, D.S., and Rushton, C.H. 2007. Trust: The foundation for team collaboration and healthy work environments. *AACN Adv Crit Care* 18(2):103–8.

Rourke, M.T. 2007. Compassion fatigue in pediatric palliative care providers. *Pediatr Clin N Amer* 54:631–44.

Rushton, C.H. 1992. Caregiver suffering in critical care nursing. *Heart and Lung* 21(3): 303–6.

———. 1995. The Baby K case: The ethics of preserving professional integrity. *Ped Nurs* 21(4):367–72.

———. 2005. A framework for integrated pediatric palliative care: Being with dying. *J Ped Nurs* 20(5):311–25.

———. 2006. Defining and addressing moral distress: Tools for critical care nursing leaders. *AACN Adv Crit Care* 17(2):161–68.

———. 2007. Respect in critical care: A foundational ethical principle. *AACN Adv Crit Care* 18(2):149–56.

———. 2009. Ethical discernment and action: The art of pause. *AACN Adv Crit Care* 20(1):108–11.

Rushton, C.H., and Adams, M. 2009. Asking ourselves and others the right questions: A vehicle for understanding and resolving conflicts between clinicians, patients, and families. *Adv Crit Care* 20(3):295–300.

Rushton, C.H., Halifax, J., and Dossey, B. 2007. Being with dying, contemplative practices for compassionate end-of-life care. *Amer Nurse Today. ANA* 2(9):16–18.

Rushton, C.H., Hogue, E.E., Billet, C.A., et al. 1993. End of life care for infants with AIDS: Ethical and legal issues. *Ped Nurs* 19(1):79–83; 94.

Rushton, C.H., Reder, E., Hall, B., et al. 2006. Interdisciplinary interventions to improve pediatric palliative care and reduce health care professional suffering. *J Palliat Med* 9(4):922–33.

Rushton, C.H., Sellers, D.E., Heller, K.D., et al. 2009. Impact of contemplative end-of-life training program: Being with dying. *Palliat and Support Care* 7(4):405–14.

Sabo, B.M. 2006. Compassion fatigue and nursing work: Can we accurately capture the consequences of caring work? *Int J Nurs Pract* 12:136–42.

Sanders, J., and Valente, S. 1994. Nurse's grief. *Cancer Nurs* 174(4):318–25.

Sinclair, H.A., and Hamill, C. 2007. Does vicarious traumatisation affect oncology nurses? A literature review. *Eur J Oncol Nurs* 11:348–56.

Singh, K. 1998. *The Grace in Dying*. San Francisco: HarperCollins.

Solomon, M.Z., Sellers, D.R., Heller, K.S., et al. 2005. New and lingering controversies in pediatric end-of-life care. *Pediatrics* 116(4):872–83.

Stamm, B.H. 2002. Measuring compassion satisfaction as well as fatigue: Developmental history of the compassion satisfaction and fatigue test. In *Treating Compassion Fatigue*, ed. C.F. Figley, pp. 107–19. New York: Brunner-Routledge.

Stanley, K.M., Martin, M.M., Michel, Y., et al. 2007. Examining lateral violence in the nursing workforce. *Issues in Mental Health Nurs* 28(11):1247–65.

Sundin-Huard, D., and Fahy, K. 1995. Moral distress, advocacy and burnout: Theorizing the relationships. *Int J Nurs Pract* 5:8–13.

Tattlebaum, J. 1989. *You Don't Have to Suffer: A Handbook for Moving beyond Life's Crises*. New York: Harper & Row.

Tiak, M. 2007. Touchstones: Tangible spiritual nourishment. *Chaplaincy Today* 23(2): 36–7.

Tiedje, L.B. 2000. Moral distress in perinatal nursing. *J Perinat Neonat Nurs* 14(2): 36–43.

Wada, K., and Park, J.2009. Integrating Buddhist psychology into grief counseling. *Death Studies* 33:657–83.

Webster, G.C., and Baylis, F. 2000. *Moral Residue in Margin of Error: The Ethics of Mistakes in Practice of Medicine*. Hagerstown, MD: University Publishing Corp.

Wilkinson, J.M. 1987. Moral distress in nursing practice: Experience and effect. *Nurs Forum* 23(1):16–29.

PART III

SPECIAL CARE ENVIRONMENTS
AND PATIENT POPULATIONS

13

Palliative Care in the Neonatal-Perinatal Period

Suzanne S. Toce, M.D., Steven R. Leuthner, M.D., M.A.,
Deborah L. Dokken, M.P.A., Anita J. Catlin, D.N.Sc., F.N.P.,
Jennifer Brown, and Brian S. Carter, M.D.

Our son, Aubrey, was diagnosed prenatally with a giant omphalocele and a ventriculoseptal defect in his heart. He was born full-term and lived for 158 days, all within the confines of the neonatal intensive care unit (NICU). His care shifted to exclusively comfort/palliative care in the last 2 weeks of his life. The one thing I can say is that even though I left without my son, my experience with the hospital and their staff is something that I will always treasure. In the midst of a horrible tragedy, his end-of-life care was done right. We were included in all decisions, treated with respect, considered part of the team, and retained a sense of control in an out-of-control situation. Extraordinary measures were taken for us to have the ending we desperately needed. The end of our son's life was amazing and beautiful, all due to the diligence of a team that was willing to think outside the box. We were allowed to take Aubrey outside, removed from the sights and sounds of the NICU, to peacefully and lovingly say goodbye to him. The hospital is a place that holds tremendous memories for us, but in the end, that was his home. The staff was his family. They will forever remain in our hearts as having provided exemplary care for our amazing little boy.

Palliative care in the perinatal period is distinct in that care is provided in a setting usually associated with the joy of welcoming a normal newborn into the family. The birth of a baby with a life-limiting condition or fetal or newborn death is in stark contrast to the expected outcome of a natural and "normal" pregnancy, labor, and delivery. Likewise, in the NICU, the reality that cure-directed treatment may fail to achieve its intended goal clashes with the expectation that cure is the norm and miracles happen every day. Perinatal palliative care goals can be applicable following the prenatal diagnosis of a lethal fetal anomaly, after the diagnosis at birth of a neonatal lethal condition, or after the failure of cure-directed treatment to reverse severe medical problems.

There are numerous opportunities for integrating palliative care concepts into care provided in the perinatal period. This will require attention to the questions addressed in this chapter:

- What is the scope of the problem?
- What are effective approaches to shared decision making so that the family's goals, values, and preferences are incorporated into the care plan while acting in the newborn's best interest, including minimizing suffering?
- For which fetuses and infants should we consider palliative care goals as primary?
- How can palliative care be implemented in the prenatal period?
- How can pain, agitation, and other symptoms at the end of life be optimally managed for neonates?
- Do existing models of care exemplify optimal neonatal palliative care?

The Scope of the Problem

Despite remarkable strides in neonatal survival, some newborns will inevitably die. Each year in the United States, there are almost 19,000 neonatal deaths (Kung et al., 2008) and more than 1 million fetal losses (Ventura, Abma, and Mosher, 2004); 9,000 additional deaths occur before the child's first birthday, after a lifelong experience of chronic illness. As neonatal and perinatal practitioners will commonly manage severe illness and death, the need to be able to do so thoughtfully and effectively is clear. Regardless of the duration of the child's life, parents want the child's existence, individual importance, and familial relationships to be recognized and valued. When done well, perinatal palliative care accomplishes this goal.

Applying hospice/palliative care concepts to neonatal care was first described in 1982 (Whitfield et al., 1982). More recently, with life-limiting diagnoses being discovered in utero, palliative care is also initiated prenatally. Clinicians practicing maternal-fetal medicine and neonatal intensive care can and should create an environment in which high tech and high touch coexist and complement each other (Marron-Corwin and Corwin, 2008).

The integration of a palliative care philosophy into the care of families faced with a diagnosis of fetal anomaly or a sick newborn requires the expansion of the goals of care in neonatology (Pierucci, Kirby, and Leuthner, 2001).

The concept of success must include supporting families to find meaning in their babies' lives, however brief (Milstein, 2005). Death itself does not represent failure; however, allowing unnecessary suffering for infants and families is a profound and, unfortunately, common failure. Prevention of suffering through the incorporation of palliative care principles into perinatal care includes attention to the physical environment, the comfort needs of the newborn, and a seamless family-centered approach, including psychosocial, emotional, and spiritual support. Palliative care facilitates collaborative decision making and advance care planning and supports the staff who are challenged by the care of these unfortunate patients and their families.

Decision Making

As with older patients, the "best interests" of the newborn remain the basis of decision making (AAP COFN, 2002, 2007; see also chap. 6). Treatments that are harmful, are not or are no longer beneficial, are ineffective, or will merely prolong the dying process should not be offered. Physicians are not obligated to provide interventions that they consider futile in terms of survival (e.g., resuscitation of a <22-week fetus or an infant with anencephaly), nor are they obligated to withhold interventions that they feel are overwhelmingly likely to be beneficial to the child (i.e., resuscitation of an otherwise-normal 28-week newborn; Paris, 2005).

PRENATAL DECISIONS

Decisions made in advance of delivery to withhold resuscitative or other measures are based on the best interests of the not-yet-born fetus, the family's values, and the input of the health care team. Such decisions are usually reserved for conditions with a high degree of prognostic and in utero diagnostic certainty (Hoeldtke and Calhoun, 2001; Leuthner, 2004; Howard, 2006; Leuthner and Jones, 2007; Marron-Corwin and Corwin, 2008). Three factors should be considered in decision making (Leuthner, 2004):

1. The certainty of the diagnosis
2. The certainty of the prognosis
3. The meaning of the prognosis to the parents

Trisomies 13 and 18, renal dysplasia with anhydramnios and associated pulmonary hypoplasia, anencephaly, and holoprosencephaly can be diagnosed with certainty in utero. Lethal forms of dwarfism, oligohydramnios associated with pulmonary hypoplasia, complex central nervous system anomalies, neurodegenerative diseases, severe complex congenital heart disease, prematurity <23 weeks, and other significant structural anomalies may have prognostic certainty, even if there is no specific diagnosis or etiology. When the fetus has a condition incompatible with prolonged extrauterine survival, alternatives to the usual disease-directed course of care, which in this context may include burdensome and potentially nonbeneficial interventions, should include palliative care as well as pregnancy termination (which may be indicated on medical grounds or personal preferences; Goldsmith, Ginsberg, and McGettigan, 1996; Leuthner, 2004; Paris, 2005). The Neonatal Resuscitation Program acknowledges that resuscitation is not always appropriate, noting that noninitiation of resuscitation in the delivery room is appropriate for infants who have *confirmed* gestation <23 weeks or birth weight <400 grams, anencephaly, or confirmed trisomy 13 or 18 (Byrne, Szyld, and Kattwinkel, 2008; Escobedo, 2008).

DELIVERY ROOM DECISIONS

Delivery room resuscitation is an unusual team sport in which the only player who never swings the bat is also the only one who can strike out. Decisions regarding appropriate resuscitation and treatment of the extremely low birth weight infant should neither be the triumph of hope over reason nor the victory of ego over uncertainty.

—*N. Finer, M.D. (Finer and Barrington, 1998)*

While it would be ideal to have prenatal discussions among the family, the obstetrician, and the pediatrician, it is not always possible. Whether because of a precipitous delivery or lack of prenatal care, at times there are inadequate data at the time of delivery to determine fetal maturity. Especially with the uncertainty of outcomes in premature infants at the limit of viability and when there are differing data and values, determination of best interests becomes challenging (Goldsmith, Ginsberg, and McGettigan, 1996; Leuthner, 2001; Mercurio, 2005; Paris, 2005; Janvier, Leblanc, and Barrington, 2008; Meadow and Lantos, 2009). Evidence-based ethics provides a framework for decision making based on outcomes (Halamek, 2003; Tyson and Stoll, 2003; Byrne, Szyld, and Kattwinkel, 2008). In cases associated with an uncertain prognosis, the family must be aware that the treatment plan depends on verification in the delivery room of the infant's condition and, to the extent possible, the gestational age (Halamek, 2003).

Resuscitation efforts will usually proceed if there is a reasonable chance of survival without severe disability, since delayed intervention will most certainly result in increased disability but not necessarily death (Goldsmith,

Ginsberg, and McGettigan, 1996; Boyle and Kattwinkel, 1999; Leuthner, 2004; Byrne, Szyld, and Kattwinkel, 2008; Escobedo, 2008). If there is a poor response to resuscitative measures (e.g., Apgar score of <3 at 15 minutes) and death or severe disability is overwhelmingly likely, parents should receive recommendations to transition to palliative goals of care. In fact, the *Neonatal Resuscitation Textbook*, fifth edition, notes that it may be appropriate to discontinue resuscitative efforts performed by competent personnel if spontaneous circulation does not return within 10 minutes (Escobedo, 2008).

Resuscitation decisions made prenatally based on birth at the limits of viability (i.e., 22–24 weeks gestation) are difficult because of limited accuracy of gestational age determination and birth weight variability at each gestational age (Boyle and Kattwinkel, 1999; AAP COFN, 2007). Early obstetrical dating (i.e., first-trimester ultrasound, certainty of the exact date of conception) is more accurate and should supersede other estimates, when available. As outcome depends on more than birth weight and gestational age, a web-based calculator is available to help provide more informative data (www .nichd.nih.gov/about/org/cdbpm/pp/prog_epbo/epbo_case.cfm); accurate estimates are critical to a decision before birth to withhold resuscitative measures. There are no data to support the notion that the appearance and "vigor" of the 23-week infant at birth have any impact on the outcome (Leuthner, 2004; Byrne, Szyld, and Kattwinkel, 2008). Several resources are available to assist the physician and other team members to provide antenatal consultation for newborns at the limit of viability (Halamek, 2003; Batton, 2009; Pont and Carter, 2009).

DECISIONS AFTER LIVE BIRTH

As the infant's condition evolves medically, so too may the family values that determine the *meaning of the outcome* for the child within the family. The factors with greatest impact on parental medical decision making are their values, especially religious beliefs, spirituality, and perceptions and definitions of hope, independent of the predicted mortality, prognosis, or other data presented to them (Boss et al., 2008). When guiding decision making, health care providers must recognize that they and parents may have different values and may view the benefits and burdens of treatment differently (Sydnor-Greenberg and Dokken, 2000; Leuthner, 2001; Racine and Shevell, 2009).

In the presence of uncertainty, decisions become value laden. Families should therefore have the primary role in determining the values guiding care goals unless they are clearly acting against societal norms and widely agreed-upon standards of care. This approach requires the willingness of the medical staff to admit to uncertainty and to disclose personal values and potential biases relevant to the decision at hand. Providing guidance and recommendations after exploring parental knowledge and values can relieve parents of the burden, or the perception of burden, of being the sole decision makers (Sydnor-Greenberg and Dokken, 2000; Leuthner, 2001; Engler et al., 2004; Weisleder, 2008; Racine and Shevell, 2009).

It is interesting to note that what caregivers perceive to be fact-based decision making may actually be value based. For instance, when physicians and nurses were queried about resuscitation of extremely low birth weight babies, decisions that respondents perceived to be based on the child's best interests did not in fact relate to known survival or morbidity data, unlike decisions for older children or adults (Janvier, Leblanc, and Barrington, 2008). It should be recognized that the cost of NICU care per life year or quality-adjusted life year gained is lower than many commonly used treatments for older children and adults. A trusting relationship, continuity of care, family meetings, frequent informal updates, and involvement of all members of the health care team facilitate a shared decision-making model (Engler et al., 2004). Most parents hope for more time to spend with their baby, whether the child's life will last minutes, days, weeks, or months, and may therefore have difficulty hearing terms such as "incompatible with life," "lethal," "fatal," "life-limiting," or "life-threatening."

Collaborative determination of the goals of care for newborns with life-limiting conditions is essential to a family-centered plan of care. Once a lethal prognosis is accepted, most families identify comfort, minimizing suffering, and maximizing time together as a family as their major goals. Other goals might be to optimize function, experience the outdoors, survive until a beloved grandparent arrives, etc. Once identified, all elements of the treatment plan should be reviewed to determine if they help achieve the goals. Goals may need to be adjusted over time as the baby's condition dictates or as the family's preferences change.

DECISIONS AFTER A TRIAL OF TREATMENT

A trial of treatment can be offered in cases of a poor but uncertain prognosis (Leuthner, 2004; Laing and Freer, 2008). Prognosis can and should be reassessed frequently based on the best available information, in conjunction with the changing condition and response to treatment of the individual infant, the physician's judgment, ongoing review of the medical literature, analysis of institutional data, and consultation with experts as needed. A decision-making process that is dynamically shared with parents by providing digestible information and frequent brief updates ensures that decisions incorporate parental values in determining the infant's best interests.

The probability of death or severe neurological impairment is difficult to predict for an individual newborn (Tyson and Stoll, 2003; Racine and Shevell, 2009). Factors that are somewhat predictive include birth weight, gestational age, gender, exposure to antenatal steroids, singleton versus multiple gestation, and acuity of illness in the first hours of life. While a high percentage of deaths in the NICU still occur in the first 72 hours after birth, there is an increasing proportion of late deaths (Meadow et al., 2004; Catlin, 2008). Opportunities to introduce the option of palliative care as the main goal of treatment can occur at any time during the hospital stay (Goldsmith, Ginsberg, and McGettigan, 1996; Stevenson and Goldworth, 1998; Boyle and Kattwinkel, 1999), including at admission, at diagnosis, when the infant's condition deteriorates, when new information indicates a grave prognosis for survival without severe disability, or when the child is not benefiting from or is unduly burdened by medical intervention. It is always difficult to deliver bad news to families, and sharing a prediction of death or severe neurological impairment for a newborn is challenging; this process requires sensitivity and often benefits from a team approach. Established strategies can be adapted for difficult conversations in the NICU setting (Izatt, 2008).

Similar to other settings, families need to be involved in decision making to the extent that they wish (Howard, 2006; see also chap. 6). Parents, especially the mother, can feel an exceptional burden and guilt when their baby is dying. Most parents do not wish to be solely responsible for difficult decisions (Engler et al., 2004; Orfali, 2004; Weisleder, 2008). Care-planning meetings (Laing and Freer, 2008) and infant progress charts have been shown to enhance parents' understanding and collaborative decision making (Penticuff and Arheart, 2005). Physicians should take a leadership role in communicating to the family that their infant is dying, and that all potentially beneficial treatments have been attempted, and strongly recommend transition to intensive palliative care (Laing and Freer, 2008).

Sometimes, parents and caregivers disagree about the proper goals of care. Health care providers may perceive the care they are providing as unduly burdensome, while parents insist on maintaining the goal of life extension, sometimes even in the face of certain death. On the other hand, occasionally parents are concerned that continuing critical care is not in the best interests of the child; if no health care provider addresses this possibility, the parents may doubt themselves and the care team. Discontinuity of care providers and inconsistency of the message exacerbate parental distress. A consistent and supportive message, including the idea of hoping for the best while planning for the worst, can make an otherwise terrible situation more bearable. The development of a trusting parent-physician partnership, created by ongoing discussions about hopes, dreams, limitations, and goals, can help the physician better guide family decisions.

DECISIONS ABOUT ARTIFICIAL NUTRITION AND HYDRATION

Amy was born precipitously at home before the midwife could arrive; at birth, Amy had an abnormal neurologic exam and abnormal vital signs. At the community hospital, her parents were grief stricken when the neurology consultant confirmed that Amy had likely suffered severe brain damage. After careful consideration, including discussion with the hospital chaplain, their own minister, and extended family, they requested cessation of mechanical ventilation. When Amy continued to breathe on her own, her parents requested discontinuation of artificial nutrition and hydration. After the hospital's legal counsel recommended against the proposed plan, arrangements were made to transfer Amy to a tertiary care center. There, intensive comfort care was continued in a regular hospital room to maximize comfort and family access. Amy's parents and her older siblings spent nearly every minute at the hospital for the next few days, holding her until she died peacefully in their arms. With coaching from the nurses and social workers, they took photographs, made a hand mold, dressed Amy in baby clothes, and celebrated her short life. They expressed their gratitude for the support that the hospital staff provided. Several months after Amy's death, her parents and three siblings attended the annual memorial service at the tertiary care center and released a balloon in Amy's memory.

As with other medical treatments, such as mechanical ventilation, decisions about providing artificial nutrition and hydration to newborns who do not have the ability to suck and swallow are based on benefits versus burdens of the treatment (Carter and Leuthner, 2003; Frader, 2007). There may be some state-based legal restrictions on withholding or discontinuing artificial nutrition and hydration, but the ethics literature supports considering this practice as equivalent to decisions about any other medical treatment. It is important to inform parents that patients do not show signs of discomfort from withholding artificial means of nutrition and hydration in these situations. Therefore, this process should not be expected to increase suffering. In fact, continuing artificial nutrition as death nears will likely increase respiratory distress. When artificial nutrition is withheld, continued provision of palliative care in the hospital or home is important over the several days (and rarely weeks) the baby may live. Lorezepam and morphine can be provided for agitation or discomfort. Moistening the lips and other mouth care can also provide comfort. The discussion of artificial nutrition and hydration can be emotional, and parental and health care team values are central to these difficult decisions. (See chap. 6 for further discussion on decision making.)

BABY DOE REGULATIONS

Providing comfort to a dying newborn is a critical goal. However, in conjunction with the Baby Doe regulations, concerns about malpractice liability have influenced physicians' attitudes toward withholding or discontinuing no-longer-beneficial interventions, even when they believe that what is being done is morally wrong (Goldsmith, Ginsberg, and McGettigan, 1996; Peabody and Martin, 1996; Boyle and Kattwinkel, 1999). The Baby Doe regulations of 1986, regarding the federal allocation of state funds for child abuse, are not laws and do not provide penalties to health care providers, health care institutions, their employees, or families for "violation." Even so, strict interpretation of the regulations by some has interfered with logical and compassionate decision making on behalf of dying infants and their families. In honoring the Baby Doe regulations, it is permitted to limit or discontinue "life-sustaining" measures when

- the baby is diagnosed with a chronic and irreversible coma (rarely diagnosed in newborns);
- treatment merely prolongs dying, is not effective, or otherwise is futile in terms of survival (common); and
- ongoing (disease-directed) treatment would be inhumane (common).

Physicians too often mistakenly feel that the regulations mandate treating until death is certain and that, as clinicians, they are placed at increased liability when "life-sustaining" treatment is discontinued. Clearly, this is not the case; while the Baby Doe regulations have been mentioned in recent court cases, no state has lost federal funding based on lack of enforcement. There is also no provision in these regulations for assertion of malpractice or loss of professional standing. Efforts to overcome the misconceptions regarding Baby Doe regulations must be pursued to prevent the loss of opportunities to provide appropriate palliative care to newborns. Of course, care providers should be aware of any state rulings that might affect their decision making.

Conflict resolution in the perinatal period is similar to that at other ages. See chapter 2 on goals, values, and conflict resolution, and chapter 6 on decision making.

Selection of Candidates for Perinatal Palliative Care

Clinicians should consider and discuss with families three general categories of indication for hospice referral or palliative care consultation (Catlin and Carter, 2002; Leuthner, 2004; Leuthner and Jones, 2007; Munson and Leuthner, 2007):

1. Newborns at the limit of viability
2. Newborns or fetuses with congenital anomalies that are incompatible with prolonged life
3. Newborns with complex and multiple birth defects or newborns with overwhelming illness not responding to medical intervention

NEWBORNS AT THE LIMIT OF VIABILITY

Angela was a 530-gram 23-week female delivered to a 25-year-old multigravid woman. After antenatal counseling, her parents had chosen to decline resuscitation if delivery occurred at less than 24 weeks' gestation. The NICU team, including the chaplain, provided "comfort care" for Angela and psychosocial and spiritual support for her family. Angela was baptized in the delivery room and spent the next hour in her family's arms until she died. Her family received information about bereavement support services in the community as well as follow-up phone calls from the care team.

There is debate in the neonatal literature about what gestational age constitutes viability, but most would agree that infants born at less than 23 weeks' gestation are "nonviable," making palliative care the standard recommendation. For babies born at 23 to 24 weeks' gestation, the low survival rates and high morbidity justify offering palliative care either as an alternative to or as part of a trial of life-prolonging interventions.

NEWBORNS OR FETUSES WITH CONGENITAL ANOMALIES THAT ARE INCOMPATIBLE WITH PROLONGED LIFE

Elizabeth was diagnosed prenatally with anencephaly. Her parents elected to continue the pregnancy and were introduced to a perinatal palliative care consultation service. The team assisted in the development of a comfort care plan for Elizabeth after birth, including remaining with her mother in labor and delivery and subsequently in the mother's room. She was provided with warm baby blankets, maternal cuddling, and oral feedings. She went home with her family on her second day of life. The palliative care team provided follow-up services. Elizabeth died at home 3 days later; her family reported that these three days were highly valued and were comfortable for all.

Included in this category would be newborns who have anencephaly, trisomy 13 or 18 with significant cardiac anomaly, lethal forms of dwarfism with pulmonary hypoplasia, and renal dysplasia with Potter syndrome.

Mallory was prenatally diagnosed with trisomy 18 with no significant heart disease. While her family felt prepared for her death, they did not feel prepared for her life. She was referred to a pediatric palliative care program at age 2 weeks, providing opportunity for extensive anticipatory guidance and advance care planning. Potential airway obstruction limited her ability to safely ride in a car seat, so the team arranged for a car bed, allowing her to participate fully in family life, including attending all of her six siblings' sporting events. The pediatric palliative care program collaborated with the community home nurse to enable optimal care at home. Except for two hospitalizations for symptom management, Mallory remained at home, where she died at 7 months of age, surrounded by her family.

These babies might include those who have severe complex congenital heart or central nervous system disease, neuromuscular and neurodegenerative diseases, lethal chromosomal anomalies without severe heart or CNS disease, and some inborn errors of metabolism.

NEWBORNS WITH COMPLEX BIRTH DEFECTS OR OVERWHELMING ILLNESS NOT RESPONDING TO MEDICAL INTERVENTION

Joshua was born at 26 weeks' gestation and was doing well off the ventilator until 3 weeks of age, when he developed fulminant necrotizing enterocolitis. The parents, who had been hoping for a good outcome, were devastated. At surgery, all of his gut was necrotic and it became clear he would not survive regardless of further medical intervention. After a discussion between the multidisciplinary team and the family, the goals of care were changed to exclusively palliative goals. Medications were adjusted to provide optimal comfort, addressing pain and agitation. Antibiotics and blood pressure medications were stopped. Still receiving ventilator support, Joshua was moved to the family care room, where he spent time with his family, including his siblings and grandparents. Six hours later, at his parents' request, he was extubated; he died in his father's arms 45 minutes later.

Provision of palliative care concurrent with attempts at life-prolonging medical intervention is appropriate for many newborns with severe but potentially correctable conditions. Palliative care and attempts to cure or prolong life are not mutually exclusive. Babies with uncertain prognoses might include infants with extreme prematurity, severe neurodevelopmental conditions (e.g., severe hypoxic-ischemic encephalopathy; Racine and Shevell, 2009), inability to survive free of parenteral nutrition (e.g., severe short gut syndrome), inability to wean off extracorporeal membrane oxygenation (ECMO), congenital diaphragmatic hernia, renal dysfunction requiring dialysis, inborn errors of metabolism, significant congenital heart disease, and other severe structural, genetic, infectious, medical, or surgical problems. In these cases, the burdens of continued life-prolonging efforts might outweigh the benefits. In cases in which death is likely or becomes inevitable or medical intervention may only prolong suffering, transition of the goals of care to the prevention of suffering should be made (Laing and Freer, 2008).

Implementation of Perinatal Palliative Care

PRENATAL PALLIATIVE CARE

Abnormal prenatal test results can lead to major parental grief responses (Leuthner and Jones, 2007). The time between recognition of a fetal anomaly by the ultrasonographer and the confirmation by the obstetrician or perinatologist can seem like a lifetime to anxious parents (Askelsdottir, Conroy, and Remple, 2008). Minimizing the wait as much as possible is critical. The parents should be provided privacy during the informing consultation, which should be done by an expert physician who is familiar with the child and able to answer parents' questions. Referral to a specialist, if needed, should be prompt. (See chap. 7 on communication for additional information.)

Prenatal palliative care is an emerging concept, which can be offered as an adjunct or alternative to pregnancy termination when the fetus has been diagnosed with a fatal condition (Hoeldtke and Calhoun, 2001; Askelsdottir, Conroy, and Remple, 2008). It is a compassionate, structured program that is based on the premise that all pregnancies, no matter their duration, and all newborns, no matter how long their life span, are of value not only to the family but also to all of us (Marron-Corwin and Corwin, 2008). Parents who choose perinatal palliative care do so for the following reasons:

- They wish to experience the life of their child, if only for a brief time.
- They understand that their baby will die prematurely but are morally opposed to termination.
- There is uncertainty of diagnosis or prognosis (Leuthner and Jones, 2007).
- They need grief and bereavement support, whether the pregnancy is terminated or not.

It has been variably reported that 20–75 percent of parents choose to continue the pregnancy to focus on the life of their child and the normal aspects of pregnancy (Peller, Westgate, and Holmes, 2004; D'Almeida et al., 2006; Breeze et al., 2007; Leuthner and Jones, 2007). Perinatal palliative care can be particularly helpful for these parents and newborns.

The interdisciplinary team assembled to provide coordinated, seamless care may include the OB provider or perinatologist, neonatologist, pediatric subspecialists (particularly geneticists), clinic nurse, social worker, chaplain, bereavement counselor, and others. The team's goal is to reduce the feelings of fear and loneliness during the pregnancy, delivery, and death and through bereavement. To alleviate anxiety and empower decision making, the team should be prepared to inform parents about the fetal diagnosis, prognosis, level of certainty, and the pros and cons of all treatment options, including perinatal hospice/palliative care (Leuthner and Jones, 2007; Kon, 2008; Marron-Corwin and Corwin, 2008). The parents should understand what the consequences or likely short- and longer-term outcomes will be with each potential treatment plan. The concurrent themes of hope and sorrow and of welcoming and mourning require sensitivity and a keen awareness among the health care professionals caring for the parents. There are many excellent resources to guide the provision of perinatal hospice and palliative care (Leuthner, 2004; Sumner, Kavanaugh, and Moro, 2006; Leuthner and Jones, 2007; Munson and Leuthner, 2007; Askelsdottir, Conroy, and Remple, 2008; Marron-Corwin and Corwin, 2008).

Anticipatory guidance and the development of a prenatal advance care plan or "Birth Plan" (see box 13.1) allow the family to have a sense of control over significant details, focus on the baby rather than the anomaly, participate in decision making, and establish an understanding of what might

Box 13.1 Elements of a Preliminary "Birth Plan"

- Name of the baby
- Fetal diagnosis and prognosis
- Goals of care
- Maternal care
  - Site of care of the mother, labor, and delivery
  - Normal birth plan requests
  - Desire for fetal monitoring and notification in event of fetal demise
  - Mode of delivery; response if fetal distress
  - People to be present at time of delivery
  - Liaison staff person to link with other family members
- Care of the baby
  - What resuscitation measures are and are not to be provided in the delivery room
  - Specific wishes, who will cut cord, bathing, dressing, rituals such as baptism
  - Site of care for the baby
  - Anticipated symptoms and management plan
  - Nutrition plan
  - Memories/mementos/pictures (such as Now I Lay Me Down to Sleep)
  - Genetic and other studies
  - Feasibility and desirability for autopsy, organ donation, funeral/memorial
  - Contingency advance care plan for a baby who can be discharged to home (see box 13.2)

Source: Adapted from Finer and Barrington, 1998; Hoeldtke and Calhoun, 2001; Catlin and Carter, 2002; Leuthner, 2004; D'Almeida et al., 2006; Gale and Brooks, 2006a; Sumner, Kavanaugh, and Moro, 2006; Haven Network, 2007; Leuthner and Jones, 2007; Munson and Leuthner, 2007; Marron-Corwin and Corwin, 2008; UNC Perinatal Hospice.

happen in the event of a live birth. It is important to involve key obstetrical and neonatal staff, to share the birth plan with all clinicians who might be involved, and to make sure that all clinicians are comfortable with the plan of care (Munson and Leuthner, 2007; Walker, Miller, and Dalton, 2008). A tour of the NICU can be helpful for many parents.

In cases in which the decision is made in advance not to attempt resuscitation, a live-born baby may be cared for in the mothers' hospital room or at home, increasing comfort and easy access to support from family, friends, or the religious community (Catlin and Carter, 2002; Leuthner and Jones, 2007).

In the case of clear lethal anomalies, the strong medical recommendation in the majority of cases should be normal vaginal delivery, without fetal monitoring, followed by palliative care. However, there are rare circumstances in which there is a high risk of intrapartum fetal demise and a request for an elective cesarean delivery at term can be considered (Leuthner and Jones, 2007; Munson and Leuthner, 2007). This should be offered only if the mother feels strongly that she must give the baby every chance to live, even at risk of enduring major surgery herself, and she states that in the absence of that opportunity she would be emotionally devastated. Similarly, early induction of delivery may be indicated in cases of maternal medical concerns such as preeclampsia, or obstetrical issues such as hydrocephalus, and likewise could be considered in select situations to enhance maternal mental health by avoiding the stress of abortion as well as that of continuing the pregnancy until term (Leuthner and Jones, 2007).

Maternal transport to the tertiary care center before delivery may be preferred if the diagnosis is uncertain, the likelihood of survival is long, or the community hospital personnel are unable or unwilling to carry out the care plan. When the plan is for an in-hospital delivery, the community hospice team should be involved in the advance care planning and can collaborate with inpatient staff to facilitate parental goals, preventing the initiation of undesired interventions.

CARE AFTER A LIVE BIRTH

Some newborn infants will survive until the time of maternal discharge; in these cases, decisions about the site and goals of ongoing infant care and death should be openly discussed. Although most infants currently die in the hospital, under the care of specialists with expertise in pain and symptom management, and with the provision of emotional and spiritual support for the family, many families may prefer care at home. There are fewer disruptions to family life (Cavaliere and Howe, 2007), and parents can attend promptly to their child's every need. At home, siblings have the opportunity to care for and bond with the baby, decreasing their feelings of helplessness, loneliness, and jealousy. Siblings of children who die at home are less withdrawn and fearful and adapt better to the loss than do siblings of children whose deaths occur in the hospital (Mulhern, Lauer, and Hoffmann, 1983; Cavaliere and Howe, 2007). Home nursing or hospice/palliative care can enable effective symptom management and provide anticipatory support, overcoming parental fears of isolation and lack of skill in providing care. Advance care planning empowers parents and fosters feelings of competency and control (Leuthner, 2004). The process begins with anticipatory guidance, including an explanation of physical changes near the time of death, the possibility of survival after discontinuation of technical interventions, the ranges of expected life span, and the need for contingency planning. Advance care planning, ideally taking into account family and community resources, operationalizes the decision making and implements the plan of care. The focus is on what can and should be done, not what is avoided; it is a process that enhances communication and promotes shared understanding. During this process, future needs are anticipated and a contingency plan developed. The advance care plan helps families live with and parent their infant in a way that is consistent with their goals and values, no matter how long the life will be. Box 13.2 delineates the elements of a neonatal advance care plan.

Unfortunately, pediatric hospice/palliative care by community providers is not currently universally available, and some community physicians may not feel comfortable with managing an infant's death (Catlin, 2007). Whether the newborn remains in the local community hospital, is transferred from a tertiary care center, or is cared for at home, collaborative consultation by the tertiary specialty center is essential to ensure that symptom assessment and management and seamless, family-centered care appropriate to a dying newborn will be provided. Continuity of care is facilitated by a written advance care plan and neonatal palliative care protocols and policies. Together with consultation and ongoing communication, these are effective tools to facilitate transitions of care (Carter and Bhatia, 2001; Pierucci, Kirby, and Leuthner, 2001; Catlin and Carter, 2002; Gale and Brooks, 2006a; Leuthner and Jones, 2007). The neonatal advance care plan is pertinent for both the infant who may die in days to weeks and the infant with a life-limiting or life-threatening condition who is still receiving some disease-directed or life-prolonging care.

PALLIATIVE CARE IN THE NICU

In the highly technical environment of the NICU, where the norm is intensive, invasive, and burdensome life-saving or life-prolonging interventions for premature infants or those with severe birth defects, integration of palliative care paradigms should be the standard of care. This is not only possible—it is imperative. Newborns and families, as well as NICU staff, benefit from palliative care. While most neonatal units consider themselves family centered and competent to care for infants with life-limiting or life-threatening conditions, there are numerous opportunities to improve the integration of palliative care concepts into the treatment of newborns. Overcoming the barriers to palliative care in the NICU requires a culture change that applies to the care of each patient and his or her family. If parents are viewed as "visitors" rather than integral members of the care team, it is difficult for them to participate in care or decision making. Understanding the value of parents as partners in the care of each child is a fundamental tenet of palliative and family-centered care. Honoring this role includes maximizing

Box 13.2 Elements of the Neonatal Advance Care Plan

- Goals of care
- Medical issues
  - Diagnosis and prognosis
  - Members of the health care team, contact information, and triggers to call for help
  - Anticipatory pain and symptom recognition and management
    - Provision of supplies and/or prescriptions as needed
  - Nutrition and hydration status and plans
  - In anticipation of death
    - Anticipatory guidance about signs of impending death
    - Clear information about likely response to resuscitation
    - Resuscitation status, what should be provided and forgone
    - Completion of POLST or DNR form (check with your own state)
    - Preferred setting of care and death
  - Other medical treatments—oxygen, symptom relief, routine preventive care
  - Monitoring, lab tests—newborn metabolic screening, bilirubin levels, diagnostic interventions, such as cord blood or fibroblast samples, DNA banking
  - Use of community services, such as home nursing or palliative/hospice care
- Family support
  - Psychosocial, emotional, and spiritual support for family, including siblings
  - Consultations—genetics, other pediatric subspecialists, chaplain, social worker, child life, etc.
  - Financial/insurance issues
  - Memories, mementos, photographs (Now I Lay Me Down to Sleep)
- Continuity of care
  - Plan for communication of preferences to current and potential care providers
  - Contact information for hospital and community-based providers
  - Indications and method for contacting preferred providers
- Plan for emergencies
  - Do you call Emergency Medical Services?
  - Whom do you call?
- At time of death
  - Who will declare death?
  - Body care, rituals, transport of the body
  - Responsibility for contacting coroner / medical examiner / health care providers
  - Preferences regarding autopsy
  - Feasibility and preferences regarding organ/tissue donation
  - Burial/cremation
  - Funeral arrangements / memorial services
  - Obtaining birth and death certificates
- Plan for bereavement support

Source: Adapted from Finer and Barrington, 1998; Hoeldtke and Calhoun, 2001; Catlin and Carter, 2002; Leuthner, 2004; D'Almeida et al., 2006; Gale and Brooks, 2006a; Sumner, Kavanaugh, and Moro, 2006; Haven Network, 2007; Leuthner and Jones, 2007; Munson and Leuthner, 2007; Marron-Corwin and Corwin, 2008; UNC Perinatal Hospice.

Box 13.3 Strategies to Optimize NICU Palliative Care

- Recognize the infant and family (including siblings) as the unit of care
- Determine goals of care with the family as an equal partner
- Help families decide the optimal setting of care
- Modify the environment to be more family and infant friendly
- Optimize pain and symptom management
- Minimize the child's suffering
- Support the unique needs of each family, including spiritual care
- Minimize family separation, enhance parental caregiving
- Support the needs of the health care providers
- Address community needs to enable effective palliative care, regardless of site
- Promote advance care planning to achieve the best outcome for patients, families, and staff
- Determine, implement, promote, and monitor best practices

---

parental access to the child; siblings and other support persons should be welcomed as well. See box 13.3 for strategies to optimize NICU palliative care. Gale and Brooks (2006b) developed an excellent summary for parents describing perinatal palliative care.

Optimization of perinatal palliative care can occur when unit and hospital leaders attend to the causes of death in their institution and make a determination regarding which infants and families will benefit from palliative care.

FAMILY CONSIDERATIONS

Any parent whose newborn requires resuscitation or admission to the NICU experiences numerous losses, including the loss of self-esteem; past losses also often surface at this time. Grief for the wished-for, healthy, term baby (Sydnor-Greenberg and Dokken, 2000) often occurs simultaneously with anticipatory grief for the impending death of the ill newborn. These families clearly need emotional, psychosocial, and spiritual support.

Posttraumatic stress syndrome is increasingly being recognized as a result of having a loved one in the ICU, regardless of patient outcome (Callahan, Borja, and Hynan, 2006). In the NICU, parents too often perceive that they have no role in parenting their child or that their presence is not welcome (Peabody and Martin, 1996). Staff can teach parents how to safely touch their infant; even most unstable newborns can tolerate gentle touch and maternal or paternal skin-to-skin ("kangaroo") care. Staff can also welcome parents by enabling and encouraging parents to provide normal baby care, such as positioning, diapering, cord care, feeding, suctioning, bathing, comforting, holding, rocking, and reading to the baby. When parents provide toys and family pictures at the bedside and tapes of their voices, it makes the NICU a more family-centered environment, benefiting both the baby and the family (Harrison, 1993; Sydnor-Greenberg and Dokken, 2000).

Family-centered care affirms the central role of the family in their newborn's care as well as the individuality of each family unit; thus, care is tailored to the needs of each family (Harrison, 1993; Sydnor-Greenberg and Dokken, 2000). Understanding the family's coping strategies requires inquiring about past losses, past experiences with health care, and cultural context. An interdisciplinary team including physicians, nurses, social workers, child-life therapists, bereavement counselors, chaplains, and others as indicated may be critical to meet all these needs. Box 13.4 suggests ways to support families and enhance their NICU experience.

Questions such as "How would you like to be involved in your baby's care?" and "What would be comfortable for you?" are good ways to start the inquiry. Inclusion in medical rounds and nursing change-of-shift report provides a clear message that parents are valued members of the care team.

Box 13.4 Means to Enhance the Parental NICU Experience

- Provide an orientation to the NICU
- Hold discussions in quiet, private rooms
- Provide information about the baby's condition and the roles of various health care providers
- Staff should support
  - Honest, open communication
  - Empowered decision making
  - Care and support for parents and the infant's siblings
  - Recognition of parents' role in the infant's care and well-being
  - Facilitation of family participation in the infant's care
  - A welcoming and comfortable physical environment
  - Spiritual support
  - A positive relationship between the family and the nurses and doctors providing care to their child
- Staff should explore parents'
  - Expectations of health care providers
  - Preferences for involvement in the care of and decision making for their ill newborn
  - Goals for their baby
  - Existing support systems
  - Values concerning death and disability

Source: Adapted from Sydnor-Greenberg and Dokken, 2000; Catlin and Carter, 2002; Brosig et al., 2007.

Attention must also be paid to the mother's physical postpartum needs, such as assessment for bleeding or infections and milk donation or lactation suppression (Moore and Catlin, 2003; Gale and Brooks, 2006a).

Parents should be supported by the care team as they work through the anticipatory grief at the diagnosis of a fetal anomaly, extremely premature newborn, or newborn with severe complex medical or surgical problems. Offering baptism, other religious rituals or traditions, and pastoral counseling can be helpful (Kobler, Limbo, and Kavanaugh, 2007). Provision of mementos, such as the newborn armband and the crib card, is important to many families (Catlin and Carter, 2002; AAP COFN, 2007). Regardless of duration of life or site of care, most parents wish to name, hold, and photograph their baby. Even in the presence of severe anomalies, parents should have the opportunity to see and hold their newborn. Sensitively pointing out the beauty of the child's normal features may be appreciated. Offering to make hand and foot prints or a 3-D casting (Jung et al., 2003) and locks of hair may also be appreciated.

Parents may have many existential questions (Catlin and Carter, 2002), often unspoken, that health care providers should anticipate and address. Because guilt, particularly on the part of the mother, is common, it is frequently helpful to review the prenatal history and specifically address whether or not the condition was preventable or might recur in future pregnancies (Catlin and Carter, 2002). Referral to a genetic counselor may be indicated and helpful. Chapter 9 addresses spiritual dimensions of palliative care.

Grief support should begin at diagnosis and continue through the pregnancy, delivery, and the life and death of the infant; further, bereavement care ideally would be offered for many months to years after the death as well (see chap. 11 on grief and bereavement for more on perinatal loss).

NICU STAFF ISSUES: GRIEF, MORAL DISTRESS, AND CONSCIENTIOUS REFUSAL

People attracted to working in the NICU environment enjoy applying their skills and energy to the care of fragile patients, seeing the babies getting better and surviving. Many may feel confused and conflicted when stopping ICU interventions and may fail to see the benefit to the child, adding guilt to their grief when a child dies. The fact that American society is largely a death-denying culture is nowhere more evident than in the NICU, presenting a barrier to the initiation of palliative care. Because of lack of training, health care providers may not be comfortable providing palliative care, assisting in decision making, breaking bad news, or asking permission for autopsy (Engler et al., 2004). Physicians, who bear much of the responsibility for directing care and treatment decisions, can find the death of a newborn particularly stressful (Catlin and Carter, 2002; Olson, 2006; Janvier, 2009), sometimes feeling that they have failed. Unfortunately, by publicizing "miracle" babies, the media contribute to denial of infant death and the public's expectation that all babies will be cured and survive (Carter and Stahlman, 2001).

At the other end of the spectrum of caregiver suffering, there may be intense moral distress when the health care provider is expected to provide care that he or she feels is futile and is contributing to the suffering of the newborn (Engler et al., 2004; Gale and Brooks, 2006a; Catlin, 2008; Janvier, 2009; Kain, Gardner, and Yaters, 2009). In some cases, this distress results from thinking that the outcome after resuscitation of an extremely premature newborn is much worse than the data suggest (Janvier, Leblanc, and Barrington, 2008). The care provider may ask, "Is the health care team doing this for the baby or to the baby?" Conversely, there may be distress when she or he is asked to participate in discontinuation of medical intervention that she or he feels is still of benefit. Additional risks for health care provider grief include feelings of loss over a long-term relationship with the patient and family that may end with the death of the newborn. Nurses bear much of the responsibility for bedside care and family interaction. In some centers, however, they may have limited involvement in the decision-making process. Whether the plan is driven by the physicians or the parents is immaterial to the degree of distress that other members of the team may feel. Feelings of helplessness, moral distress, and spiritual suffering have been frequently reported in nurses but may be seen among all health care professionals (Catlin et al., 2001; Catlin, 2008). Some organizations have policies that allow staff to excuse themselves from providing care in cases of *extreme* religious or moral distress. The standard in the obstetrical field is that conscientious refusals are limited if there is an imposition of religious or moral beliefs on families, care of the patient would be negatively affected, refusals are based on misinformation, or inequalities in care are created (ACOG, 2007). In general, conscientious refusals should be accommodated only if there are no interruptions in patient care. Physicians are obligated to provide full, unbiased information to families and must refer the patient to another care provider if they, in good conscience, cannot provide the requested care (ACOG, 2007).

Staff support is most effective when provided by trained and experienced coworkers. In addition, some NICU personnel may appreciate spiritual support (Catlin et al., 2001), while others find meaning in helping families create memories or participating in end-of-life rituals, such as bathing, taking pictures, and holding the baby (Engler et al., 2004). Education and training in neonatal palliative care principles, cultural differences, and bereavement care may reduce stress, but offering staff other support is necessary as well (Catlin and Carter, 2002; Engler et al., 2004; Gale and Brooks, 2006a; Epstein, 2008). Some centers have responded to this need with implementation of formal neonatal palliative care courses, monthly palliative care rounds, interdisciplinary mortality review, small-group discussion, and/or formal debriefing (Whitfield et al., 1982; Reddick, Catlin, and Jellinek, 2001; Catlin and Carter, 2002; Gale and Brooks, 2006a), during which reactions to the death and review of both the good and the problematic aspects of the care are discussed. Debriefing as a team after the death of a baby can be a productive way of learning and of improving the team's skills, knowledge, cohesion, and confidence. When success in the provision of perinatal care is redefined to include orchestration of peaceful deaths for dying newborns and their families, the staff can derive a great sense of professional and personal fulfillment in providing perinatal palliative care.

END-OF-LIFE CARE IN THE NICU

While excellent palliative care can be provided in the NICU setting, the critical care environment itself may not be conducive to the provision of excellent palliative care (Catlin and Carter, 2002; Brosig et al., 2007). Noxious environmental stimuli result in neonatal behaviors indistinguishable from pain responses and may contribute further morbidity and suffering; thus, minimization of noise, light, sleep interruptions, and other negative stimuli for the infant and the family is an important goal, which may require transfer to a more peaceful location.

LOCATION OF DEATH

If the newborn is likely to die before discharge, relocation of the patient and family to a family or parent care room should be considered, allowing the baby to remain on life support for a time if desired, surrounded by parents and extended family. The supportive environment created by staff members who are expert in perinatal palliative care is more important than the physical location of care (Catlin and Carter, 2002; Leuthner, 2004). With proper preparation, nurses in the mother-baby unit or pediatric floor can provide excellent palliative newborn care. In some hospitals, a quiet room is available outside of the NICU. Whatever the setting, family access to their newborn, sleep rooms for parents, privacy, quiet, and support by the current team of health care providers represent crucial elements of optimal care (Sydnor-Greenberg and Dokken, 2000; Brosig et al., 2007).

If the newborn has been transferred to the tertiary care center, back transfer to the community hospital or transition to home may be possible. Parents should be fully informed and supported in deciding the preferred site of care; some may desire the death to occur at home. See box 13.2 for the components of a neonatal advance care plan. Regardless of location, such patients and families deserve competent caregivers who are sensitive to the specific needs of the newborn patient and the unique aspects of perinatal loss for the family.

DEATH IN THE NICU

In many intensive care nurseries, more than 70 percent of deaths occur after the discontinuation or withholding of no-longer-beneficial treatment (Wall and Partridge, 1997; Pierucci, Kirby, and Leuthner, 2001; Buus-Frank, 2006). Although the definition of a "good death" is child and parent specific, some strategies help the family define the preferred circumstances of their child's death (Pearson, 1997). Several recent reviews describe the use of palliative care consultation and protocols in the NICU, assisting staff to focus not on what cannot be done ("cure" the baby, prevent death, spare the family anguish, etc.) but on what *can* be done (provide compassion, comfort, warmth, humane care, provide for a "good death," etc.) (Carter and Bhatia, 2001; Pierucci, Kirby, and Leuthner, 2001; Catlin and Carter, 2002; Leuthner, 2004; Gale and Brooks, 2006a). Palliative care consultation in the NICU has been shown to decrease invasive and unduly burdensome interventions, decrease the length of stay in the NICU without increasing the mortality rate, decrease the use of nonbeneficial cardiopulmonary resuscitation, and increase the involvement of chaplains and social workers (Pierucci, Kirby, and Leuthner, 2001). Currently, such consults occur most often when it is clear the infant will die. Ideally, formal palliative care consultation or palliative care principles should be introduced soon after admission or diagnosis.

TREATMENT AFTER A DECISION TO
FORGO CRITICAL CARE INTERVENTIONS

Regardless of other aspects of care, the care team must provide continual assessment and management of pain and other physical symptoms as well as coordination of the plan of care. All paralytic agents should have been discontinued as far in advance as possible to allow for assessment of pain and dyspnea (Burns et al., 2000; Catlin and Carter, 2002). Treatments not consistent with the new goals of care, such as vital signs monitoring, lab tests, mechanical ventilation, transfusions, and artificial nutrition and hydration, may be discontinued after discussion with the family. Discontinuation of artificial nutrition and hydration can prevent noisy gurgling. Nevertheless, maintaining reliable intravenous access or a nasogastric tube is useful for the administration of analgesic, anticonvulsant, sedative, or other symptom-relieving medication as needed.

Emotional and spiritual support for the family is intensified. Health care providers should prepare parents for their child's likely physical changes as death nears, such as abnormal respiratory patterns, including gasping and dyspnea, and indications for interventions, such as oxygen or morphine (Leuthner and Jones, 2007). The ranges of the child's likely length of survival should be discussed (Catlin and Carter, 2002; Leuthner, 2004). The health care team should remain continuously accessible. Contingency plans should be made in case of unexpected duration of survival, usually including home- or hospital-based palliative care / hospice services (see box 13.5).

When the family is ready for mechanical ventilation to be discontinued, the infant's endotracheal tube should be suctioned and preparation for intensive management of symptoms ensured. All alarms should be silenced and monitors removed. Analgesics and sedatives should be titrated to relief. It is common for children to experience increased pain, agitation, and dyspnea after extubation, requiring increased doses of medication (Burns et al., 2000). The providers' clear intent to treat symptoms, but not to hasten death,

---

Box 13.5 Options to Present to Parents in Preparation for Discontinuation of NICU Technology

- Do you want to hold your baby before, during, and/or after extubation, or not at all?
- Do you want to be alone, or would you like family, friends, and/or specific health care providers to be present?
- Are there any special rituals or arrangements for the baby that we need to facilitate?
  - Baptism / last rites / other religious needs
  - Presence of a cleric from your own congregation or other
  - Help with arranging family visitation (i.e., visa, jail furlough)
- How do you want to celebrate your child's life?
  - Would you like to bathe him/her?
  - Would you like to dress him/her?
  - Do you want to take photos, make hand or foot molds or prints?
- If you want to have the maximum amount of information possible, I can discuss the benefits associated with autopsy and accommodations that can be made as needed to honor your beliefs.
- I have discussed your infant's condition with the local tissue transplant consortium and can make a referral if you wish

---

should be communicated to parents and other members of the health care team and documented in the medical record.

Documentation about end-of-life events should include content of the discussion and decisions made with the family. Do-not-resuscitate/allow-natural-death orders should be unambiguous regarding treatment and comfort measures. After discontinuation of NICU interventions, the baby will usually die peacefully within minutes to hours. Most parents prefer to hold the child at this time and some prefer to be surrounded by loved ones; others prefer solitude. There should be no restriction on the duration of time the family can remain with the infant, even after the death; most parents are ready to leave within 2–3 hours after the death.

Discussion with the parents about tissue and organ donation and autopsy is important and may even be required in some jurisdictions. The newborn is rarely a suitable donor for tissues other than the cornea, cartilage, or heart valves. This limitation may change in the future with non-heart-beating donor protocols. The regional transplant organization can be a resource concerning tissue donation and can provide up-to-date answers to other donor-related questions. Cord or newborn blood and skin or other tissue samples that are important to diagnose genetic or metabolic conditions should be collected and sent for analysis (Leuthner, 2004; Munson and Leuthner, 2007).

Autopsy continues to provide valuable insights into the cause of the newborn's death as well as possible genetic conditions that may be of importance to family reproductive planning (Battaglia, 2003; Leuthner, 2004; Brosig et al., 2007; Leuthner and Jones, 2007; Munson and Leuthner, 2007; Marron-Corwin and Corwin, 2008). Autopsy results may validate decisions to discontinue NICU interventions, alleviating guilt, assisting with grieving, and supporting feelings of altruism. When cultural or religious prohibitions exist, autopsy can be modified to accommodate those beliefs. For example, the organs can be left in situ, obtaining only core biopsies; the organs can be replaced in their usual location after being sampled; the autopsy can be limited to the main organ of interest, etc.

After declaring death, in addition to filling out the death certificate and any other required paperwork, the physician should contact the referring obstetric and pediatric physicians concerning the death of the baby. An appointment for postdeath follow-up, including review of any autopsy results, should also be arranged with the family. Many families value such a conference, typically held 6–12 weeks after the infant's death. The content should be planned in advance (Gold, 2007; Meert et al., 2007; Laing and Freer, 2008). Important topics for this conference are listed in box 13.6.

Bereavement support is further discussed in chapter 11.

Box 13.6 Topics for Postdeath Follow-up Conference

- Pertinent pregnancy events
- The clinical course, including the moments surrounding death, with reassurance that the infant was comfortable throughout (when true)
- Autopsy results and other new clinical information/interpretation, translated into layman terms
- Any genetic and reproductive findings, especially the likelihood of recurrence in future pregnancies of the parents or close relatives
- Questions the parents may have
- Assessment of the need for referral to a grief and bereavement support service
  - Are the parents and siblings getting adequate and not excessive sleep?
  - Are they eating and maintaining their weight?
  - Do they discuss their baby with each other?
  - Are they receiving good support from friends, family, or other groups?
  - How are the siblings doing at home and in school?
  - How are the parents handling sibling grief?
- Acknowledgment that grief is a lifelong experience that gets easier with time
- Invitation for the family to memorial services, if offered

Source: Adapted from Laing and Freer, 2008.

Management of Pain, Agitation, and Symptoms at the End of Life

PAIN

Assessment and management of pain is standard of care and an ethical and professional imperative. Poor understanding of pain in newborns, especially in premature babies, ignorance of medications, and prejudices against the use of opioids for fear of addiction and hastening death are barriers to appropriate pain management.

> Infants never cry without legitimate cause: Having as yet no speech, they show their trouble by crying, screaming, anger, and restlessness.
> —Omnibonus Ferrarus (about 1577)

Newborns, even those who are extremely premature, experience, perceive, and remember pain (Anand and Craig, 1996; Anand, 2001). Pain results in physiologic, metabolic, and behavioral changes, although a lack of behavioral response does not mean that the newborn is not in pain (Scanlon, 1991; Anand and Craig, 1996; Lynn, Ulma, and Spieker, 1999; Anand, 2001; AAP COFN, 2006). There are long-term negative consequences of newborn pain, including alterations of stress responses (Grunau, Holsti, and Peters, 2006; Walker et al., 2009). Untreated, severe, or prolonged pain increases neonatal mortality and morbidity. The effects of pain on the infant's neurodevelopment remain unclear.

Regular use of appropriate tools for assessing pain and other symptoms will aid caregivers to assess and manage pain in neonates (AAP COFN, 2006; Anand, 2007a; Ranger, Johnston, and Anand, 2007). As premature infants may have blunted behavioral responses, clinicians should use an assessment tool adapted specifically for premature infants; several acute pain scales have proven useful in assessing pain in term and preterm neonates (Lawrence et al., 1993; Krechel and Bildner, 1995; Stevens et al., 1996; Anand, 2007a; Ranger, 2007). One such scale is the Neonatal Pain, Agitation, and Sedation Scale (N-PASS; Hummel et al., 2008; see table 13.1). Use of a pain scale should be incorporated into routine nursing assessment, to be done with vital signs, with procedures, and after interventions. Procedure-related pain, including that associated with surgery and discomfort associated with ventilation, is a common experience in the NICU. In addition, newborns may experience pain when handled, positioned, suctioned, having a nasogastric tube inserted, and undergoing other procedures. Ideally, painful stimuli will be prevented or limited.

An international consensus statement on the appropriate pharmacologic and nonpharmacologic analgesic interventions for neonates (table 13.2) was published in 2001 (Anand, 2001). Nonpharmacologic interventions that modify mild pain include swaddling, positioning, non-nutritive sucking, holding with skin-to-skin contact, and oral provision of milk or sucrose (Lynn, Ulma, and Spieker, 1999; Anand, 2001; AAP COFN, 2006; Golianu et al., 2007; Axelin et al., 2009; Johnston et al., 2009). In fact, for some routine procedures such as oral suctioning, glucose plus holding was shown to be superior to opioids in managing the procedure-related discomfort (Axelin et al., 2009). When avoidance is not possible, nonpharmacologic methods prove inadequate, or if pain is severe, pharmacologic analgesia must be provided. It is critical that health care providers understand the unique dosing and safety issues relevant to analgesic drug administration in newborns (Lynn, Ulma, and Spieker, 1999; AAP COFN, 2006; Anand, 2007b; Young and Mangum, 2010). Cardiorespiratory monitoring of the newborn and the availability of trained staff may be needed.

Pain related to bedside procedures, such as chest tube insertion, can usually be managed by infiltration of the affected area with buffered local anesthetics such as lidocaine, with or without systemic analgesics (Scanlon, 1991;

Table 13.1 N-PASS: Neonatal Pain, Agitation, and Sedation Scale

Assessment criteria	Sedation −2	Sedation −1	Normal 0	Pain/Agitation 1	Pain/Agitation 2
Crying/ irritability	No cry with painful stimuli	Moans or cries minimally with painful stimuli	Appropriate crying; not irritable	Irritable or crying at intervals; consolable	High-pitched or silent-continuous cry; inconsolable
Behavior state	No arousal to any stimuli; no spontaneous movement	Arouses minimally to stimuli; little spontaneous movement	Appropriate for gestational age	Restless, squirming; awakens frequently	Arching, kicking; constantly awake or arouses minimally/no movement (not sedated)
Facial expression	Mouth is lax; no expression	Minimal expression with stimuli	Relaxed; appropriate	Any pain expression intermittent	Any pain expression continual
Extremities tone	No grasp reflex; flaccid tone	Weak grasp reflex; decreased muscle tone	Relaxed hands and feet; normal tone	Intermittent clenched toes, fists, or finger splay; body is not tense	Continual clenched toes, fists, or finger splay; body is tense
Vital signs HR, RR, BP, SaO2	No variability with stimuli; hypoventilation or apnea	<10% variability from baseline with stimuli	Within baseline or normal for gestational age	↑ 10%–20% from baseline SaO2 76%–85% with stimulation—quick ↑	↑ >20% from baseline SaO2 <75% with stimulation—slow ↑ out of sync with vent

Source: Adapted from Hummel and Puchalski, 2002.
Note: Premature pain assessment: Add 3 if <28 weeks corrected age; add 2 if 28–31 weeks corrected age; add 1 if 32–35 weeks corrected age.

Lynn, Ulma, and Spieker, 1999; Anand, 2001, 2007b; AAP COFN, 2006). Lidocaine-prilocaine 5 percent (EMLA) can be safely applied topically 1 hour in advance of procedures such as lumbar puncture, venipuncture, and insertion of a peripheral intravascular catheter. Use of an indwelling catheter or venipuncture to obtain blood is much less painful than heel lance; the clinician should strongly consider these alternatives when appropriate. Unfortunately, EMLA does not eliminate pain associated with heel-lance procedures (Lynn, Ulma, and Spieker, 1999; Anand, 2001), and safety of EMLA for premature babies has not been determined.

The limited data available suggest that nonsteroidal anti-inflammatory drugs and acetaminophen may be helpful to treat mild to moderate pain and as an adjunct to opioid medications. Data on ibuprofen in the neonate are limited (Lynn, Ulma, and Spieker, 1999).

Opioids are effective for moderate to severe pain, for procedures, during surgery, for postprocedural pain, and for medical conditions that are painful, such as necrotizing enterocolitis (Anand, 2001, 2007b). However, morphine is not as effective for postoperative pain and other acute pain as once thought. Alternatives include fentanyl and methadone. There are fewer data about the use of ketamine in newborns. The opiate dose may need to be adjusted as the pharmacokinetics in the newborn, and especially the premature newborn, are different from those in older infants. Opioids are usually given orally and by intermittent or continuous intravenous infusion. While it is possible to give infants opioids intramuscularly, subcutaneously, sublingually, and rectally, there are few data concerning safety in neonates. In general, intramuscular injections should not be used; they have a high burden, including unnecessary pain, unpredictable pharmacokinetics, potential for the development of a hematoma, and risk of nerve injury. Continuous infusions result in less variation in drug levels and are preferred if long-term use is necessary. For infants who have no existing intravenous line, sublingual administration of medication is usually used when rapid onset of analgesia is desired. Health care provider ignorance and inappropriate fears of addiction, tolerance, dependence, and adverse effects such as respiratory depression (incidence probably less than 1%) unfortunately continue to contribute to inadequate dosing of pain medications in patients of all ages (AAP COFN, 2006). These concerns are indications for education, vigilance, monitoring, and the availability of skilled and knowledgeable personnel, rather than inappropriate withholding of medication. Effective doses of medications should be titrated to the relief of discomfort, even as death approaches. Inadequate dosing of analgesics to avoid the appearance of hastening death is inexcusable.

Table 13.2 Suggested approaches to analgesic management

Procedure	Prevent, limit, use alternative	Swaddling, tucking, holding	Nonnutritive sucking	Sucrose/milk	Topical anesthetic	Injection anesthetic	NSAID	Opioid	Other
Heel stick	Consider venipuncture, umbilical catheter								Use automated lancet
Venipuncture, IV insertion									
PICC insertion									
Peripheral cutdown			Consider					Consider	
Umbilical catheter placement				Consider					
Lumbar puncture					Consider				
SQ or IM injection	IV if possible					Consider	Consider if multiple		

Procedure					
Non-life-threatening intubation	Atropine, sedative or analgesic, paralytic				
ETT suctioning		Consider continuous			Consider
NG/OG suctioning					
Chest tube insertion		Strongly consider		Strongly consider	
Circumcision	Mogen less painful than Gomco		Consider before and after	Dorsal penile nerve or ring block	
Ongoing analgesia for routine care and procedures		Consider continuous for ventilated baby	Consider		Consider
Postoperative	Reduce environmental stress	Continuous	Consider		

Source: Adapted from Anand, 2001.
Note: Shading indicates applicable intervention.

Muscle relaxants have no analgesic or anxiolytic properties and should not be used alone if the baby is experiencing pain (Anand, 2001; AAP, Committee on Fetus and Newborn, 2006).

STRESS AND AGITATION

In the absence of pain, when stress is unavoidable and nonpharmacologic measures are insufficient, sedatives and anxiolytics may be required (AAP COFN, 2006). Table 13.3 lists these and other medications commonly used in neonatal palliative care. As with opioids, physiologic tolerance and dependence result from long-term use of sedatives and anxiolytics. Thus, if use is no longer required, these medications must be tapered. Of the benzodiazepines, midazolam is approved for use in neonates and is preferred for intermittent use over long-acting benzodiazepines, such as diazepam. The potential for intranasal administration may also make midazolam a preferred short-term anxiolytic. Because of a paucity of data concerning long-term constant use in premature infants and concern about neurologic sequelae, midazolam cannot be recommended as a routine continuous sedative in the NICU (Anand, 2001). Because of a high potential for adverse effects such as cardiorespiratory depression and possible neurologic complications, close monitoring is required when using these agents; their potential dangers may be exacerbated in combination with opioids. Chloral hydrate, a hypnotic sedative, may be used in the short term, is well studied, and appears to be safe. In summary, the assessment and treatment of pain, stress, and anxiety in the neonate should be routine in the NICU.

ANTICIPATORY MANAGEMENT OF SYMPTOMS FOR HOME DISCHARGE

Some newborns survive long enough to be discharged home, despite the discontinuation or withholding of critical care interventions. Families of these infants will need the support of hospice/palliative care services, optimally provided by professionals skilled in neonatal as well as palliative care. This care may include elements of normal newborn care, such as cord care, bottle- or breast-feeding, and diaper changes, but often requires more, as in the case of artificial means of feeding, which some parents may prefer. While the medical goal for nutrition and hydration is typically growth and maturation, in palliative care the goal is comfort for the infant and parents. If artificial nutrition is chosen, families should be counseled not to expect "normal" volumes of intake and that, as death nears, nutrition and hydration needs will decrease and ongoing use of artificial nutrition and hydration may exacerbate respiratory distress (Catlin and Carter, 2002; Carter and Leuthner, 2003).

Clinicians should anticipate other symptoms, such as dyspnea, nausea, and seizures, in the care of the dying neonate and give them prompt attention when they occur. Poor skin integrity can be treated with lotions. Dry mouth can be improved with glycerin swabs, and petroleum jelly may help dry lips. These symptoms may be particularly challenging as the baby is dying. Because seizures are generally distressing to parents, oral anticonvulsants should be provided to treat seizures or as a contingency if seizures are likely. For newborns who have congenital heart disease associated with congestive heart failure, oxygen, morphine, oral digoxin, and furosemide may effectively prevent or relieve respiratory distress. Before discharge home, clinicians should anticipate symptoms, develop a plan, educate parents and other caregivers, write prescriptions, and obtain medications. In addition, they should provide contact information to answer any questions or respond to emergencies.

Model Programs

One model for community-based palliative care for children with life-limiting conditions is FOOTPRINTS^{SM} (Toce and Collins, 2003). Advance care planning and documentation, care coordination, and a continuity physician from the tertiary care center ensure seamless, community-based care after discharge. Nearly all community caregivers in the Saint Louis area, including physicians, nurses, and EMS providers, agreed to follow the advance care plan developed with the family. Program staff members provide education about pediatric palliative care to the community health care providers at the time of the baby's transition from hospital to home.

In 2003, the Hospice of the Florida Suncoast, in Clearwater, Florida, implemented a perinatal loss doula service to provide birthing and bereavement support to mothers and families affected by an impending perinatal death. Services are available 24 hours a day, 7 days a week. Professional doulas, trained as hospice volunteers with a specific focus on perinatal loss, attend the labor and births of women who have full knowledge that their pregnancy will result in either a stillbirth or an infant who will not survive long. The doula's role is to "mother the mother." The doula stays with the mother throughout her labor and birth and for as long as requested afterward, anticipating needs and helping with hellos and goodbyes. She provides a continuous presence of emotional comfort and reassurance and acts as a

Table 13.3 Medications for neonatal palliative care

Drug	Category	Starting dose (per kg)	Route and interval	Comments
Acetaminophen	Analgesic Antipyretic	20–25 mg load 12–15 mg 30 mg load 12–18 mg	PO once PO PR once PR Interval q 6 hr term q 8 hr 32–36 weeks q 12 hr <32 weeks	Inhibits prostaglandin synthesis. Reversible liver dysfunction at high doses.
Chloral hydrate	Sedative, hypnotic	25–75 mg	PO, PR per dose	Bradycardia, gastric irritation, irritability after a single dose. After prolonged use: indirect hyperbilirubinemia; CNS, respiratory, and myocardial depression; arrhythmias, ileus, bladder atony. Do not use if significant hepatic and/or renal disease.
EMLA (lidocaine-prilocaine 5%)	Topical anesthetic	1–2 g	Topical, 1 hr before procedure; cover with occlusive dressing	Methemoglobinemia with prolonged use, not effective for heel lance procedures. Skin must be intact. Safety in premature infants not shown.
Fentanyl	Opioid analgesic	0.5–4 mcg 1–5 mcg/kg/hr	IV (IM) q 2–4 hrs Continuous IV	Respiratory depression, hypotension reversed by naloxone. Stiff chest more likely with bolus; reversed by naloxone. Urinary retention. Fewer GI effects than morphine. Tolerance with prolonged infusion.
Furosemide	Diuretic	1–2 mg	IV, PO, IM q 12 hrs, q 24 hrs in premature	Hypokalemia, hypochloremia, hypercalciuria

Drug	Classification	Dose	Route/Frequency	Comments
Glycopyrrolate	Anticholinergic drying agent	4–10 mcg 40–100 mcg	IV, IM q 3–4 hrs PO q 6–8 hrs	
Lorazepam	Benzodiazepine sedative, anxiolytic, anticonvulsant	0.05–0.1 mg	IV q 4–8 hrs	Respiratory and CNS depression, hypotension reversed by flumazenil. May potentiate phenobarbital. Limited data in neonates.
Methadone	Opioid analgesic	0.05–0.2 mg	IV, PO q 12–24 hrs	Long duration of action, ileus, delayed gastric emptying.
Metoclopramide	Antiemetic Promotility	0.033–0.1 mg	IV, PO, IM q 8 hrs	May improve feeding tolerance. Dystonic reactions at high doses. Watch for irritability or vomiting.
Midazolam	Benzodiazepine sedative, anxiolytic	0.05–0.15 mg 0.01–0.06 g/kg/hr 0.25 mg 0.2–0.3 mg 0.2 mg	IV, IM q 2–4 hrs Continuous IV, PO Intranasal Sublingual	Respiratory depression, myoclonus, hypotension reversed by flumazenil. Decrease dose if concurrent opioids. Use with caution, particularly in the premature infant.
Morphine	Opioid analgesic, decreases dyspnea	0.05–0.2 mg 0.2–0.5 mg 0.01–0.02 mg/kg/hr	IV, IM, SC q 2–4 hrs PO q 4–6 hrs, IV infusion	Respiratory depression, hypotension reversed by naloxone. Decreases GI motility. May also be given rectally and sublingually.
Naloxone	Opioid antagonist	0.1 mg 0.001 mg/kg/hr	IV, IM, SC, per ET IV infusion	May precipitate discontinuation if prolonged opioid use.
Sucrose 12%–25%	Analgesic	Pacifier dipped, up to 2 ml	PO 2 min before procedure	Stimulates endorphins. Fewer safety data in premature infants.

Source: Adapted from Young and Mangum, 2008; Taketomo, Hodding, and Kraus, 2009.

liaison with the hospital staff, ensuring that the family can see and hold their infant if they choose. The infant is presented to the mother in soft clothing that is hand stitched by hospice volunteers. Each family receives a memory box that includes photographs, ink footprints, and a permanent mold with the imprint of the infant's hands and feet, as well as books and pamphlets to help guide bereavement. The doula provides follow-up contact with the mother for a full year, if requested, to ensure that bereavement needs are being met and that the family is making a healthy adjustment to the loss. Additionally, the Hospice of the Florida Suncoast offers the entire family unit anticipatory grief and bereavement counseling provided by specially trained hospice counselors for as long after the birth as requested.

The Fetal Concerns Program at Children's Hospital of Wisconsin provides a complete range of care when pregnancy is complicated by maternal or fetal health concerns. A collaborative team includes obstetricians, neonatologists, pediatric and surgical subspecialists, and a nurse coordinator. Services include medical diagnostics and counseling, fetal therapies, and the continuum of palliative care services. The program supports the concept of grief work and building hope from diagnosis onward. The goal is to integrate medical information into the family's life in addition to providing other support services, such as child-life therapy for siblings, spiritual counseling through chaplains, lactation consultation, social work, and financial counseling as necessary. Support continues from prenatal diagnosis through birth until the family transitions to using community resources, whether via the Children's Hospital Clinics or a home hospice/palliative care program (Leuthner and Jones, 2007).

Deeya Perinatal Hospice at Children's Hospital of Minnesota is available for parents whose fetus is diagnosed with a life-threatening condition. The program individualizes services to each family, offering medical, emotional, and spiritual support. The program supports families from pregnancy through bereavement. Children's Hospital of Minnesota also offers the Karuna Pediatric Palliative Care Program and Pediatric Hospice.

Conclusion

If newborns and their families are to receive optimal family-centered care, the application of palliative care principles is necessary. Clinicians and staff members across all pertinent disciplines can cooperate to provide an environment in the obstetrical clinic, the delivery room, the nursery or mother's room, the NICU, home, and other settings of care. Palliative care principles can be integrated into the entire trajectory of care, regardless of whether the treatment goal is cure, prolongation of life, or exclusively palliation. Treatment must always be in the best interests of the newborn, consistent with the goals and preferences of the family, compassionate, and humane. Care should focus on not only the physical comfort of the baby but also the emotional, psychosocial, and spiritual needs of the entire family, including (especially) siblings and grandparents. The process can begin prenatally with the identification of fetal conditions that may limit the life or function of the newborn. There is a need for further research to ensure that evidence-based, ethically sound, multidisciplinary, family-centered decision making before and after birth will become the standard for infants who have potentially fatal outcomes. Bereavement support should be provided to enable families to integrate the loss into their lives and to return to a functional existence (see chap. 11 on grief and bereavement). Finally, health care professionals working with infants who die should care for themselves and their colleagues so that they may continue to provide compassionate care for all high-risk newborns and their families.

References

American Academy of Pediatrics, Committee on Fetus and Newborn (AAP COFN). 2002. Perinatal care at the threshold of viability. *Pediatrics* 110:1024–27.
———. 2006. Prevention and management of pain in the newborn: An update. *Pediatrics* 118:2231–41.
———. 2007. The noninitiation or withdrawal of treatment for high-risk newborns. *Pediatrics* 119:401–3.
American College of Obstetricians and Gynecologists (ACOG). 2007. ACOG Committee Opinion no. 385: The limits of conscientious refusal in reproductive medicine. *Obstet Gynecol* 110:1203–8.
Anand, K.J. 2001. Consensus statement for the prevention and management of pain in the newborn. *Arch Pediatr Adolesc Med* 155(2):173–80.
———. 2007a. Pain assessment in preterm neonates. *Pediatrics* 119:605–7.
———. 2007b. Pharmacologic approaches to the management of pain in the neonatal intensive care unit. *J Perinatol* 27:S4–11.
Anand, K.J., and Craig, K.D. 1996. New perspectives on the definition of pain. *Pain* 67:3–6.
Askelsdottir, B., Conroy, S., and Remple, G. 2008. From diagnosis to birth: Parents' experience with expecting a child with congenital anomaly. *Adv Neonatal Care* 8: 348–54.
Axelin, A., Salantera, A., Kirjavainen, J., et al. 2009. Oral glucose and parental holding preferable to opioid in pain management in preterm infants. *Clin J Pain* 25:138–45.
Battaglia, J. 2003. Paying our last respects: The neonatal autopsy as continuing care and ethical obligation. *Neonatal Intensive Care* 16:36–39.
Batton, D., AAP Committee on Fetus and Newborn. 2009. Clinical report—antenatal

counseling regarding resuscitation at an extremely low gestational age. *Pediatrics* 124:422–27.

Boss, R., Hutton, N., Sulpar, L., et al. 2008. Values parents apply to decision-making regarding delivery room resuscitation for high-risk newborns. *Pediatrics* 122:583–89.

Boyle, R.J., and Kattwinkel, J. 1999. Ethical issues surrounding resuscitation. *Clin Perinatol* 26:779–92.

Breeze, A., Lees, C., Kumar, A., et al. 2007. Palliative care for prenatally diagnosed lethal fetal abnormality. *Arch Dis Child Fetal Neonatal Ed* 92:F56–58.

Brosig, C., Peirucci, R., Kupst, M., et al. 2007. Infant end-of-life care: The parents' perspective. *J Perinatol* 27:510–16.

Burns, J.P., Mitchell, C., Outwater, K.M., et al. 2000. End-of-life care in the pediatric intensive care unit after the forgoing of life-sustaining treatment. *Crit Care Med* 28:3060–66.

Buus-Frank, M. 2006. Sometimes a time to be born is also a time to die. *Adv Neonatal Care* 6:1–3.

Byrne, S., Szyld, E., and Kattwinkel, J. 2008. The ethics of delivery-room resuscitation. *Sem Fetal/Neonatal Med* 13:440–47.

Callahan, J.L., Borja, S.E., and Hynan, M.T. 2006. Modification of the Perinatal PTSD Questionnaire to enhance clinical utility. *J Perinatol* 26:533–39.

Carter, B., and Leuthner, S. 2003. Ethics of withdrawing/withholding nutrition in the newborn. *Semin Perinatol* 27:480–87.

Carter, B.S., and Bhatia, J. 2001. Comfort/palliative care guidelines for neonatal practice: Development and implementation in an academic medical center. *J Perinatol* 21:279–83.

Carter, B.S., and Stahlman, M.T. 2001. Reflections on neonatal intensive care in the U.S.: Limited success or success with limits? *J Clin Ethics* 12(3):215–22.

Catlin, A. 2007. Home care for the high-risk neonate: Success or failure depends on home health nurse funding and availability. *Home Healthcare Nurse* 25:131–35.

———. 2008. Extremely long hospitalizations of newborns in the United States: Data, descriptions, dilemmas. *Adv Neonatal Care* 8:125–32.

Catlin, A., and Carter, B. 2002. Creation of a neonatal end-of-life palliative care protocol. *J Perinatol* 22(3):184–95.

Catlin, E.A., Guillemin, J.H., Thiel, M.M., et al. 2001. Spiritual and religious components of patient care in the neonatal intensive care unit: Sacred themes in a secular setting. *J Perinatol* 21:426–30.

Cavaliere, T., and Howe, T. 2007. Should neonatal palliative care take place at home, rather than the hospital? *MCN* 12:270–71.

D'Almeida, M., Hume, R., Lathrop, A., et al. 2006. Perinatal hospice: Family-centered care of the fetus with a lethal condition. *J Am Phys Surg* 11:52–55.

Engler, A., Cusson, R., Brockett, R., et al. 2004. Neonatal staff and advanced practice nurses' perceptions of bereavement/end-of-life care of families of critically ill and/ or dying infants. *Am J Crit Care* 13:489–98.

Epstein, E. 2008. End-of-life experiences of nurses and physicians in the newborn intensive care unit. *J Perinatol* 28:771–78.

Escobedo, M. 2008. Moving from experience to evidence: Changes in US Neonatal

Resuscitation Program (NRP) based on International Liaison Committee on Resuscitation review. *J Perinatol* 28:S35–40.

Finer, N.N., and Barrington, K.J. 1998. Decision-making in delivery room resuscitation: A team sport. *Pediatrics* 102:644–45.

Frader, J. 2007. Discontinuing artificial fluids and nutrition: Discussion with children's families. *Hastings Cent Rep* 37(1):1 p following 48.

Gale, G., and Brooks, A. 2006a. Implementing a palliative care program in a newborn intensive care unit. *Adv Neonatal Care* 6:37–53.

———. 2006b. A parents' guide to palliative care. *Adv Neonatal Care* 6:54–55.

Gold, K. 2007. Navigating care after a baby dies: A systematic review of parent experiences with health providers. *J Perinatol* 27:230–37.

Goldsmith, J.P., Ginsberg, H.G., and McGettigan, M.C. 1996. Ethical decisions in the delivery room. *Clin Perinatol* 23:529–50.

Golianu, B., Krane, E., Seybold, J., et al. 2007. Non-pharmacological techniques for pain management in neonates. *Semin Perinatol* 31:318–22.

Grunau, R., Holsti, L., and Peters, J. 2006. Long term consequences of pain in human neonates. *Semin Fetal Neonat Med* 11:268–75.

Halamek, L. 2003. Prenatal consultation at the limits of viability. *NeoReviews* 4:e153–56.

Harrison, H. 1993. The principles for family-centered neonatal care. *Pediatrics* 92:643–50.

Haven Network. 2007. Family Birth Plan. www.thehavennetwork.org/birthingplan.asp (accessed September 22, 2009).

Hoeldtke, N., and Calhoun, B. 2001. Perinatal hospice. *Am J Obstet Gynecol* 185:525–29.

Howard, E. 2006. Family-centered care in the context of fetal abnormality. *J Perinat Neonat Nurs* 20:237–42.

Hummel, P., and Puchalski, M. 2002. N-PASS. www.n-pass.com/assesment_table.html (accessed September 22, 2009).

Hummel, P., Puchalski, M., Creech, S.D., et al. 2008. Clinical reliability and validity of the N-PASS: Neonatal pain, agitation and sedation scale with prolonged pain. *J Perinatol* 28:55–60.

Izatt, S. 2008. Educational perspective: Difficult conversations in the neonatal intensive care unit. *NeoReviews* 9:e321–25.

Janvier, A. 2009. I would never want this for my baby. *Pediatr Crit Care Med* 10:113–14.

Janvier, A., Leblanc, I., and Barrington, K. 2008. The best interest standard is not applied for neonatal resuscitation decisions. *Pediatrics* 121:963–69.

Johnston, C., Filion, F., Campbell-Yeo, M., et al. 2009. Enhanced kangaroo mother care for heel lance in preterm neonates: A crossover trial. *J Perinatol* 29:51–56.

Jung, A., Milne, P., Wilcox, J., et al. 2003. Neonatal hand casting method. *J Perinatol* 23:519–20.

Kain, V., Gardner, G., and Yaters, P. 2009. Neonatal Palliative Care Attitude Scale: Development of an instrument to measure the barriers to and facilitators of palliative care in neonatal nursing. *Pediatrics* 123:e207–13.

Kobler, K., Limbo, R., and Kavanaugh, K. 2007. Meaningful moments: The use of ritual in perinatal and pediatric death. *MCN* 32:288–95.

Kon, A.A. 2008. Healthcare providers must offer palliative treatment to parents of neonates with hypoplastic left heart syndrome. *Arch Pediatr Adolesc Med* 162: 844–48.

Krechel, S., and Bildner, J. 1995. CRIES: A new neonatal pain measurement score. Initial testing of validity and reliability. *Pediatr Anesth* 5:53–61.

Kung, H., Hoyert, D., Xu, J., et al. 2008. Deaths: Final data for 2005. *National Vital Statistics Report* 56:95–102.

Laing, I., and Freer, Y. 2008. Reorientation of care in the NICU. *Semin Fetal Neonat Med* 13:305–9.

Lawrence, J., Alcock, D., McGrath, P., et al. 1993. The development of a tool to assess neonatal pain. *Neonatal Network* 12:59–66.

Leuthner, S., and Jones, E.L. 2007. Fetal Concerns Program: A model of perinatal palliative care. *MCN* 32:272–78.

Leuthner, S.R. 2001. Decisions regarding resuscitation of the extremely premature infant and models of best interest. *J Perinatol* 21:1–6.

———. 2004. Fetal palliative care. *Clin Perinatol* 31:649–65.

Lynn, A.M., Ulma, G.A., and Spieker, M. 1999. Pain control for very young infants. *Contemp Pediatr* 16:39–66.

Marron-Corwin, M., and Corwin, A. 2008. When tenderness should replace technology: The role of perinatal hospice. *NeoReviews* 9:e348–52.

Meadow, W., and Lantos, J. 2009. Moral reflections on neonatal intensive care. *Pediatrics* 123:595–97.

Meadow, W., Lee, G., Lin, K., et al. 2004. Changes in mortality for extremely low birth weight infants in the 1990's: Implications for treatment decisions and resource use. *Pediatrics* 113:1223–29.

Meert, K.L., Eggly, S., Pollack, M., et al. 2007. Parents' perspectives regarding a physician-parent conference after their child's death in the pediatric intensive care unit. *J Pediatr* 151:50–55.

Mercurio, M. 2005. Physicians' refusal to resuscitate at borderline gestational age. *J Perinatol* 25:685–89.

Milstein, J. 2005. A paradigm of integrative care: Healing with curing throughout life, "being with" and "doing to." *J Perinatol* 25:563–68.

Moore, D.B., and Catlin, A. 2003. Lactation suppression: Forgotten aspect of care for the mother of a dying child. *Pediatr Nurs* 29(5).

Mulhern, R., Lauer, M., and Hoffmann, R. 1983. Death of a child at home or in the hospital: Subsequent psychological adjustment of the family. *Pediatrics* 71: 743–47.

Munson, D., and Leuthner, S. 2007. Palliative care for the family carrying a fetus with a life-limiting diagnosis. *Pediatr Clin North Am* 54:787–98.

Olson, M. 2006. Beginnings and endings. *Arch Pediatr Adolesc Med* 160:770–71.

Orfali, K. 2004. Parental role in medical decision-making: Fact or fiction? A comparative study of ethical dilemmas in French and American neonatal intensive care units. *Social Science and Medicine* 58:2009–22.

Paris, J. 2005. What standards apply to resuscitation at the borderline of gestational age? *J Perinatol* 25:683–84.

Peabody, J.L., and Martin, G.I. 1996. From how small is too small to how much is too much. *Clin Perinatol* 23:473–89.

Pearson, L. 1997. Family-centered care and the anticipated death of a newborn. *Pediatr Nurs* 23(2):178–82.

Peller, A., Westgate, M., and Holmes, L. 2004. Trends in congenital malformations, 1974–1999: Effect of prenatal diagnosis and elective termination. *Obstet Gynecol* 104:957–64.

Penticuff, J.H., and Arheart, K.L. 2005. Effectiveness of an intervention to improve parent-professional collaboration in neonatal intensive care. *J Perinat Neonat Nurs* 19:187–202.

Pierucci, R.L., Kirby, R.S., and Leuthner, S.R. 2001. End-of-life care for neonates and infants: The experience and effects of a palliative care consultation service. *Pediatrics* 108(3):653–60.

Pont, M., and Carter, B. 2009. Maternal and neonatal characteristics of extremely low birth weight infants who die in the first day of life. *J Perinatol* 29:33–38.

Racine, E., and Shevell, M. 2009. Ethics in neonatal neurology: When is enough, enough? *Pediatr Neurol* 40:147–55.

Ranger, M., Johnston, C., and Anand, K. 2007. Current controversies regarding pain assessment in neonates. *Semin Perinatol* 31:283–88.

Reddick, B.H., Catlin, E., and Jellinek, M. 2001. Crisis within crisis: Recommendations for defining, preventing, and coping with stressors in the NICU. *J Clin Ethics* 12(3):254–65.

Scanlon, J.W. 1991. Appreciating neonatal pain. *Adv Pediatr* 38:317–33.

Stevens, B., Johnston, C., Petryshen, P., et al. 1996. Premature infant pain profile: Development and initial validation. *Clin J Pain* 12:13–22.

Stevenson, D.K., and Goldworth, A. 1998. Ethical dilemmas in the delivery room. *Semin Perinatol* 22(3):198–206.

Sumner, L., Kavanaugh, K., and Moro, T. 2006. Extending palliative care into pregnancy and the immediate newborn period: State of the practice of perinatal palliative care. *J Perinat Neonat Nurs* 20:113–16.

Sydnor-Greenberg, N., and Dokken, D. 2000. Coping and caring in different ways: Understanding and meaningful involvement. *Pediatr Nurs* 26:185–90.

Taketomo, C.K., Hodding, J.H., and Kraus, D.M. 2009. *Pediatric Dosage Handbook*, 16th ed. Ohio: Lexicomp.

Toce, S., and Collins, M. 2003. The FOOTPRINTS model of pediatric palliative care. *J Palliat Med* 6:989–1000.

Tyson, J., Parikh, N., Langer, J., et al. 2008. Intensive care for extreme prematurity—moving beyond gestational age. *NEJM* 352:1672–81.

Ventura, S., Abma, J., and Mosher, W. 2004. Estimated pregnancy rates for the United States, 1990–2000: An update. *National Vital Statistics Report* 52:1–12.

Walker, L., Miller, V., and Dalton, V. 2008. The health-care experiences of families given the prenatal diagnosis of trisomy 18. *J Perinatol* 28:12–19.

Walker, S.M., Franck, L.S., Fitzgerald, M., et al. 2009. Long-term impact of neonatal intensive care and surgery on somatosensory perception in children born extremely preterm. *Pain* 141:79–87.

Wall, S.N., and Partridge, J.C. 1997. Death in the intensive care nursery: Physician practice of withdrawing and withholding life support. *Pediatrics* 99(1):64–70.

Weisleder, P. 2008. Physicians as healthcare surrogate for terminally ill children. *J Med Ethics* 34:e8.

Whitfield, J.M., Siegel, R.E., Glicken, A.D., et al. 1982. The application of hospice concepts to neonatal care. *Am J Dis Child* 136:421–24.

Young, T.E., and Mangum, B. 2010. *Neofax, 2008.* Montvale, NJ: Thomas Reuters.

Additional Resources

Deeya: www.childrensmn.org/Web/Hospice/008384.asp

FOOTPRINTS^SM: www.footprintsatglennon.org

Grieving for Babies: www.grievingforbabies.org

Initiative for Pediatric Palliative Care. 2003. An Initiative of the Center for Applied Ethics at Education Development Center, Inc. www.ippcweb.org/curriculum.asp

Now I Lay Me Down to Sleep photographers: www.nowilaymedowntosleep.org

Perinatal Hospice. Website maintained by bereaved parent Amy Kuebelbeck; includes resources for parents and health care providers as well as listings of perinatal hospices: www.perinatalhospice.org

RTS Bereavement training programs: http://bereavementservices.org/

UNC Perinatal Hospice: www.mombaby.org/index.php?c=1&s=57

14

Palliative Care in the Pediatric Intensive Care Setting

Kathryn Weise, M.D., M.A., Marcia Levetown, M.D.,
Carol Tuttle, and Stephen Liben, M.D.

Integrating the principles of palliative care into the pediatric intensive care unit (PICU) environment can be challenging because of physical, organizational, philosophical, and training issues specific to this setting. However, children receiving care in the PICU and their families have at least as much need for comprehensive child-centered care, control of symptoms, and anticipatory guidance as children in less acute hospital care areas or in the home. Although the upheaval resulting from admission to a high-intensity unit after an acute or chronic deterioration can make the management of symptoms and psychosocial support for the patient, family, and staff seem less immediately relevant than other critical care measures, it is important to institute these approaches as soon as possible after admission.

Issues discussed in this chapter include the following:

- The value of palliative care in the PICU
- Specific aspects of the delivery of palliative care in the PICU
- Management of symptoms
- Forgoing or discontinuing no-longer-beneficial or unduly burdensome treatment
- Care after discharge from the PICU or death

The field of pediatric palliative care is relatively new compared to pediatric critical care medicine. Because of the common misconception that palliative care is indicated only at the end of life, attempts to integrate palliative care approaches may sometimes be perceived as antithetical to the mission of critical care practice (Boldt, Fouza, and Himelstein, 2006; Docherty, Miles, and Brandon, 2007). However, because many aspects of palliative care may be useful to patients and families throughout a chronic illness, it is incumbent on critical care practitioners to recognize the value of palliative care for their patients and families. At times, the palliative medicine practitioner has a role to play in transforming the culture of the PICU from an environment full of intense, focused, and often invasive care toward one in which collaborative and educational approaches with PICU staff help all concerned to succeed in incorporating attention to communication, symptom control, psychosocial and spiritual support, and advance care planning while attending to the realities of critical care practice.

Gaining the trust of the ICU staff through inquiry and education about critical care and demonstrating respect for and recognition of the expertise, humanity, and intense struggles of critical care specialists will enable a collegial relationship between the palliative care specialist and the PICU team. The relationship will be sustained by a collaborative approach, consisting of ongoing mutual learning, consistent presence, effective and respectful communication, and bidirectional support. Ideally, the palliative care provider will help ICU staff realize that palliative care is most effective when the team is given the opportunity to offer the staff and family support and advice before the terminal stage is reached, to facilitate discussions of goals of care, and to develop a sustaining and therapeutic relationship with the family.

Effective collaboration between palliative care and PICU teams in institutions requires careful attention to program setup. Several models of providing palliative care in the PICU exist (Carter, Hubble, and Weise, 2006). Examples include teams that are able to accept patients onto a palliative care service on the ward and continue to follow them in the PICU, consult-only services that function in multiple areas of the hospital, and services that provide both inpatient and outpatient continuity of care. Composition of the team may vary among institutions, often utilizing the expertise of physicians, nurses, and multiple ancillary support personnel with formal or informal ties to the service. Integration of the team into the ICU works best when there is acknowledgment of the benefits of concurrent palliative and disease-directed care by both intensivist and palliative care providers, as well as agreed-on goals for collaboration, regular communication, and regular exchange of training regarding the other's methods and philosophies of care. Discussions about goals of care require open-mindedness among palliative care and critical care staff alike as a child's illness evolves; uncertainty about prognosis exists in many cases. Appropriate goals may realistically include making plans to optimize life in addition to preparing for potential death.

Together with models of clinical care delivery, early and ongoing bidirectional education is a key ingredient to successful PICU / palliative care collaboration. Models of inclusive transdisciplinary education have been successfully adapted for pediatric palliative care and are available on the web (e.g., Initiative for Pediatric Palliative Care at www.ippcweb.org, Society of Critical Care Medicine iCritical Care Podcasts at LearnICU.org). In addition to formal training programs, there is a need for ongoing "informal" education, using "teachable moments" occurring just before and after a patient encounter. For example, a quick debriefing of professionals after a family-staff meeting provides an opportunity for ongoing education. Care in future cases may be optimized by answering questions such as, "Did we miss any opportunities for communication in this meeting?" and "How could we have better understood and addressed all of the issues that were brought up explicitly or implicitly?" It may be helpful for palliative care professionals to view each consult as an opportunity not only to improve the care of children and families in the ICU but also to deepen understanding of how to enhance their own skills in providing palliative care within the ICU.

The Value of Palliative Care in the PICU

EPIDEMIOLOGY OF PEDIATRIC DEATH

More than 50,000 children die in the United States each year. Causes of death in infancy (under 1 year of age) include congenital defects, complications of prematurity, sudden infant death syndrome (SIDS), and trauma, including unintentional injury and homicide. Between the ages of 1 and 24 years, approximately 60 percent of deaths result from trauma, while the remaining 40 percent are due primarily to cancer, congenital anomalies, and metabolic defects (Martin et al., 2008). Many of these children live their entire lives in the shadow of an early death, often visiting the PICU on multiple occasions. The increasing frequency of complex, chronic conditions of childhood being managed in the PICU and the difficulties of navigating our specialized health care system set the stage for fragmentation of care. In response, an integrated, realistic, family-centered, clearly communicated and holistic care plan to ensure the best quality of life for the patient and family is increasingly the desired standard of care for these children by providers, case managers, the medical home, and accreditation agencies.

At the other end of the spectrum, injury and acute critical illness in previously healthy children usually prompt initial resuscitative measures in emergency and ICU settings. Unfortunately, many of these children will die in these locations, despite vigorous efforts to preserve or prolong their lives (Feudtner et al., 2002; Garros, Rosychuk, and Cox, 2003; Carter et al., 2004; Copnell, 2005; Brandon, Docherty, and Thorpe, 2007). Death rates among

PICUs are widely variable, depending on patient mix and other factors. Incorporation of palliative care approaches should be considered early in the course for children at high risk for dying and may be valuable beyond discharge if the child survives (Meert, Thurston, and Sarnaik, 2000; Carter, Hubble, and Weise, 2006; Truog, Meyer, and Burns, 2006; Truog et al., 2008).

Families stricken with sudden, unexpected illness or injury in a previously healthy child may react with anxiety, anger, disbelief, or other understandable behaviors that require patience and compassion from health care providers. The lack of a preexisting relationship with caregivers bearing bad news puts additional stress—for families and medical professionals—on an already difficult situation. Careful attention to communication, emphasizing clarity, simplicity, and repetition, as well as providing time and support for second opinions, may help families accept a poor outcome. Consultation with trusted family members, and, when possible, passage of time, may also help families cope with an unfolding tragedy. The palliative care team, when well informed about the medical condition and prognosis of the child and in close communication with the members of the ICU team, can provide a valuable service to the child, family, and ICU staff.

> Jackie was an infant in foster care when she came to live with us, and then we were able to adopt her shortly before she died. She had a chromosomal duplication, causing her to be blind, deaf, developmentally delayed, and with a partial cleft palate. She had trouble gaining weight, so she had a gastrostomy tube for feeding. She was constantly sick with respiratory issues, ear infections, and episodes of vomiting. Three days before she was to have corrective cleft-palate surgery, Jackie suddenly became very ill, resulting in an ambulance transport and admission to the PICU. An emergency echocardiogram showed that there was an unidentified mass entangling her lungs, heart, and great arteries. The debate began: What was it? Cancer, or a benign tumor? Operable or not? Everyone had a different opinion and no one could say for sure, so how were we to know what to do next? Would she survive?
>
> Jackie was trached and was soon put on a ventilator because the mass, which was growing and compressing her lung, could not be resected. Four months after admission to the PICU, we took her home, to an uncertain future and a roller coaster ride of appointments and hospital stays. There was not a palliative care team at the hospital during Jackie's life, which involved chronic problems and a sudden arrest that led to her death in the hospital.

Later, after a palliative care service was developed, we fostered KJ, an infant with a severe brain injury and multiple related problems. Through him, we learned firsthand how he and our family could benefit from their services both in the PICU and afterward. KJ died peacefully at home.

CHRONIC LIFE-THREATENING CONDITIONS

A disproportionate number of children in the PICU with acute life-threatening illness are those with chronic underlying health conditions, and many will die in this setting (Zawistowski and DeVita, 1994; Dosa, Boeing, and Kanter, 2001; Feudtner et al., 2002; Carter et al., 2004; Copnell, 2005; Brandon, Docherty, and Thorpe, 2007). Anticipatory guidance for families of children living with chronic, life-threatening conditions can lay the groundwork for avoiding death in the ICU setting. However, variable courses of health and illness, as well as perceptions of an uncertain prognosis, may prompt escalation of interventions in the face of acute deterioration of the chronically ill child (Davies et al., 2008; Liben, Papadatou, and Wolfe, 2008).

Ideally, the family of a chronically ill patient with a progressive, likely fatal condition would be provided information clearly and gradually, preferably in an outpatient setting. Effective communication is tailored to the child's condition and the family's value system, orchestrated when possible by a trusted physician coordinating care for the patient (Wharton et al., 1996; AAP, 2005; Hammes et al., 2005; Tulsky, 2005; Baker et al., 2008; Mack and Wolfe, 2008). Content of ongoing communication should include the projected trajectory of the child's chronic illness and symptoms that may develop; reasonable interventions available for life extension; the likely effectiveness and outcomes, including anticipated benefits and burdens; family prioritization of goals and outcomes; preferences for location of care; and plans for symptom management. Discussions held *before* a child becomes unstable can help a family develop informed preferences and develop an associated coordinated plan of care, helping to avoid pressured decisions at the end of life (Bartel et al., 2000; Meert, Thurston, and Sarnaik, 2000; Baker et al., 2008; Mack and Wolfe, 2008). Parents state that the opportunity for advance care planning provides them with comfort and assurance that their child received proper care (Wharton et al., 1996; Hammes et al., 2005).

Too often, however, these anticipatory discussions do not occur and the ICU staff and consultants are left to help families address important decisions during a crisis situation. Thankfully, patient and compassionate communication can lead to improved satisfaction with the process even in an acute setting (Tulsky, 2005; Truog, Meyer, and Burns, 2006; Feudtner, 2007). Various members of the health care team may play a leading role in initiating such discussions. Ideally, the patient's medical home providers will be contacted to continue their involvement in designing and implementing a viable care plan (AAP, 2005).

ENHANCING AWARENESS OF PALLIATIVE CARE PRINCIPLES IN THE PICU SETTING

In the high-technology ICU environment, efforts have traditionally been oriented toward either cure or return to the previous baseline level of function. Sacrifices in terms of physical and psychosocial suffering have been traditionally accepted in exchange for these goals in the critical care setting. However, the twin goals of life prolongation and minimization of suffering are not mutually exclusive. The palliative care principles of family-centered care, effective and empathetic communication, and limitation of suffering are broadly applicable in the ICU setting regardless of the child's outcome.

Additionally, when it becomes clear that the child is not likely to survive, palliative goals become the foundational elements of the care plan. Unfortunately, many pediatric professionals, in the ICU and elsewhere, have not received training in comprehensive symptom assessment and control, communication skills, family dynamics during the grieving process, bereavement care, or self-care (Forbes et al., 2008). When clinicians are not exposed to such issues during training, a lack of appreciation of the importance of these concerns often results. Thus, for critical care professionals to better understand and appreciate what palliative care may have to offer patients and families, a process of ICU professional-directed education and validation may be needed. Table 14.1 reviews several general benefits of concurrent inclusion of palliative care into the care of children in the ICU. Specific skills applicable in this setting include the following:

- Prevention, assessment, and management of distressing symptoms, including sleep disturbance, constipation, anxiety, and feelings of abandonment
- Facilitation of sibling involvement before and after the death of the ill child
- Empathetic, respectful, and bidirectional communication with families, with particular attention to the words used when discussing prognosis and care at the end of life
- Facilitation of family-centered death

- Bereavement care
- Self-care for health care providers and creation of mutual support opportunities

Other interventions that may benefit critically ill children who have a high likelihood of death, but that are often not available in the ICU setting, include child life, integrative therapies (music, pet, massage, etc.), and regularly scheduled family meetings with non-ICU team members. Creative solutions to make these opportunities available can often be accomplished. Sometimes legitimate concerns prevent such choices, however. To avoid disappointing patients and families, the clinician should offer only confirmed available options rather than make suggestions that cannot be fulfilled.

After one particularly trying hospital stay, we were eager to take Jackie home. We were close to being able to finalize the adoption, which would allow us to act as her parents, rather than deferring all medical decisions to the county. My other daughter, Amanda, was helping us bring Jackie home.

Within two miles of home, Amanda shouted that something was wrong. Jackie was turning blue despite her ventilator being on. Amanda dialed 911, while I started CPR and tried to keep Amanda calm. When EMS arrived, they stabilized her enough to life-flight her back to the PICU. You really don't mind going 200 miles an hour, hundreds of feet in the air, when you think your child is dying.

As the Life Flight team and I literally ran through the halls to the PICU, my mind was empty and I was still running on adrenaline. Suddenly, I was given a straight back chair and told to sit in it. It faced the room where they were all scrambling around Jackie, trying to assess and stabilize her. I began to process the tragic event. What was happening to Amanda? Still an adolescent, she needed me; I needed to comfort her for her sake as well as mine. I hadn't had time to support or explain anything to my husband, just asked him once again to leave work, rush to the hospital, and now deal with all the problems this crisis placed on our home life and our other children. That's when the tears started; I now had to put into words what I didn't want to believe was happening. I knew the doctors and nurses who had taken care of her before, but they were busy trying to save her. There was nobody else to help me think through what to do next, like I had later when a palliative care team helped me with KJ.

Table 14.1 Value-added benefits of concurrent critical care and palliative care

Skill	Intensive care team role	Palliative care team role	Value added by palliative care team
Identify patients fitting criteria for palliative care	Recognize criteria for palliative care among acute and chronically ill children	Round regularly in PICU; suggest patients who could benefit from PC services and/or offer care suggestions; provide background information on patients known to the service before PICU admission (course of illness; previously developed goals of care; effective prior symptom management approaches)	Collaborative problem solving for individual patients and families; ongoing education of all involved staff about palliative approaches that can be integrated into ICU environment; continuity of care for patients and families known to palliative care service
Address immediate care needs	Acute stabilization within accepted standards of care; address family needs during crisis	Recognize contributions of skilled intensivists; anticipate evolving medical and psychosocial needs of family and staff; obtain additional medical and social information pertinent to care of the child and family; augment spiritual and psychosocial family support	Additional insights into prior goals and care needs of the child; ability to spend additional time with family and staff to discuss mutually agreed-on goals of care; validation of trust in ICU team
Develop and refine evolving goals of care	Address prognosis based on changing physiological indicators; recognize uncertainty and its effect on family and staff; choose treatments appropriate to the prognosis; strive for clear communication with family about treatment recommendations and choices	Strive to understand changing physiology pertinent to prognosis and treatment in order to collaborate in development of goals of care; reinforce mutually agreed-on messages; attend family meetings; provide avenue for communication between ICU staff	Vantage point allows recognition of splitting of staff groups and/or family based on differing goals, opportunity to mitigate these behaviors when possible; recognition of dynamics that may lead to limiting family's choices of care paths; ability to educate staff

		and family when ICU staff less available; recognize that some patients will improve in spite of a dire prognosis	and family about ethical issues pertaining to limitation or discontinuation of no-longer-beneficial treatment as an alternative
Treat adverse symptoms	Maintain adequate pain control and sedation to achieve goals of care; recognize changing medication and environmental needs as the illness and treatments evolve	Remain informed of changing treatments and their impact on comfort; provide information about patient's prior medication needs (if known); provide suggestions for adjunctive pain or anxiety management techniques that can be used in the PICU setting (additional medications and dosing; nerve blocks; relaxation techniques)	Familiarity with adjunctive treatment modalities including additional medications and nonpharmacologic treatments; skill in considering impact of patient's illness and symptoms on family and in working with family to enhance patient's comfort
Excellent communication with patient (when possible) and family	Trained to synthesize and communicate information from multiple sources and subspecialists; environmental barriers to communication with family may exist (e.g., multiple teams rounding and speaking with family; little uninterrupted time to spend with each family; often cast in the role of "bearer of bad news"); clearly communicate when treatments have become ineffective or unduly burdensome relative to benefits	Trained to synthesize information from diverse sources, and to communicate this well to families; may have more uninterrupted time to spend listening to family to hear their concerns and discern gaps in understanding or misconceptions; may have a prior history with family that adds to trust; risk of adding to confusion exists if team does not seek information about what medical changes or conversations have occurred in their absence	Opportunity to help PICU staff and family understand misconceptions; opportunity to help family process information about child's course; generally well versed in developmental issues that affect patient and sibling understanding; opportunity to coordinate ancillary supports for family; opportunity to promote continuity with primary care provider, other subspecialists, home care providers

(continued)

Table 14.1 (cont.)

Skill	Intensive care team role	Palliative care team role	Value added by palliative care team
Facilitate changes in goals and treatment as the illness evolves	Recognize and institute changes in treatment appropriate to phase of illness; during limitation of treatments, relay that care priority has become comfort, rather than giving family impression that care is being stopped; maintain supportive, communicative role with family; if treatment is discontinued, arrange time and use resources that will best support the patient's comfort and support family through the event; provide information about what will happen at time of death (uncertain time course; anticipated physical changes) and after death (paperwork; usefulness of autopsy)	Remain involved in anticipatory discussions of goals of care; inform PICU staff of new knowledge gained by team; share expertise about options for transition to comfort medications that can be used outside of the PICU environment for patients who will be discharged; acknowledge that intensivists may feel, and may in fact be, skilled in end-of-life care; add to rather than usurp role of intensivist who has developed a positive relationship with family and wants to be involved during limitation or discontinuation of treatment in the PICU; assist with practical tasks/after-death paperwork as needed; in some instances, facilitate discontinuation of treatments/interventions and administer comfort medications	Opportunity to help refine goals of care by assisting in staff and family meetings; ability to acknowledge and validate discomfort PICU physician, nursing, respiratory staff may have in discussing end-of-life issues with families; ability to support staff through difficult cases; ability to assist family with memory making; ability to assist with practical tasks around discontinuation and death, as needed by PICU staff; if desired by PICU staff, can facilitate discontinuation and symptom management to free ICU staff to attend to other patients

Coordination of discharge	Choose appropriate discharge venue for surviving patients (acute care ward; rehabilitation facility; inpatient hospice; home with hospice care)	Suggest or assist choice of discharge venue based on knowledge of regional facilities, family preferences or capabilities; offer options for transitioning medications; assist in coordination of home-going arrangements for durable medical equipment or symptom control measures	Prior collaboration with care facilities outside of the PICU environment; ability to provide continuity of care that will help family transition to another site of care; possible prior experience with family's strengths and limitations in home-based care
Bereavement care	Acknowledge family's loss and ongoing nature of bereavement; provide follow-up visit to discuss case and autopsy (if done)	Provide anticipatory care for families of surviving children who have now lost function and for families who will experience the death of a child; initiate involvement of hospice services if accepted by the family; provide contacts to support family after death	Opportunity to provide ongoing follow-up with family, including telephone contact, home visits, hospital memorial services; opportunity to augment supportive services to staff

Specific Aspects of Palliative Care in the PICU

COMMUNICATION ABOUT THE PICU
ENVIRONMENT AND ABOUT THE PATIENT

The ICU is an unfamiliar environment for most children and families, and one in which the potential for conflict over decision making exists among team members and between the team and the family (Studdert et al., 2003). The experience of a child and family admitted to a busy, highly technical environment peopled by unfamiliar medical staff engaged in unfamiliar activities is predictably overwhelming, anxiety provoking, and often depressing (Azoulay et al., 2005; Carvalho and Fonseca, 2008). Lautrette et al. (2007) have shown that there may be up to a 70 percent incidence of post-traumatic stress disorder (PTSD) among family members of patients in the ICU, regardless of patient outcome. Information needed to help families adjust to the environment includes the following:

- Types of ICU personnel, their function, and how to distinguish them
- ICU monitors, alarms, and devices
- Hospital resources available outside the ICU
- How questions can be answered and by whom

A family confronted by unwelcome news in an unfamiliar environment will benefit from establishing the identity of and trust in the staff caring for their child. The rapid development of a therapeutic relationship can be enhanced by endorsement of the ICU staff and their capabilities by trusted long-term caregivers and by good communication among the ICU team and family. Crucial elements of staff communication include the following:

- introductions, explanations of roles, and titles of caregivers from various disciplines;
- demonstration of knowledge of the child's past medical history;
- clear explanations of new devices or medications currently in use or that may be anticipated;
- explanations of diagnostic or supportive measures to be anticipated;
- prediction of the near-term course;
- explanations of how the family can participate in the care of the child in the ICU environment;
- offers to work with siblings or help parents work with them to understand what is unfolding in an age-appropriate way;

- acknowledgment of prognostic uncertainties; and
- an explanation of communication patterns in the unit.

Information from the family that is immediately useful in providing care for the child includes

- who is currently present, and their relationship to the child;
- identity of and contact numbers for the child's usual health care providers;
- advance care plans or content of previous discussions in the case of a chronically ill child;
- the name the child/family prefers to use;
- how each family member present prefers to be addressed;
- effective comfort measures used in past illnesses;
- whom the family wishes to be included (or not included) in the information loop;
- how best to effectively communicate within the group, including how much specific medical information to share with whom;
- explanations of the child's care provided at home and family preference for continuing to provide certain components of that care in the ICU;
- siblings' ages and names, and who is caring for them while the critical illness is evolving; and
- any specific cultural or spiritual traditions that need to be respected during care and communication.

COMMUNICATING CHANGES IN STATUS

If it becomes clear that the child will not recover or that burdens of treatment have come to outweigh benefits to the child, this must be communicated clearly and consistently to the family. Because different subspecialists caring for a child in the ICU round at different times, the family may seek or receive information from multiple professionals, often hearing different interpretations of the child's trajectory of illness. This phenomenon can result in the family receiving mixed messages (Weise, 2004), which is consistently reported as a source of distress (Meert, Thurston, and Sarnaik, 2000; Contro et al., 2002; Meyer et al., 2002; Sharman, Meert, and Sarniak, 2005). Further, families understandably focus on the most positive information they hear, which masquerades as denial and may interfere with goal-directed decision making. Parents are better able to accept their child's declining health and likely death when they have been included in brief, frequent, understandable, and compassionate updates on the child's condition. When possible, a consistent physician or nurse communicator, who is able to synthesize the information from various specialists and caregivers, can be a relief to confused and overwhelmed families. Such an approach may ultimately improve families' adaptation to the child's demise (Mosenthal et al., 2008). In contrast, news that is perceived as a sudden change in prognosis may predictably result in shock, anger, and lack of acceptance.

Effective mechanisms to enhance consistency in communication include the following:

- Involving the bedside nurse, respiratory therapist, social worker, key subspecialists, and parents in daily rounds
- Providing a communication notebook for families and staff to record questions as they occur
- Striving for consistency in messages given to the family by designating primary communicators as much as possible
- Conducting regular and inclusive family meetings when any major change occurs, using the phone or Internet to include critical decision makers who cannot be physically present
- Providing information that is as free of jargon as possible, discussed in a fashion that is responsive to emotional and informational needs
- Including known and trusted health care providers who can assist the family to understand and process information

The language used when discussing end-of-life care in the ICU may contribute to the discomfort and ethical concerns of families and health care providers. For example, it is important to be clear that when death from an underlying disease is inevitable, the child dies from the illness, rather than from discontinuation of clinical interventions that are no longer effective or are disproportionately burdensome. It may also help families and staff to cope with changes in goals of care if they understand that discontinuing no-longer-beneficial treatment is ethically equivalent to not starting futile interventions, although this may not be deemed true within all religious or cultural traditions. Further, it can be reassuring for families and staff to realize that the child was given every opportunity to benefit from existing medical knowledge, but that it is now clear that he was too ill to recover; the emphasis, therefore, is appropriately shifting to ensuring the child's comfort.

Numerous tests were done on Jackie, and the results were not encouraging. Jackie's neurologist either seemed to be immune to our devastation or perhaps felt as helpless as we did, rushing out of the PICU room after delivering the results of the EEG: "No brain activity."

We watched as our little girl's fingers started to swell, then her hands and feet, and most heartbreaking of all, her face. She no longer looked like our Jackie. It was obvious that there was no hope of recovery.

How do we know what to do? The doctors are giving gentle suggestions, skirting around "The Question." I know they aren't God, but they've seen more than I. Couldn't just one of them have said she's going to die and soon, without the euphemisms? Or am I refusing to truly hear them because I don't want them to be right? Both my husband and I have a strong faith in God and are willing to accept His will in this matter. How does a family without faith find any comfort at a time like this?

When it becomes clear that treatment is failing to achieve the hoped-for result, the physician's responsibility is to inform the family of this fact. This can be done compassionately, expressing regret for the inability of the medical staff to change the outcome, and listening to the family's stated and implied concerns about what may happen next. Reassurance about the team's commitment to continuing care, to the priority of the child's comfort, and to support of the family remains important and is an obligation of both the ICU and the palliative care teams.

In preparation for discontinuation of critical care interventions, the child, family, and staff may be comforted by

- gathering friends and family members who will be supportive;
- dressing the child in his or her usual clothing, playing the child's favorite music, reading the child's favorite stories, reviewing the child's life using scrapbooks and photo albums, and telling funny or poignant stories about the child;
- addressing spiritual needs by offering to assist in the observance of any rituals, prayer, poems, readings, or songs or inviting spiritual leaders to be present;
- eliciting cultural or personal rituals important to the child and family, and facilitating them when possible;
- making mementos for the family, including siblings, by offering such items as a mold of the child's hand, handprints of the child on the same page as that of a surviving sibling, or offering family or professional photography. Child-life or psychology care may benefit siblings during this phase by addressing age-specific fears.

Jackie did not need much pain medication toward the end because she was in a deep coma and did not seem to be aware of the commotion in the ICU. KJ's more chronic brain injury also made him unaware of his surroundings. However, when we took him home to pass away in a quiet environment, we had medications available through hospice and felt comforted that if he needed something as his breathing got worse, it would be available.

Assessment and Management of Symptoms in the PICU

PAIN MANAGEMENT

Many PICU specialists are well versed in managing acute pain using opioids and intravenous nonsteroidal agents and may be comfortable with escalating doses within "standard" ranges in opioid-naïve patients, especially when ventilation is being supported. They may be less comfortable with escalating to the higher dose ranges sometimes needed in patients who have been on opioids long term or with using adjunctive agents that are not part of the usual ICU medications. There may also be physiological barriers to escalating systemic pain medications in the hemodynamically unstable patient who is not imminently dying. For these reasons, the palliative care team can play a crucial role in ensuring adequate symptom and pain control.

Intensivists and ICU nurses who are experienced in managing symptoms at the time of death may be comfortable with the "principle of double effect," while others less experienced may be reluctant to respond to signs of pain or air hunger with appropriate opioid doses (Burns et al., 2000). Trainees, newer staff, and family members may benefit from anticipatory discussion, bedside guidance, debriefing, and formal education to avoid conflating symptom management with an intention to shorten life. Concerns about addiction, defined as continued use despite self-harm, are unwarranted. Physiologic dependence resulting in withdrawal symptoms may develop if the medication is suddenly stopped or the dose drastically reduced; this is unrelated to addiction. Staff and families may need to be educated to understand these differences. In the child who recovers from the acute illness and painful symptoms, careful weaning from opioids may be done. Such weaning is not usually warranted in the terminally ill child with persistent pain, unless side effects of opioids are unmanageable and other effective agents can be substituted.

Children who have chronic illness, a prolonged hospitalization, multiple procedures, or an ongoing painful condition may have received a number of analgesic agents before or during the ICU admission. In such cases, staff members who have worked with the patient previously, as well as certain patients themselves and their parents, may be invaluable sources of information about approaches to pain management that have been effective in the past and those to be avoided. They may be able to provide guidance on unpleasant side effects particular to that child. Similarly, the palliative medicine provider who has a history with the child may be able to offer insights that will be valuable to the managing team in the PICU.

Because enteral medications may be poorly absorbed or contraindicated in acutely ill patients, intravenous forms of pain medications are often administered in the ICU setting. These may include potent opioids such as morphine, fentanyl, hydromorphone, and methadone. Pain management and hemodynamic stability may be optimized in the critically ill patient by using infusions rather than intermittent dosing, or by using adjuvant agents and cautious sedation.

The ICU environment includes many stimuli, some noxious, that may make pain management and sedation especially challenging. Ambient noise levels, frequent vital sign assessments, intrusive alarms, mechanical ventilation with endotracheal tube suctioning, painful procedures, frequent bedside rounds, and parental anxiety all add to the potential need for sensitivity to environmental controls and may call for higher dosing or additional medications. Rarely, paralytic agents are required to maintain the child's oxygenation or hemodynamic stability. Paralytics may make assessment of pain or anxiety more difficult, although vital sign changes often alert the clinician to these symptoms. Additionally, assumptions can be made regarding the pain associated with invasive procedures, and pain management should be modified and escalated accordingly.

As in other settings, the clinician should thoroughly investigate the source of pain to guide treatment. It is important to recognize that as an illness evolves, new pathology may develop, potentially causing pain that may be difficult for the patient to communicate. For example, the intubated, sedated patient may develop painful abdominal distension from a physiologically benign cause such as constipation or from a more ominous condition such as typhlitis. Evaluation, treatment, and symptom management differ markedly for each entity, guided by the skilled clinician.

Pain scales developed for use in the PICU setting include the COMFORT Scale, FLACC, and the Children's Pain Checklist (Stevens et al., 1996; van Dijk et al., 2000; Breau et al., 2002; Voepel-Lewis et al., 2002). None of these scales is without its challenges—especially for children who have chronic illness and/or pain—making consistent observation by those familiar with the particular child an important aspect of pain management throughout the PICU stay.

Sedation at the end of life may relieve intractable suffering when all other avenues for relief have been attempted by skilled caregivers (Quill and Byock, 2000). Symptoms other than pain may require the use of sedative or hypnotic agents. Such conditions as delirium, severe anxiety, dyspnea, or intractable seizures may respond well to specific agents such as benzodiazepines, barbiturates, phenothiazines, butyrophenone, propofol, or antihistamines. As with opioids, certain drugs may worsen hemodynamic instability in the critically ill patient; therefore, dosing must be carefully chosen and monitored in the patient for whom cardiovascular stability remains a goal of care. Literature describing palliative sedation (aka sedation to unconsciousness) in children is not extensive; nevertheless, palliative sedation may be beneficial to children (Kenny and Frager, 1996; Postovsky and Ben Arush, 2004; Postovsky et al., 2007).

> If you have not experienced the death of a child, you want someone to walk you through it. Why is it so hard for our culture to speak of death? Is it because most people today die in a hospital with their rules and regulations, rather than experiencing it quietly, peacefully, and privately at home with loved ones around until the end? You feel like a specimen on a slide, sitting at your child's bedside. Are you being judged if for a moment you chuckle at a TV show or if you sob uncontrollably? Will they ask you to leave? You need a "Best Friend" to be there, to see that you eat and rest, to help absorb all the medical "stuff" they throw at you, to listen to your fears and problems related to family separation and practical concerns, and to reassure you that you CAN hang in there.
>
> One day toward the end, I was exhausted and Adam, an RN, knew it. He first gave me permission and when I refused, insisted ever so gently that I lie in bed and hold and cuddle Jackie. That created more work for him as he moved wires, hoses, tubes, and IV lines so I could gather her in my arms and hold her tight. What a precious memory that gentle and caring man gave me that day. Thank you, Adam.

Forgoing No-Longer-Beneficial or Unduly Burdensome Treatment

ADVANCE CARE PLANNING AND FORGOING INTERVENTIONS

As an illness evolves, specific ICU interventions may become more burdensome than beneficial, spurring an adjustment of the goals of care away from a primary focus on life prolongation to give more weight to the goal of achieving comfort. Diverse medical staff experiences and beliefs, family dynamics, and a child's developmental age and awareness may challenge the ability for all to agree on consistent goals. Careful communication among team members and with the family, allowing concerns of diverse stakeholders to be addressed, is important to ensure a consistently supportive environment for all involved.

When appropriate, limitation of additional medical interventions while maintaining comfort and current treatments may be a first step toward changing the plan of care. This may include deciding not to escalate ventilator settings or blood pressure medications (pressors), for example, while continuing pain medications and other comfort measures. Therapies that are inconsistent with goals of care or that will be ineffective should not be offered. Often, discussion of the lack of benefit of CPR and associated "resuscitative measures" may accompany conversation about not escalating therapy and may be tailored to the language used at the institution (e.g., "do not resuscitate," "do not attempt resuscitation," or "allow natural death"). Misperceptions about the effectiveness of CPR in life-threatening conditions should be proactively addressed with family and staff (Diem, Lantos, and Tulsky, 1996; Topjian, Berg, and Nadkarni, 2008). It is important to pair discussion of limitation of nonbeneficial interventions with reassurance that other care for the patient does not stop and will include aggressive symptom control, ongoing availability of support staff and visits from family and friends, observation of rituals important to the patient and family, and spiritual support when desired. In some cases, transfer to another care setting outside of the ICU may be possible and of great comfort to the patient and family (Quill, 1995; Meert, Thurston, and Sarnaik, 2000; Meert et al., 2008).

The clinician should discuss the need to adjust comfort medications in an anticipatory fashion with the family and among the staff to address potential concerns about increasing doses in response to changing symptoms. ICU staff may be willing to encourage family members to hold a child while still ventilated if it can be done without dislodging supports; this may comfort both the child and the family members.

Parents and children may be haunted by thoughts of limiting medical intervention now or at a future date, especially if the discussion is framed as whether or not "the family wants to limit life support." No family wishes to stop effective treatments that will help their child survive. Instead, the skilled clinician will inform the parents that the child is too ill to survive no matter what is done and that the ICU interventions have all been tried to give him or her the best chance to make it. The family's love, heroic efforts, and anguish must be acknowledged explicitly and supportively (Levetown, 2008).

> One of Jackie's doctors became a favorite because he was always willing to explain his actions, what he was ordering and why, and to answer my questions, despite his overwhelming workload. Toward the end, as I told him I thought I should give Jackie "permission" to go if she needed to, she suddenly "crashed." He "called a code," working fervently to stabilize her, though I could see in his eyes that he didn't think she would make it. Oh how I wanted to tell him it was okay to stop all efforts and that I was at peace with doing so! Though he was greatly affected by Jackie's near-death event, he gave us time to call Dad to ensure that the family was together when the end came.
>
> Years later, when KJ came along, a palliative care team met with us in the ICU and helped us to understand what we could do to keep him comfortable and to avoid ICU stays that wouldn't help him in the long run. They worked with us to make a plan for what we thought was best for him, helped the social service agency understand his long-term needs, and worked alongside us and the hospice team once we got him home. We were able to adapt his care to what seemed to help him, rather than just doing things to him because they could be done.

DISCONTINUATION OF NO-LONGER-BENEFICIAL OR UNDULY BURDENSOME INTERVENTIONS

A decision to forgo no-longer-beneficial or unduly burdensome interventions occurs in 20–55 percent of terminally ill children who die in PICUs in North America and Europe (Devictor, Latour, and Tissieres, 2008). When considering this choice, parents place high priority on quality of life, likelihood of improvement, and their perceptions of their child's pain and suffering (Meyer et al., 2002). Given these considerations and others, enhancing comfort may become preferable to continuing interventions with little hope of improving the quality or meaningful length of life. Benefits for the patient and family may include an ability to restore the child's appearance and personhood, creating memories of last moments without medical equipment, alarms, and uncomfortable examinations. Discontinuing technical interventions is best done in a controlled, planned time frame that allows family and staff to ready themselves, gathering those the family would like to have present and maximizing staff attention in an unpredictable situation. Minimizing distractions or interruptions of involved staff and avoiding laughter in the hallways outside the room or other unwelcome intrusions may help mini-mize bad memories. Most families prefer to choose the time of discontinu-ation; in other cases, they may rely on staff regarding when to discontinue mechanical ventilation or pressor therapy.

Some families may need time to make final arrangements before the discontinuation of ICU interventions in order to be able to leave the hospi-tal without logistical delays after their child's death. Examples include funeral home choice, discussion of organ donation or donating remains for science, and autopsy. Most critical care physicians are aware of federal and local regulations pertaining to these issues; discussion may be facilitated by social workers, chaplains, and other personnel trusted by the family as well. It is important to recognize that even if a family does not want to consider autopsy during the stressful time near the end of a child's life, the decision not to proceed cannot be undone. Because autopsy results may answer lin-gering questions about why the child died, may help with family planning for parents and siblings, and may allow for an altruistic contribution to scientific knowledge, staff should become comfortable with offering autop-sies in a supportive, affirming, and compassionate fashion, simultaneously addressing families' concerns. Except when under the jurisdiction of the medical examiner, the approach to autopsy or obtaining postmortem diag-nostic tissue sampling can be adapted to accommodate personal or religious beliefs.

Discontinuation of unwanted or ineffective treatment can be done grad-ually (e.g., weaning pressor agents to allow hypotension to ensue) or more abruptly (e.g., a planned extubation in anticipation of death). Either ap-proach can be made more understandable, for family and staff, by talking in advance about what can be expected. Significant preparation of family and less-experienced staff is needed, because a dying child, even while being kept comfortable, will change in appearance. A child changing color from pink to cyanotic or gray, for instance, can be disturbing for parents as well as staff. Similarly, reflexes and automatisms such as an agonal gasp or a "Lazarus sign" at the time of death may be alarming. Anticipating and addressing these possibilities in a kind but explicit way may reassure the family that these are reflexive events near the time of death, rather than signs of pain or distress.

Uncertainty regarding the length of time over which death may occur necessitates careful preparation as well. Families invariably ask, "How long?" In rare cases, some children continue to survive after compassionate extuba-tion, and plans must then be made to transition them to other care settings. More commonly, death does occur but may take longer than anticipated. This can lead families to question their decisions, and increased support during this time is crucial. Not uncommonly, once the decision is made to discontinue interventions, families experience conflicting emotions—wanting their child's suffering to be over once the difficult choice has been made, yet feeling intense guilt at wanting their child's life to end. The services of a palliative care team can be helpful to augment ICU staff support during times like these, as often the presence of a consistent, compassionate caregiver who can provide ongoing explanation and reassurance is beneficial.

Discontinuation of mechanical ventilation is a common practice near the time of death in the PICU environment and may be associated with a decrease in agitation after the removal of the endotracheal tube (Levetown et al., 1994). There is no evidence that weaning the ventilator provides greater comfort for the patient than does extubation. However, dyspnea after extubation is uncomfortable for the child, family, and caregivers, necessitating advance preparation to meet the goal of comfort at the end of life. Measures to minimize distress include stopping intravenous fluid administration, suctioning the endotracheal tube before extubation, and administering medications to treat observed symptoms. Opioids are effective for the management of air hunger and can be easily titrated to comfort if the child is frequently observed. Benzodiazepines can alleviate anxiety. Health care providers and family should understand in advance that treating symptoms of discomfort at the end of life is ethically preferable to allowing suffering. The experience and thoughtful deliberation of clinicians and ethicists are reflected in the literature concerning this practice. It is important to understand that symptom management with life-support discontinuation is ethically acceptable even at the risk of unintentional hastening of death (Truog et al., 2001). However, it may be reassuring to note that there is evidence indicating a statistically longer duration of life after extubation that is accompanied by aggressive symptom control, perhaps related to the increase in comfort (Partridge and Wall, 1997). On the other hand, administration of paralytic agents before extubation is not acceptable because it masks most symptoms, making it difficult to effectively treat discomfort. Experts recommend reversing paralytic agents already in use if termination of mechanical ventilation is planned (Truog et al., 2000, 2001).

Some staff members may be uncomfortable with direct participation in certain dimensions of care, such as discontinuation of support or palliative sedation. This should be honored, both to respect the provider and to avoid adding to a family's stress by instilling doubt about decisions that have been made. All staff members should be encouraged to express their views in a professional manner and should be able to opt out of direct care of any patient and family if unable to meet their needs for personal, religious, or any other reasons.

> We were extremely grateful that another doctor who had taken care of Jackie often was on duty the night we made the heart-wrenching decision to take her off of the ventilator. What I really wanted was to be alone with just my husband and Jackie, with us holding each other as the vent was turned off. But it seemed like many of the people who cared for Jackie were there and there were tears in their eyes as Jackie slipped from this life to the one in heaven.

For Jackie's family, having consistent, trusted caregivers among the PICU staff afforded familiarity and support for difficult decisions surrounding the sudden event that resulted in her death. However, uncertainty about her prognosis before this event and lack of advance care planning may have made the decision-making process more difficult for both Jackie's family and the medical caregivers.

Care after Discharge from the PICU or Death

Discharge of the palliative care patient to another level of care may occur in some situations, such as the chronically ill or acutely injured child who recovers sufficiently to allow this transition. The palliative care provider can assist in these arrangements, whether it is to a regular nursing care area, a rehabilitation facility, an inpatient hospice, or home. Depending on the situation, discussion of an out-of-hospital do-not-resuscitate order may be desirable, to avoid the need to make all the same decisions again and to best guide care in the event of further decline or death in the home or school setting (Kimberly et al., 2005; Berkowitz and Morrison, 2007). This advance care planning will help providers within the community adhere to well-thought-out goals of care if the ICU and/or palliative care team takes an active role in communicating the events that have occurred in the hospital and the decisions and expectations of the family for ongoing care. Often, it may be necessary to collaborate with community-based caregivers and potentially school officials to effect the family's wishes and protect the child from unwanted interventions, while assuring his or her best quality of life. Ongoing contact by the palliative care team may ease future transitions in care by offering continued discussion and support for the child and family.

When children do die, families benefit from acknowledgment of their loss and from meeting with PICU staff after a period of time has passed

(Meert et al., 2008). Information to be discussed at such a meeting includes the following:

- Review and explanation of events leading to the child's death
- Review of autopsy results if available
- Discussion of risks to present and future other children
- Thorough and honest explanations and answers to their lingering questions
- Help finding ways to explain events leading to the child's death to family members and friends

Parents value the opportunity to express gratitude or complaints about the PICU experience (Meert et al., 2008). Interventions also of value in a bereavement meeting include assessing the need for support for siblings or for professional help for the family, providing an opportunity to visit the unit where a child died if desired, and recognition by the staff of signs of "pathological" grief (Cook, White, and Foss-Russell, 2002). The grieving process may be prolonged and complex, even for families with strong coping skills, and unanswered questions may complicate the grief process (Oliver and Fallat, 1995). Staff are also deeply affected by the death of a child and need support from each other and sometimes from specialists as well (Lee and Dupree, 2008).

Conclusion

Critical care practice will be more effective and valuable to patients and families by embracing the tenets of palliative care in its everyday approaches. When the specialized communication and symptom management skills offered by palliative care practitioners are available, they can benefit patients, families, and critical care staff. A collaborative and respectful relationship between the palliative and critical care teams is the key to ensuring that the patient has access to the best that both disciplines have to offer. Such a relationship will enhance professional satisfaction for all involved in the care of children in the PICU. Integration of palliative care into the team in a trust-building fashion is of paramount importance, to avoid the perception that palliative care is useful only at the time of death. A palliative care approach can begin before or during admission to the PICU, depending on the circumstances of the child's illness, and should continue after discharge or death.

References

American Academy of Pediatrics, Committee on Children with Disabilities (AAP). 2005. Care coordination in the medical home: Integrating health and related systems of care for children with special health care needs. *Pediatrics* 116:1238–44.

Azoulay, E., Pochard, F., Kentish-Barnes, N., et al. 2005. Risk of post-traumatic stress symptoms in family members of intensive care unit patients. *Am J Resp Crit Care Med* 11:987–94.

Baker, J.N., Hinds, P.S., Spunt, S.L., et al. 2008. Integration of palliative care practices into the ongoing care of children with cancer: Individualized care planning and coordination. *Pediatr Clin N Amer* 55:223–50.

Bartel, D.A., Engler, A.J., Natale, J.E., et al. 2000. Working with families of suddenly and critically ill children: Physician experiences. *Arch Pediatr Adolesc Med* 154: 1127–33.

Berkowitz, I., and Morrison, W. 2007. Do not attempt resuscitation orders in pediatrics. *Pediatr Clin N Amer* 54:757–71.

Boldt, A.M., Fouza, Y., and Himelstein, B.P. 2006. Perceptions of the term palliative care. *J Pall Med* 9(5):1128–36.

Brandon, D., Docherty, S.L., and Thorpe, J. 2007. Infant and child deaths in acute care settings: Implications for palliative care. *J Palliat Med* 10(4):910–18.

Breau, L.M., Finley, G.A., McGrath, P.J., et al. 2002. Validation of the non-communicating Children's Pain Checklist—post-operative version. *Anesthesiology* 96:528–35.

Burns, J.P., Mitchell, C., Outwater, K.M., et al. 2000. End-of-life care in the pediatric intensive care unit after the forgoing of life-sustaining treatment. *Crit Care Med* 28(8):3060–66.

Carter, B.S., Howenstein, M., Gilmer, M.J., et al. 2004. Circumstances surrounding the deaths of hospitalized children: Opportunities for pediatric palliative care. *Pediatrics* 114(3):e361–66.

Carter, B.S., Hubble, C., and Weise, K.L. 2006. Palliative medicine in neonatal and pediatric intensive care. *Child Adolesc Psychiatr Clin N Am* 15(3):759–77.

Carvalho, W.B., and Fonseca, M.C.M. 2008. Pediatric delirium: A new diagnostic challenge of which to be aware. *Crit Care Med* 36(6):1986–87.

Contro, N., Larson, J., Scofield, S., et al. 2002. Family perspectives on the quality of pediatric palliative care. *Arch Pediatr Adolesc Med* 156:14–19.

Cook, P., White, D.K., and Foss-Russell, R.I. 2002. Bereavement support following sudden and unexpected death: Guidelines for care. *Arch Dis Child* 87:36–39.

Copnell, B. 2005. Death in the pediatric ICU: Caring for children and families at the end of life. *Crit Care Nurs Clin N Amer* 17:349–60.

Davies, B., Sehring, S.A., Partridge, J.C., et al. 2008. Barriers to palliative care for children: Perceptions of pediatric health care providers. *Pediatrics* 121(2):282–88.

Devictor, D., Latour, J.M., and Tissieres, P. 2008. Forgoing life-sustaining or death-prolonging therapy in the pediatric ICU. *Ped Clin N Amer* 55:791–804.

Diem, S.J., Lantos, J.D., and Tulsky, J.A. 1996. Cardiopulmonary resuscitation on television: Miracles and misinformation. *N Engl J Med* 334:1604–5.

Docherty, S.L., Miles, M., and Brandon, D. 2007. Searching for "the dying point": Providers' experiences with palliative care in pediatric acute care. *Pediatr Nurs* 33(4):335–41.

Dosa, N.P., Boeing, M., and Kanter, R.K. 2001. Excess risk of severe acute illness in children with chronic health conditions. *Pediatrics* 107:499–504.

Feudtner, C. 2007. Collaborative communication in pediatric palliative care: A foundation for problem-solving and decision-making. *Pediatr Clin N Amer* 54:583–608.

Feudtner, C., Christakis, D.A., Zimmerman, F.J., et al. 2002. Characteristics of deaths occurring in children's hospitals: Implications for supportive care services. *Pediatrics* 109(5):887–93, e361–66.

Forbes, T., Goeman, E., Stark, Z., et al. 2008. Discussing withdrawing and withholding of life-sustaining medical treatment in a tertiary paediatric hospital: A survey of clinician attitudes and practices. *J Paediatrics and Child Health* 44:392–98.

Garros, D., Rosychuk, R.J., and Cox, P.N. 2003. Circumstances surrounding end of life in a pediatric intensive care unit. *Pediatrics* 112:e371.

Hammes, B.J., Klevan, J., Kempf, M., et al. 2005. Pediatric advance care planning. *J Pall Med* 8:766–73.

Kenny, N.P., and Frager, G. 1996. Refractory symptoms and terminal sedation of children: Ethical and practical management. *J Palliative Care* 12:40–45.

Kimberly, M.B., Forte, A., Carroll, J.M., et al. 2005. Pediatric do-not-attempt-resuscitation orders and public schools: A national assessment of policies and laws. *AJOB* 5(1):59–65.

Lautrette, A., Darmon, M., Megarbane, B., et al. 2007. A communication strategy and brochure for relatives of patients dying in the ICU. *N Engl J Med* 357(2):203.

Lee, K.J., and Dupree, C.Y. 2008. Staff experiences with end-of-life care in the pediatric intensive care unit. *J Pall Med* 11(7):986–90.

Levetown, M., AAP Committee on Bioethics. 2008. Communicating with children and families: From everyday interactions to skill in conveying distressing information. *Pediatrics* 121:e1441–60.

Levetown, M., Pollack, M.M., Cuerdon, T.T., et al. 1994. Limitations and withdrawals of medical intervention in pediatric critical care. *JAMA* 272:1271–75.

Liben, S., Papadatou, D., and Wolfe, J. 2008. Pediatric palliative care: Challenges and emerging ideas. *Lancet* 371:852–64.

Mack, J.W., and Wolfe, J. 2008. Early integration of pediatric palliative care: For some children, palliative care starts at diagnosis. *Curr Opin Pediatr* 18:10–14.

Martin, J.A., Kung, H.-C., Mathews, T.J., et al. 2008. Annual summary of vital statistics, 2006. *Pediatrics* 121:788–801.

Meert, K.L., Briller, S.H., Schim, S.M., et al. 2008. Exploring parents' environmental needs at the time of a child's death in the pediatric intensive care unit. *Pediatr Crit Care Med* 9(6):623–28.

Meert, K.L., Thurston, C.S., and Sarnaik, A.P. 2000. End-of-life decision-making and satisfaction with care: Parental perspectives. *Pediatr Crit Care Med* 1(2):179–85.

Meyer, E.C., Burns, J.P., Friffith, J.L., et al. 2002. Parental perspectives on end-of-life care in the pediatric intensive care unit. *Crit Care Med* 30(1):226–31.

Mosenthal, A.C., Murphy, P.A., Barker, L.K., et al. 2008. Changing the culture around end-of-life care in the trauma intensive care unit. *J Trauma* 646:1587–93.

Oliver, R.C., and Fallat, M.E. 1995. Traumatic childhood death: How well do parents cope? *J Trauma* 39:303–8.

Partridge, J.C., and Wall, S.N. 1997. Analgesia for dying infants whose life support is withdrawn or withheld. *Pediatrics* 99:76–79.

Postovsky, S., and Ben Arush, M.W. 2004. Care of a child dying of cancer: The role of the palliative care team in pediatric oncology. *Pediatr Hematol Oncol* 21(1):67–76.

Postovsky, S., Moaed, B., Krivoy, E., et al. 2007. Practice of palliative sedation in children with brain tumors and sarcomas at the end of life. *Pediatr Hematol Oncol* 24(6):409–15.

Quill, T.E. 1995. When all else fails. *Pain Forum* 4(3):89–91.

Quill, T.E., and Byock, I.R. 2000. Responding to intractable terminal suffering: The role of terminal sedation and voluntary refusal of food and fluids. *Ann Intern Med* 132:408–14.

Sharman, M., Meert, K.L., and Sarniak, A.P. 2005. What influences parents' decisions to limit or withdraw life support? *Pediatr Crit Care Med* 6:513–18.

Stevens, B., Johnston, C., Petryshen, P., et al. 1996. Premature infant pain profile: Development and initial validation. *Clin J Pain* 12:13–22.

Studdert, D.M., Burns, J.P., Mello, M.M., et al. 2003. Nature of conflict in the care of pediatric intensive care patients with prolonged stay. *Pediatrics* 112:553–58.

Topjian, A.A., Berg, R.A., and Nadkarni, V.M. 2008. Pediatric cardiopulmonary resuscitation: Advances in science, techniques and outcomes. *Pediatrics* 122:1086–98.

Truog, R.D., Burns, J.P., Mitchell, C., et al. 2000. Pharmacologic paralysis and withdrawal of mechanical ventilation at the end of life. *N Engl J Med* 342:508–11.

Truog, R.D., Campbell, M.L., Curtis, J.R., et al. 2008. Recommendations for end-of-life care in the intensive care unit: A consensus statement by the American Academy of Critical Care Medicine. *Crit Care Med* 36:953–63.

Truog, R.D., Cist, A.F.M., Brackett, S.E., et al. 2001. Recommendations for end-of-life care in the intensive care unit: The Ethics Committee of the Society of Critical Care Medicine. *Crit Care Med* 29:2332–48.

Truog, R.D., Meyer, E.C., and Burns, J.P. 2006. Toward interventions to improve end-of-life care in the pediatric intensive care unit. *Crit Care Med* 34(11 Suppl): S373–79.

Tulsky, J.A. 2005. Beyond advance directives: Importance of communication skills at the end of life. *JAMA* 294:359–65.

van Dijk, M., de Boer, J.B., Koot, H.M., et al. 2000. The reliability and validity of the COMFORT scale as a postoperative pain instrument in 0- to 3-year-old infants. *Pain* 84:367–77.

Voepel-Lewis, T., Merkel, S., Tait, A.R., et al. 2002. The reliability and validity of the Face, Legs, Activity, Cry, Consolability observational tool as a measure of pain in children with cognitive impairment. *Anesth Analg* 95:1224–29.

Weise, K. 2004. Finding our way. *Hastings Center Report* 34(4).

Wharton, R.H., Levine, K.R., Buka, S., et al. 1996. Advance care planning for children with special healthcare needs: A survey of parental attitudes. *Pediatrics* 97:682–87.

Zawistowski, C.A., and DeVita, M.A. 2004. A descriptive study of children dying in the pediatric intensive care unit after withdrawal of life-sustaining treatment. *Pediatr Crit Care Med* 5(3):216–23.

15

Palliative Care in the Home, School, and Community

Susan M. Huff, R.N., M.S.N., Stacy F. Orloff, Ed.D., L.C.S.W., A.C.H.P., Janice Wheeler, Ed.D., and Lee Ann Grimes

The benefits of home are many. In an interview after the death of their 2-year-old son at home, Mike and Gail Bielanin stated, "We wouldn't have done it any other way. Being at home, away from those hospital walls, that cold steel crib, all those residents coming in every day . . . compared to sitting in our own comfy chair, our own living room, eating our own food, with our kitty, mom and dad and brother and grandma and grandpa all together. . . . It didn't make sense to be anywhere else. . . . The Essential Care Team came whenever we needed them, even at 2 or 3 in the morning. When his pain got worse, the nurse came; when something went wrong with the IV pump, the nurse came. When Bryce felt left out or needed someone to help with school work, his child-life specialist came. Everyone should have this care in their town."

In an ideal world, every infant, child, or adolescent facing a life-limiting condition and his or her family would be afforded a choice to receive care at home, supported by a pediatric palliative care team. Despite having the technology to deliver safe care at home and the availability of improved educational resources for pediatric palliative care, access to home-based pediatric palliative care programs remains poor. Infants, children, and adolescents in the United States who are diagnosed with life-limiting conditions will most often die in the hospital, not at home; few comprehensive pediatric palliative care programs exist. Acute care institutions are beginning to recognize the need for hospital-based pediatric palliative care services; studies suggest that if parents were prepared and could choose, they would prefer to receive end-of-life care for their child at home (Collins, Stevens, and Cousens, 1998; Dussel et al., 2009).

Each child and family has a unique response to a life-threatening diagnosis, and every child's home and family situation is different. In the absence of a willing, competent, and supportive family member, home-based care options are difficult to effect, even with a palliative care or hospice team available 24 hours a day. Flexibility in the delivery of pediatric palliative care is critical and should include the option to transition back to the hospital or to an alternative setting, such as a respite facility, a hospice inpatient unit, or a long-term care facility.

This chapter addresses the following:

- The benefits of home- and community-based palliative care for children living with life-threatening conditions, their parents, their siblings, and the larger community
- Emerging standards and models for pediatric palliative care
- Challenges teams encounter in providing care at home
- Effective means of promoting the availability of home care for children living with life-threatening conditions

In 1983, there were 1,400 hospices in the United States; only 4 of these accepted children as patients. Today there are approximately 4,000 member hospices of the National Hospice and Palliative Care Organization, and 10 percent accept children (Carroll, Torkildson, and Winsness, 2007; Friebert, 2009). Unfortunately, related in part to the higher cost of care for children compared to adults, as well as having less expertise in caring for them, most of these programs care for only a few children a year, serving an annual average of 10 pediatric patients. There are about 50,000 pediatric deaths annually, yet only 5,000 children receive hospice services each year (Friebert, 2009).

Some larger pediatric hospice programs in Florida, Ohio, New York, Virginia, and Colorado serve an average daily census of between 50 and 100 pediatric patients. Larger hospices can afford to support a greater pediatric census, as the payments for caring for children are often supplemented by revenues derived from providing adult patient care. In addition, these hospices are often the only hospice in the area because of a certificate-of-need system in the jurisdiction (Huang, Thompson, and Shenkman, 2008).

Palliative care organizations with large pediatric populations have been successful in obtaining referrals for patients soon after diagnosis and are highly integrated into acute care hospitals, university settings, and children's hospitals. In 2001, NHPCO's Children's Advisory Council, better known as the Children's Project on Palliative/Hospice Services (ChiPPS), estimated that on any given day more than 8,000 children are eligible for hospice services (NHPCO ChiPPS, 2001). The imbalance of need for and receipt of pediatric palliative and hospice services is the result of many different barriers, which ChiPPS and other national organizations have worked hard to resolve over the last 10 years.

Initiatives to Expand the Capacity of Pediatric Palliative and Hospice Home Care

The number of children dying at home has increased for children living with chronic, life-threatening conditions (see table 15.1). Feudtner, Christakis, and Connell (2000) documented an increase in the number of home deaths between 1983 and 2003 among this population. Children who have chronic, complex, irreversible conditions, if otherwise qualified, are eligible for long-term care through state Medicaid waiver programs. These programs provide families with shift nursing at home; most states also allow access to hospice services as part of the waiver. The support from palliative care and hospice care teams enables children to remain at home with their families during the last weeks and months of life, avoiding unwanted and expensive hospitalizations.

Pilot palliative care programs for children in both acute care and home care settings are currently being developed. Seven states have approved demonstration models in collaboration with state Medicaid departments, reallocating funding to incorporate palliative and hospice care as essential elements of care for children living with life-threatening conditions, starting at diagnosis and continuing through bereavement for the survivors. Florida and Colorado are currently admitting patients; New York and California initiated enrollment in 2010. Legislation entitled "The Children's Program of All-Inclusive Care Act" was introduced by Senator Moran and Children's Hospice International (CHI) as a federal bill to prevent the need for each state to apply individually for such Medicaid waivers (CHI, 2009). The Center to Advance Palliative Care (CAPC) launched two training sites in 2009 to assist in the more rapid development of viable new pediatric palliative

Table 15.1 Death at home among children who have chronic conditions

Age group	1989 (%)	2003 (%)
Infants through age 1	4.9	7.3
1–9	17.9	30.7
10–19	17.9	32.2

Source: Adapted from Feudtner et al., 2007.

care programs, to help existing palliative and hospice care programs develop pediatric expertise, and to assure the goal of accessible, competent care for children living with life-threatening conditions and their families.

Models and Standards of Care

Successful pediatric palliative care programs have demonstrated that an integrated model, combining care across all systems, including community-based care such as home care and hospice, is ideal (Carroll, Torkildson, and Winsness, 2007; Friebert and Huff, 2009; Knapp et al., 2009). Palliative care should begin when a life-threatening condition is diagnosed; it should be available to the sick child and the family throughout the illness and should continue through bereavement. Many programs providing care for children who have chronic needs "graduate" children and families from palliative care, providing alternative levels of support until more intensive palliative care is needed again. This need is often indicated by a relapse or exacerbation of symptoms, frequent hospital admissions, or the need for new treatments at home. Integrated models take a family-centered approach to providing services, encouraging coordination and clear communication among the child (as age and preference allows), family, and all care providers. Coordination of care includes communication with all parties responsible for the care of the child. This may include the primary physician, specialists, acute care team, home care or hospice team, school, community, friends, and family.

The conceptual model of integrated pediatric palliative care is shown in figure 15.1 (NHPCO ChiPPS, 2001), representing family-centered care encompassed by a holistic philosophy that addresses the spiritual, physical, practical, and psychosocial domains of care. Vital elements for the development of helpful and viable pediatric palliative care programs are engagement in research, advocacy, and education, as well as the identification and promulgation of quality outcomes measures and standards.

In the past two decades, three sets of standards for pediatric palliative care programs have been published, including one by Children's Hospice International (1993) and one by the National Consensus Project (2004) (Carroll, Torkildson, and Winsness, 2007). The most recent set of standards, entitled "Standards of Practice for Pediatric Palliative Care and Hospice," available at www.nhpco.org/pediatrics, was promulgated by NHPCO (2009) and is the first set of standards to incorporate and acknowledge hospice regulations and to recognize the shared principles of both hospice and palliative care. Safe, high-quality, comprehensive pediatric care in a supportive atmosphere is the primary goal of home-based palliative and hospice care

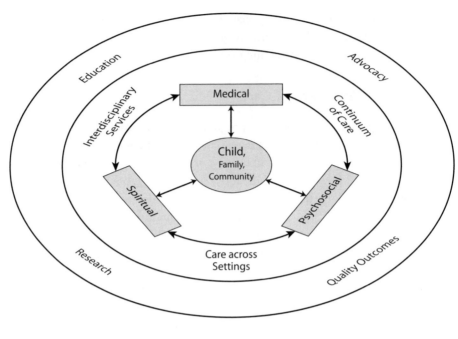

Figure 15.1. A conceptual model of integrated pediatric palliative care representing family-centered care encompassed by a holistic philosophy that addresses the spiritual, physical, practical, and psychosocial domains of care across the care continuum. *Source*: NHPCO ChiPPS, 2001

programs for children. Standards support organizations and caregivers by giving "best practice" examples. Hospice and palliative care programs that implement these standards will achieve the goal of consistently delivering high-quality pediatric care to their patients and families.

The training, experience, and expertise of the team are essential in pediatric clinical care. All direct care providers should be explicitly trained in pediatric principles, and programs should attempt to implement the nationally promulgated standards of care and best practices. Building programs around the standards will also support the staff providing care. Organizations choosing to implement NHPCO Standards of Care will (1) identify specific medical, psychosocial, spiritual, educational, developmental, and emotional needs of children of all ages and their families; (2) improve the pediatric palliative care knowledge and skills of all caregivers; (3) provide staff support to all team members; and (4) expand services and develop partnerships with community providers (Friebert and Huff, 2009).

Composition of the Team

All published pediatric palliative care standards call for care provided by an interdisciplinary team, which includes the child and family as integral members. The skills and support of different disciplines and volunteers are critical to the optimal care of the child and family, contributing to the effective functioning of the team. There can be many different disciplines working on a palliative care team, including caregivers working in the hospital and those in community settings. Comprehensive pediatric teams may be composed of members of the disciplines listed in table 15.2.

Nursing is a core discipline for any palliative care team. Nurses must be available to the patient and family 24 hours a day, 7 days a week, both via phone and for home visits as needed. Physician on-call support is also required; a pediatric physician trained in palliative care should be available to work with the team and all primary physicians caring for the child. The social worker or counselor may work primarily with the children in the family and/or with the adult family members. They provide psychosocial support through individual or family counseling, assist with financial problems and concrete practical needs, provide referral to community resources, and coordinate communication with the acute care teams.

Table 15.2 Examples of interdisciplinary team members

Art therapist	Pharmacist
Bereavement counselor	Physical, occupational, speech therapist
Chaplain or pastoral care worker	Physician
Child-life therapist	Psychologist
Dietitian	Social worker
Doula	Teacher
Music therapist	Volunteer
Nurse	

Pastoral care also represents a core discipline in all hospice settings. Pastoral care associates or chaplains are a tremendous resource to all members of the family, often bridging communication between the family and their priest, minister, rabbi, or other cleric. Spiritual support should be offered to the patient and all family members. Many families have a difficult time understanding what a chaplain or a pastoral care worker will "do." Often this service is misconstrued as supporting one religious affiliation or another. Sometimes simply encouraging the chaplain to accompany the nurse on a visit will allow an improved understanding of the nature and benefit of spiritual support and may lead to an invitation for the chaplain to come again. Simple visits can lead to valuable conversations, lending depth of meaning to the illness experience for all. Spiritual care providers also often provide support to the palliative care team, as individuals or as a group.

Perhaps uniquely important in the care of children living with life-threatening conditions and their families is care provided by art or music therapists and certified child-life specialists. These disciplines provide individual therapeutic interventions to the affected children. They also provide the opportunity for families, siblings, and the sick child to share time in a group setting. Their interventions can improve communication between family members, improve patient and family coping skills, and provide opportunities for creative self-expression and memory making, all of which lead to the increased well-being of the patient and family.

Finally, home health aides, volunteers, and respite caregivers are valued members of the home care team. Home health aides support families by providing personal care for the ill child. An example is the provision of morning hygiene care followed by getting meals ready for the day so the parents can help their other children get ready for school. Volunteers often run errands for the family, babysit siblings, help with homework, perform household chores, do yard work, or cook meals. Team members of different disciplines can visit simultaneously. One may attend to the sick child, while the other meets with siblings or spends time alone with a parent.

Successful Coordination of the Transition from Hospital to Home

The majority of referrals to a home care program occur while the child is in the hospital. Clear communication is a key element of success when coordinating care between hospital and home. The transition to home, sometimes occurring after spending weeks in the hospital, is an important, difficult, and sometimes fearful time for ill children and their families. The home care team should take this opportunity to make an initial assessment, tapping into the knowledge of the inpatient staff, child, family, and medical record to ensure the continuity of goals and plan of care and to assure that the child's and family's essential needs can be met at home. One tactic that helps build trust and confidence for families transitioning between settings is to have the referring inpatient service providers introduce the home care team as "partners in care" or as "an extended part of our team." Such a personal introduction establishes the foundation for building a solid relationship between the new team and the child and family. Ideally, members of the home care team will meet the child and family before discharge from the hospital.

Attempting to integrate the normal demands of life and schedules and to recreate life as it was before the diagnosis can be overwhelming for families. Easing the burdens of the demands brought on by the illness is a large part of the charge to the palliative care team. Assigning a coordinator for families' transitions between hospital and home has been a key element of successful service delivery for many pediatric hospice and palliative care programs. The coordinator's main responsibility is to provide reliable and effective communication and coordination across systems (Carroll, Torkildson, and Winsness, 2007). The scope of duties of the coordinator may include the following:

- Conducting the initial assessment with the child and family
- Reviewing findings with the team
- Scheduling the discharge planning meeting
- Obtaining insurance authorizations
- Coordinating all clinical care needs, including durable medical equipment, IV medications, etc.
- Completing parent teaching and return demonstrations
- Providing follow-up to the inpatient team
- Coordinating any outpatient clinic visits
- Engaging the primary care pediatrician
- Coordinating with the school and emergency medical services (EMS) as relevant, especially with regard to out-of-hospital do-not-resuscitate (DNR) orders

The needs at home vary with the innate personalities and capacities of the affected child and family, including the child's diagnosis, medical needs, and life expectancy. When first meeting the family, critical considerations include finding out the pace and elements of the medical treatment plan. The overall approach depends on whether the child has just been diagnosed or is further along in the illness trajectory, whether the child is receiving disease-directed treatment, and whether remission is possible. Does the child have a chronic condition with exacerbations and remissions, as well as a history of multiple hospital admissions? Is a slow and steady deterioration of the child's condition expected? Is this a referral for end-of-life care? Is the child's life expectancy days, weeks, months, or years? Palliative care teams must adjust to these differences, as well as understand and adapt to family values, communication and cultural preferences, and the decisions families make with respect to care.

An important question to ask of children and families is how they define "quality in their lives." In other words, what is important to them as individuals, as a family, and what drives their decision making? Simply asking "How can we help you?" or "What keeps you awake at night?" can assist in identifying families' most pressing needs. The palliative care team is there to assist the family, the child, and any siblings with returning to their home amidst the chaos of chronic illness. Families must learn to balance caring for the sick child with tending to the other aspects of their lives. If a child and the family want to remain home, a successful team will work to make this happen, even in the most challenging of circumstances. A team must always evaluate the safety of the home environment and provide the child and family with alternatives, should care at home become too difficult.

Ensuring a safe and effective discharge is the goal when the child is ready to go home. When families trust their team and perceive consistent support, they find the strength to care for their child at home. Frequent and reliable home visits, encouragement, and the availability of support any time of the day or night will enable most parents to become confident and competent care providers.

The initial assessment should begin with a discussion regarding the current plan of care, including answers to the following questions:

- Have there been previous discussions with the family related to prognosis and goals of care?
- Has the child been present during these discussions?
- What is the family structure?
- Who makes decisions within the family?
- What is the insurance coverage?
- Who will be the primary caregiver at home?

Additional components of the assessment should include a history of the illness, current medications, physical needs, psychosocial and developmental needs, and family communication patterns. Religious affiliations, spiritual assessment, school, community, and social network needs are also identified.

Meeting Patients' and Families' Needs in the Home Care Setting

The frequency of home visits made by the nurse, social worker, chaplain, volunteer, or other team members will vary based on the child's and family's needs. Many programs have defined levels of care, with home visits ranging in frequency from daily to monthly, depending on the physician's orders, the particular discipline, and the unique needs of each child and family.

Family-centered care is a core principle embedded into standards of care for children living with life-threatening conditions. The child and family are an integral part of the palliative care team. What does this mean to the team caring for the child at home? First, when the child returns home, the parents, family members, or guardian(s) take primary responsibility for the child's care; the interdisciplinary team functions as a supplement to that care. Therefore, the care provided must not only meet the medical or clinical needs of the sick child but also "fit in" (as best the medical plan will allow) with the way the family functions. Here are some examples of how to include children and families in choices at home:

- Teach additional family members how to work an IV pump and set up antibiotic doses, as backup for the parents.
- Suggest changes in medication regimens to less frequent dosing (e.g., every 12 to 24 hours when possible) so the child can return to school or otherwise leave the home and so parents can sleep through the night.
- Give the child a choice between liquid and pill forms of medications.
- Engage the adolescent to change his or her own dressings and be responsible for taking needed medications as is reasonable.

Such invitations and actions engage the child or family member to be an active participant in designing the care plan for home. When children and families are engaged as valued members of the team, trust develops, helping to support a positive relationship that, among other benefits, enhances adherence to the agreed-on care plan.

Managing Grief and Loss in the Home Care Setting

Addressing anticipatory loss, helping families cope with grief, and facilitating healthy bereavement are essential components of palliative care. Grief and bereavement counselors may be introduced to the family before the death of their child. Several program models provide consistent grief counselors to work with the child and family throughout the illness and after the death of the child. Parents often appreciate this consistency of personnel, as they long to speak to people who knew and valued their child. In a Canadian study, bereaved parents perceived flexible and continuous counseling and bereavement services provided by the treating hospital as necessary for a successful transition into community services. Continued contact with hospital staff after the loss was also noted to be helpful in healing (D'Agostino et al., 2008). Given practical issues, however, bereavement support varies substantially between communities and programs. Hospice teams are required to offer continued support for at least 13 months after a death; many programs offer support for much longer. Group intervention and bereavement camps are also offered in many communities. Bereavement camps are available across the United States, many offering financial assistance to enable attendance. The NHPCO ChiPPS website provides a listing of bereavement resources for children and families.

Clinical Challenges

Children who are cared for in home, school, and community settings have a wide array of medical conditions, some of which are rare. Caring for such children requires a well-planned effort in cooperation with the family and the various health care teams and agencies in the community, particularly the school, when relevant. The child's parents are often experts on the child's specific condition and should be welcomed and respected as partners in determining the goals of care and in creating a feasible and desirable care plan.

The family must keep current medication records, especially when the child receives care in multiple settings. When medications are changed, the family and all caregivers, particularly the physicians, should immediately receive an updated copy of the current regimen. Parents should keep the medication record in a consistent place, preferably one that lends itself to being available quickly in case of an unanticipated trip to the hospital. At every nursing or therapy visit, medication lists should be reconciled. Nurses should physically look at the medication bottles and pill caddies, reviewing the route, dose, frequency, any changes made by the family, and any perceived side effects. Parents should be able to accurately verbalize the medication regimen, understand potential side effects, and know what to do in the event of a side effect or adverse drug reaction. Medications prescribed by different specialists should be coordinated to avoid competing mechanisms of action, other dangerous interactions, or unnecessary side effects, as well as to ensure a practical administration schedule. This task is eased tremendously by the use of a single pharmacy for all of an individual patient's medications, when possible.

Pain management and symptom control are vital in the home and are a priority for patients and their families. Parents fear that their child will suffer uncontrollable pain, and they need to be reassured that effective symptom control is possible at home. Children, no matter what age, wish to return home to engage as much as possible in normal activities; they don't want pain to stand in their way. Engaging in play and social, artistic, or sporting activities; reading; returning to school; attending parties; visiting grandma on weekends; and participating in gym class bring meaning and quality to a child's life.

Many troubling symptoms afflict children living with life-threatening conditions, including psychological symptoms and disorders such as anxiety and depression. Symptoms are commonly underreported, both because children wish to protect their parents from the emotional pain of their illness progression and impending death and because of methodological problems in pediatric palliative care delivery (Carr-Gregg et al., 1997; Collins et al., 2000; Wolfe et al., 2000). Symptoms are most reliably detected when there is a deliberate attempt to elicit reports of symptomatic concerns. Thus, the nursing team should be well versed in the existing symptom assessment tools for children of various ages, as well as the common symptoms associated with the child's condition. Assessment of pain and symptoms should be completed as a priority on every nursing visit. Using the model of "transdisciplinary care," if another provider becomes aware of symptom distress of any sort, he or she should report this to the nurse at a minimum and should intervene during the visit if the individual possesses the skills to do so. Early recognition and effective treatment of pain and symptoms contributes to successful home care management.

Pain and other symptoms are more effectively managed when the parents and child are in control of the medications and treatment. The home care team should anticipate symptom distress and educate the parents, other caregivers, and the child as appropriate on what to look for, how to treat it, and when to call for help.

Parents and children will have many questions regarding the administration of opiates when and if this therapy is recommended. Common questions will include side effect management, concerns about addiction, tolerance, respiratory depression, and the fear of giving the "last dose." These are covered in detail in chapter 7. The interdisciplinary team should be educated on how to best answer the patients' and families' questions and concerns, with attention to consistency of message. Adolescents are famous for asking every member of the team the same question to see how many different answers they get. The importance of trust between the patient, family, and team cannot be overstated; when the team is unified and consistent, families have increased confidence in receiving care at home.

The nurse should ensure the availability of emergency treatment for symptom distress and should monitor and anticipate dosing needs for all hours of the day and night. Medications should be well stocked prior to weekends and holidays, as pharmacy response may be unreliable at those times. It also is a good idea to be aware of the closest 24-hour pharmacies and to ensure that they carry the medications needed by the patient. However, medications needed by children living with life-threatening conditions are often only available at specialty compounding pharmacies, which typically have limited hours, hence the need for anticipatory refill orders. While many infusion companies do support families in home care with 24-hour pharmacies, there is still an understandable lag time for the pharmacist to receive the order, mix the medications, and have them delivered to the house. The best approach is to closely assess the patient, teach the family how to assess for pain, and plan ahead with the physician for pain and other expected symptoms. Recognizing that families are not trained medical care providers, follow the KISS (keep it simple) principle at home. Complicated regimens or treatment modalities may set families up to fail, resulting in unwanted hospital admissions. When a new treatment is started, during exacerbations of pain or other symptoms, and when medications are being titrated to effect, palliative care teams must increase the intensity of patient monitoring. The frequency of nursing visits and communication between physicians and the team should increase at this time.

Pain crises are emergencies that can be managed in the home with a qualified team that has the capacity for a rapid response. Titration to pain relief may require on-site nursing and/or physician care. Some programs have physicians or nurse practitioners that make visits at home. In anticipation of symptom crises, palliative care programs should consider creating comfort kits to place in the home, consisting of medications to address common symptoms, customized for the individual child, with explicit written instructions. Comfort care kits often include acetaminophen, concentrated morphine drops, lorazepam, and rectal diazepam. The use of these medications and their mode of administration should be reviewed periodically with the parents and any other in-home providers. Comfort kits are a great help to the family, providing assurance that there are immediately available options for problems that arise in the middle of the night. Parents should be instructed to always make a call to the nurse and discuss symptoms before administering medications from the comfort kit.

Massage, play, music, art, guided imagery, behavior modification techniques, tai chi, meditation, and relaxation are examples of nonpharmacologic, complementary modalities that many children and families want to incorporate into their plan of care. Many are proven successful adjuncts to pharmacologic treatment, and the home care team should support the use of such modalities in the absence of known, significant harms.

Many parents fear being alone with their child when the death occurs. No member of any team can promise to be present at a child's death. Preparing a parent for what to do and what to expect when death occurs, even if this includes staying on the phone until a member of the team arrives, has proven to be helpful.

Addressing the Child's Needs

Children's needs are determined by their developmental capacity and specific diagnosis. Infants have different needs than toddlers, school-age children, or adolescents. The need to learn, to play, to be loved and fed, to grow, and to experience the world does not stop when a life-threatening illness strikes a child. Children who can verbalize their wishes should be asked about their preferences regarding participation in decision making and the development of the care plan. School-age children and adolescents should be active participants in planning the goals of care at home as well as other settings. While this does not happen immediately or ever in some family systems, it is a goal that the palliative care team should continually work toward.

The child's need to be normal and to continue to accomplish developmental tasks is more easily met when in familiar surroundings, among parents, siblings, pets, and friends. A complete psychosocial assessment of the child includes questions regarding the desire to return to school and his or her physical capacity to do so.

The interdisciplinary team can play an essential role in assisting the ill child to return to school, a common desire. The patient, family, school personnel, and classmates all need preparation in advance of the child's return. For hospitalized children, this transition is frequently facilitated by the social work team or child-life specialist. However, children receiving home care do not always receive such help. Palliative care programs should develop strategies to assist children healthy enough to return to school, if it is their desire, even if it is only for a portion of the school day. Returning to school is not always an easy process for the affected child or the siblings. The interdisciplinary team can help by either providing counseling or engaging the school counselors to help. At a minimum, the counselor should address issues of social and behavioral adjustment, especially when the child has a chronic illness. When a child is hospitalized or remains at home for several months, most school-related activities come to a standstill. However, school life continues as usual for classmates, making it dually difficult for the ill child to maintain friendships and to reconnect when he or she does return to school.

Assisting ill children and their classmates in the school setting is one important function home care teams can tackle. The classroom teacher may look for guidance in sharing information with classmates regarding the diagnosis, treatment, and possible return to school. Topics often discussed by home care teams in the school setting (with permission of the parents, of course) include what to expect as far as the child's appearance, behavior, and activity level, how to provide support while avoiding negative interactions and experiences, and any needed discussions related to death. Home care teams should be prepared for the "Is he going to die?" question. Someone always knows an aunt or grandfather or someone who died of "cancer," for instance, and children will ask these questions outright, especially children in primary and middle school grades. Teachers do not always feel competent to discuss these issues with their students and welcome assistance from health care providers. Discomfort with the subject matter may prevent some teachers from addressing the subject at all, leaving classmates to wonder and worry alone. Some schools have specific classroom programs regarding chronic illness; these programs often reassure students they did nothing to cause the child's illness, give them permission to ask questions and express fears, and discuss the opportunity to visit their sick classmate at home.

Children often experience changes as a result of some treatment that make school reentry a challenge. These changes may be physical in nature, such as alterations in appearance, skin color, and weight; hair loss; and decreased energy levels. Or there may be cognitive and behavioral changes such as impaired learning abilities, difficulty with impulse control, altered communication patterns, or personality changes. Children treated with radiation and chemotherapy for leukemia or brain tumors can exhibit long-term deficits, including changes in verbal function, processing speed, attention, and complex problem solving. Young age at diagnosis and being female were found to be risk factors (Buizer, de Sonneville, and Veerman, 2009; Lofstad et al., 2009). It is not uncommon for children who have exhibited these changes to repeat a grade level. Although reentry may be difficult, children are able to overcome these differences with additional support and return to the classroom.

> It is so nice to be at home with my family. Friends can come over, and it's just best to be home with your own things.
> —Grace, age 18

Grace was diagnosed with osteosarcoma—cancer in the bone—at 16 years of age. She received disease-directed treatment for 22 months, including a bone marrow transplant, before realizing she was not going to be cured of her cancer. During the last several months of her life, Grace needed multiple medications for pain and symptom control, as well as intravenous nutritional support. Despite her medical needs, she was able to stay home, surrounded by family, friends, and her beloved pets, because she had a pediatric palliative care team helping her family care for her. A few months before her death, Grace agreed to be in an educational film about palliative care at home to "help others understand how important it is for kids." Shortly after that, she presided from her wheelchair as her high school's prom queen. Her election demonstrates the degree of compassion often manifested when the school and community are given the opportunity to support children and families facing a life-threatening illness. Grace's presence at Homecoming reminded everyone that she was indeed living, even in the face of her impending death. School friends, teachers, neighbors, and the community as a whole had a strong desire to be helpful and continually sought ways to be supportive.

Grace's social networking included videos, e-mails, Facebook, personal letters, handmade cards, and "singing" telegrams. Many close friends continued to call daily and make personal visits. Grace kept a large jigsaw puzzle in her bedroom, laughingly insisting to all her guests, "If you're going to come over to see me, you have to be willing to put a piece in the puzzle." Her friends enjoyed the challenge, and this simple task helped the teens feel at ease while visiting. One friend remarked, "Sometimes I don't know what to do or say. But I can always find a piece to add to the puzzle."

As the holiday season drew near, the youth group from Grace's church gathered on her front lawn. Although too weak to come to the door, Grace could hear the caroling voices filling the evening air with joyful song, and she welcomed the bedside delivery of special gifts from her church.

Despite the unimaginable tragedy of watching her die, Grace's family had a positive and meaningful experience together because of their choice to care for her at home and their good fortune to be able to access a palliative care program willing to serve their collective needs.

Open and clear communication based on the child's ability to understand is critical. The child's wishes regarding treatment and hospitalization must be considered; they should always have the opportunity to return to the acute care setting if indicated and desired. There may also come a time when the child requires treatments or new medications to control symptoms that may not be easily delivered or even feasible in the home setting. At such times the team must consider the psychosocial and physical benefits versus burdens of such therapies and discuss alternatives with the physician and family. A short stay in the hospital with a return to home may be appropriate for several reasons; this may also serve as an opportunity for respite for the family. Both the family and the ill child should receive sensitive, open-minded support to help them reach the decisions that are best for the child and family unit. They can do this only when free from pressure or guilt-inducing words or actions.

Addressing Families' Needs

Church members delivered meals, and volunteers from the palliative care program ran errands for Grace's family. At the suggestion of the social worker, her younger sister, Rachel, was frequently included in activities and outings with family and friends. Rachel enjoyed these outings immensely; movie nights and visits to the park or zoo were simple pleasures that gave her an opportunity for companionship, fun, individual attention, and a release from the "sick house" while her parents cared for Grace at home.

Healthy children are affected in both the short and the long term by the death of a sibling. They often have questions and concerns of their own and may benefit from interventions throughout the illness experience as well as at the time of death. Early studies suggest that children experiencing the death of a sibling may suffer guilt and are at risk for adjustment disorders, often becoming withdrawn or exhibiting "acting out" behaviors (Brown and Sourkes, 2006). In studies of siblings of cancer survivors, siblings showed higher levels of posttraumatic stress disorder than the cancer survivors themselves. Sibling adjustment to serious illness in the family is markedly affected by parental coping, financial resources, marital stress, disruption to family life, and sibling-parent communication (McSherry et al., 2007). Factors placing siblings at risk for bad outcomes after the death of a sibling are not well documented. Lauer et al. (1983) found that children whose sibling died at home exhibited a positive adjustment after the death; they had had the opportunity to render care while receiving support and felt prepared, reporting close family relations after the death. Children whose sibling died in the hospital report being ill prepared and isolated, feeling disconnected from the death. Sibling outreach is often lacking in institutions and in support groups. In fact, the emotional needs of siblings are met to a lesser extent than the needs of other family members (McSherry et al., 2007).

Tim is a 17-year-old high school senior. His brother David is 15 years old and has a rare abdominal cancer. Both brothers attend the same high school. Although not missing as much school as his brother, Tim was absent quite a bit, affecting his classroom performance. The boys' mother asked the home care social worker to meet with Tim to assess what the school issues were. Tim revealed he was constantly getting "drilled by his friends" about details of David's illness and treatment and that staying out of school was the easiest way to avoid them all. He was distressed regarding what to say and was not sure with whom he could share this information. The social worker helped him find answers to these questions, collaborating (with permission) with his guidance counselor. Tim's school attendance and performance improved substantially as a result of this intervention. Excellent family-centered palliative care includes interventions that support the entire family as well as the sick child.

It is not unusual for classmates of the healthy sibling to feel uncomfortable and uncertain about how to communicate their concern, leading to avoidance behaviors and increasing the healthy sibling's sense of isolation and abandonment. Thus, sibling-focused school intervention by the palliative care team may be beneficial when the patient is nearing the end of life.

Grandparents may be the primary caregivers of the ill child and/or a primary support to the parents. A grandparent once said, "This hurts twice.

We hurt for our children, because they are our children, and we hurt for the grandchild we lost." Grandparents' burden of loss is unique. Increased use of alcohol or drugs and suicidal ideation have been documented among grieving grandparents. Knowledge of how to best support grandparents' well-being after the death of a grandchild is limited; this topic warrants further study (Youngblut et al., 2010).

A care plan developed with the parents to anticipate and meet the child's and family's specific needs is essential if the parents are to survive the demands of 24-hour caregiving. Although home care gives parents the benefit of control with regard to schedules and unlimited access to their child, the stress of providing care, coordinating and often transporting the child for treatments, interacting with insurance carriers, meeting responsibilities at work, attempting to maintain their marriage, and caring for their other children can be overwhelming. Palliative care team members and volunteers can help by providing assistance with medical treatments, pain and symptom control, financial concerns, emotional support, counseling, and respite care. Volunteers can play important roles in relieving stress and adding to a family's quality of life by running errands, grocery shopping, transporting siblings to or from school, tutoring, cleaning, making meals, babysitting, adapting the house to the child's special needs, or assisting with yard work. These services are invaluable to families caring for sick children at home. Parents are also challenged by the consistent need to perform complex medical tasks, such as suctioning a tracheostomy tube, emptying the accumulated condensate in ventilator tubing, setting up enteral tube feedings every night, and administering intravenous medications. As rewarding as it is to have the child and family united at home, it is exhausting. Palliative care teams enable home care to become a realistic option when they address these practical and recurring needs using the resources of the team and the community.

Recognizing the difficulties and challenges for families in not only learning clinical and technical tasks but also sustaining the care day in and day out, respite care is an important program asset, when available. Respite care enables the family to renew themselves, devote time to their relationships with each other, and safeguard their own physical and mental health. However, most parents need significant coaxing to leave their ill child's side for even a few hours. It is important for the team to affirm that respite care is not selfish, but rather a necessity to keep the parent healthy. Coordinating respite care can be a difficult task for the provider. Parents cite difficulty in continuity of caregivers, service organization, communication, and relinquishing control as factors leading to dissatisfaction with respite care (Eaton, 2008).

Community Support

> Each encounter with Grace was an active and effective way for members of the school and community to respond to and later remember their young friend. When she died in early January, a large number of students and teachers attended Grace's memorial service. The following day, teachers allowed time for students to talk and share memories. Students dedicated the school yearbook to Grace, and graduation was held in her memory.

If school, service clubs, and faith and various community organizations are a part of the family's social community, and if the family wishes for them to remain an integral part of their life, these organizations should be included as part of the caregiving team. With permission from the child and family, the palliative care team can work with these organizations to ensure valued support.

Sometimes the child's classmates will make "get well" or "thinking of you" cards, helping the ill child know he or she has not been forgotten. Such an act is meaningful to the ill child, while not too overwhelming for healthy classmates. Social networking sites enable teens to create web pages about themselves, describing their treatments, daily ups and downs, and the experience of being sick. This virtual communication has brought the world of individual experiences to a whole new level of sharing, with the potential for peer and family support from anywhere in the world.

Classmates themselves may need support to cope with a friend's illness and possible death. School-based activities may include group support; palliative/hospice teams can collaborate with schools to provide group support for students during the instruction day. In some communities, comprehensive grief and bereavement programs outside of schools provide group support at no cost; faith-based communities also commonly provide a vehicle for support. If the family belongs to a synagogue, church, or mosque, the congregation's youth or teen groups may offer counseling and support to family members and friends of the child and siblings.

If good rapport has been established and the patient's family is in agreement, the psychosocial member of the palliative/hospice team should provide school-based intervention when the child dies. School systems may have designated community bereavement support providers for students who experience loss; pediatric palliative care programs should take care to integrate with and supplement these services as needed.

Children and their families may have connections with community service groups such as the Boy Scouts, Girl Scouts, Junior League, or Jr. Knights of Columbus, as well as belonging to other social groups, such as athletic teams or artistic groups. Service groups in particular frequently want to assist the family by fundraising or offering to do volunteer work. Helpful activities to suggest include helping with yard work or grocery shopping, child care, tutoring the siblings, taking them on outings, or raising money for the family's out-of-pocket expenses through food drives, car washes, bake sales, or raffles. If needed, the psychosocial team can serve as the contact, coordinating the efforts of the service groups and serving as a liaison to the affected family. National groups with local chapters, such as the Candlelighters Childhood Cancer Foundation, American Cancer Society, Leukemia/Lymphoma Society, and Compassionate Friends, all offer family resources.

The Special Significance of Out-of-Hospital DNR Orders in Home Care

Parents have a legal right to make a decision with or for their child to forgo nonbeneficial attempts at cardiopulmonary resuscitation. The intent of an out-of-hospital (OOH) DNR order is to limit interventions such as intubation, cardioversion, cardiac pacing, and attempts at cardiopulmonary resuscitation, which are unlikely to benefit a child who is terminally ill from disease that has noncardiac etiology. OOH-DNR statements are medical orders signed by legal guardians and physicians, directing EMS not to follow their usual protocols. It is helpful to provide recommendations in advance regarding what the EMS provider can do if called—such as administer morphine for respiratory distress or pain, anticonvulsants for seizures, and the like. An OOH-DNR order does not mean "do nothing" in the event of an emergency. It does not prevent the administration of oxygen and medications to manage pain and other distressing symptoms; the goal is always to maximize comfort and minimize adverse outcomes.

Parents should arrange a meeting with the school before the child's return to the classroom to inquire about the school's policies regarding OOH-DNR orders and to advocate that their child's and family's wishes be honored (Mercurio et al., 2008). It is not uncommon for a member of the palliative team to join the parents for this meeting. Education of school personnel (and sometimes the school board), collaboration with the school nurse and local EMS, and an action plan in the event of an arrest are needed to effect an OOH-DNR order in the school setting.

It is helpful in all cases and required in others that the written OOH-DNR order be kept in the home and at school at all times. The team must educate the family regarding how to use the OOH-DNR order and how to communicate their wishes clearly when at home, at school, or out at community events (Carroll, Torkildson, and Winsness, 2007). This is best facilitated when the parents, pediatrician, potential EMS responder, and school personnel have a clear understanding of the goals of care and the nature of potential events leading to a 911 call. In addition, the school nurse or other potential emergency responder should be educated about and have the means to address any anticipated symptom distress. A reliable phone tree is an essential element of the OOH-DNR plan. Agreeing in advance about where to take the child in the event of a collapse and what to say to bystanders is also helpful.

In a national survey of 81 prominent public school districts across the United States, 80 percent did not have policies or procedures related to OOH-DNR orders in the school; 76 percent reported that they either would not honor an OOH-DNR order or were not sure if they could. In addition, the survey noted discrepancies between school board policies and state laws. Only a handful of states explicitly authorize EMS providers to honor advance directives for children (Kimberly et al., 2005).

Equally concerning are situations in school and the community when no OOH-DNR order is in place. Many children who have chronic conditions attend school without the benefit of a palliative care program. Interviews with school nurses and paraprofessionals point to unique and challenging issues in caring for children who have complex special health care needs or progressive disease in the school setting.

Children with severe birth defects, cerebral palsy, vital organ dysfunction, or other maladies may not be enrolled by parents in the public education setting when they reach school age. However, without adequate support, parents are likely to tire physically, mentally, and emotionally over time from the challenge of providing 24-hour care. A real-world example of the tragedies that can unfold follows:

> Jessica was diagnosed with cerebral palsy at birth; her mother was unable to work outside the home because of Jessica's care demands, and her father became the sole income support for a family of six. Jessica's mother believed that someday her daughter would be miraculously healed. No DNR order was ever put into place at home.
>
> At age 9, Jessica was enrolled in Life Skills classes at the public

school. She is described by her school-based caregiver as "mentally not observant, able to occasionally laugh and make noises, unable to speak." Jessica is confined to a wheelchair, and staff must use a wagon to position her. She frequently sleeps through most of the school day. The school nurse and paraprofessional staff members wear radios to facilitate immediate contact in case of an emergency. When asked why Jessica is in this care setting, school personnel are perplexed, questioning the educational benefit Jessica is receiving. What is more, her frequent absences affect attendance numbers and reduce state funding for the school, while her special transportation needs add financial burden to the school district. "The public school unfortunately sometimes becomes a babysitter," explains the school nurse. "I manage 620 junior high students each day. In addition, I have the responsibility of managing Jessica's care, which includes frequent suctioning and a feeding tube. It's extremely stressful. Without a DNR, I have to be ready to resuscitate her at any moment." She laments, "Caring for Jessica puts all our students at risk."

This situation highlights another role of schools in the lives of ill children. Clearly, respite care is a great need. Saddling the schools with this task seems inefficient at best in situations such as Jessica's.

Death at Home

Effective and empathic physician communication and early involvement of home care services increase the likelihood of the child dying at home. When discussion regarding end-of-life care takes place, physicians should actively seek parent and child input on planning the location of death. When parents have the opportunity to be a part of the planning, most choose home. Parental preparedness is associated with higher quality end-of-life care, less parental regret about the location of death, and fewer invasive procedures at the end of the child's life (Collins, Stevens, and Cousens, 1998; Dussel et al., 2009).

In a study of families caring for their child with cancer who died at home, several families discussed the need for better preparation for the death and for better understanding of what to do after the death (Sirkia et al., 1997). The palliative care team should educate families about what to expect at the time of death. Parents and children need concrete guidance and should not be surprised by the child's decreasing energy and alertness, declining appetite, poor urine output, or cool extremities. In one study of cancer patients during the last week of life, the loss of mental and physical energy was the most distressing aspect of a child's impending death for parents—most likely simply because they were not forewarned (Pritchard et al., 2008). Families want and need to know how to recognize impending and actual death but find it difficult to ask. Details such as changes to expect in breathing patterns, mood, appetite, energy, level of consciousness, color, skin temperature, and urinary and stool output are all areas that should be discussed sensitively and in person with families; it may additionally help to present this information in writing. Providing families reading material that is specific to infants, children, and adolescents is a must; do not give families a pamphlet addressing the impending death of an adult in preparation for their child's demise. Hospice organizations with well-developed pediatric programs are often generous about sharing the information they have developed for pediatric patients. Funeral homes also carry literature and videos that can assist teams with providing information to families.

The team should decide when to initiate conversations about events near and at the time of death; this is a difficult task that demands great sensitivity and patience. Families differ in the way they prefer to receive and process information. The tactic of introducing the topic, leaving written information for parents to read, and following up with opportunities for questions and further discussion can be helpful. By not waiting until the death is too near, the team can facilitate the common adolescents' desire to participate in planning the celebration events that will occur after their deaths. Some write their own eulogies, pick the music and bible readings for their celebration mass, or videotape messages to family and friends.

Families are reassured if they are prepared for the tasks ahead. The topic of the care of the body after death, including any religious or cultural rituals or practices and the role of siblings and other family members in washing, bathing, and dressing the child's body, should be addressed. They also need to know when and how to contact the funeral home, what role the palliative care team will play in assisting with this, and what is required to prepare for burial or various religious celebrations. Having a viewing of the body at home in lieu of a funeral parlor is a practice that is coming back into favor; however, many families do not know that this may be an option (Gonzalez and Hereira, 2008).

In some jurisdictions, if the death occurs at home, even when hospice is involved, it becomes a crime scene. As such, the sheriff is obligated to come to the home and conduct an investigation. Cultivating a relationship with the relevant judge or justice of the peace, child protective service agency, and the sheriff's office in such locations may prevent such traumatic events for families. If it is not avoidable, explaining to the family in advance what will take place and remaining at their side to corroborate their "story" and advocate for their humane care are critical activities for the care team.

Bereavement Care

Grace's sister and family received visits from the palliative care team after Grace died. Rachel attended a bereavement camp for siblings, and the family was offered bereavement counseling after Grace's death.

Grief and bereavement services are critical to families. Many hospices and grief centers offer bereavement support for families whose children died, regardless of participation in a hospice program; because 25 percent of pediatric deaths each year result from trauma, this service is of great benefit to the community. There are local chapters of national support groups such as Candlelighters Foundation and Compassionate Friends in many communities. Online support may also be helpful for some families. Grief counselors who are not familiar with the death of children and its impact on parents and siblings are not particularly effective in meeting many parents' needs. If more intensive assistance than the hospice can provide is required, appropriate referrals should be made. (See chap. 11 on grief and bereavement.)

Conclusion

The field of palliative medicine is only beginning to evolve. Pediatric palliative care has been waiting to emerge from its cocoon and transform into a butterfly for many years. The first pediatric palliative care programs in the United States were created more than 20 years ago, and today, although we are getting closer to improving access for children and families, there is still much to learn and many barriers to overcome to ensure the widespread availability of comprehensive and excellent palliative care for children living with life-threatening conditions and their families, particularly in the home setting.

It is possible to provide comprehensive and compassionate family-centered palliative care for children in any setting, including the home, school, and community. Pediatric palliative care should be a part of a unified plan starting from the time of diagnosis, through the trajectory of the illness and into bereavement. Important barriers to the development of such programs include funding and proper reimbursement of services. This problem lies within the structure of our health care system in the United States. Pilot programs and demonstration models are currently being tested in several states, with outcomes data pending. Research is required to demonstrate evidence-based needs and to assist with cost-effective solutions. In the meantime, the views of children living with life-threatening conditions and their families are clear: care at home is an option that is highly valued and needed.

References

Brown, M.R., and Sourkes, B. 2006. Psychotherapy in pediatric palliative care. *Child Adolesc Psychiatr Clin NA* 15:585–96.

Buizer, A.I., de Sonneville, L.M.J., and Veerman, A.J.P. 2009. Effects of chemotherapy on neurocognitive function in children with lymphoblastic leukemia: A critical review of the literature. *Pediatr Blood and Cancer* 52(4):447–54.

Carr-Gregg, M.R., Sawyer, S.M., Clarke, C.F., and Bowes, G. 1997. Caring for the terminally ill adolescent. *Med J Australia* 166:255–58.

Carroll, J.M., Torkildson, C., and Winsness, J.S. 2007. Issues related to providing quality pediatric palliative care in the community. *Pediatr Clin NA* 54(5):813–27.

Children's Hospice International (CHI). 2009. The Children's Program of All-inclusive Care Act. www.chionline.org (accessed April 19, 2010).

Collins, J.J., Byrnes, M.E., Dunkel, I.J., et al. 2000. The measurement of symptoms in children with cancer. *J Pain Symptom Manage* 19:363–77.

Collins, J.J., Stevens, M.M., and Cousens, P. 1998. Home care for the dying child. A parent's perception. *Australian Fam Phys* 27:610–14.

D'Agostino, N.M., Berlin-Romalis, D., Jovcevska, V., et al. 2008. Bereaved parents' perspectives on their needs. *Palliat Support Care* 6(1):33–41.

Dussel, V., Kreicbergs, U., Hilden, J.M., et al. 2009. Looking beyond where children die: Determinants and effects of planning a child's location of death. *J Pain Symptom Manage* 37(1):33–43.

Eaton, N. 2008. "I don't know how we coped before": A study of respite care for children in the home and hospice. *J Clinical Nurs* 17(23):3196–204.

Feudtner, C., Christakis, D.A., and Connell, F.A. 2000. Pediatric deaths attributable to complex chronic conditions: A population-based study of Washington State, 1980–1997. *Pediatrics* 106:205–9.

Feudtner, C., Feinstein, J.A., Satchell, M., et al. 2007. Shifting place of death among children with chronic conditions in the United States. *JAMA* 297(24):2725–32.

Friebert, S. 2009. Facts and figures on pediatric palliative and hospice care. National Hospice and Palliative Care Organization, Alexandria, VA. www.nhpco.org/files/public/ChiPPS/Pediatric_Facts-Figures.pdf (accessed April 19, 2010).

Friebert, S., and Huff, S. 2009. National Hospice and Palliative Care Organization Newline. NHPCO's Pediatric Standards: A key step in advancing care for America's children, pp. 9–13. Alexandria, VA: NHPCO.

Gonzalez, F., and Hereira, M. 2008. Home-based viewing after death: A cost-effective alternative for some families. *Am J Hospice and Palliat Care* 25(5):419–20.

Huang, C., Thompson, L.A., and Shenkman, E.A. 2008. Partners in Care: Together for Kids: Florida's model of pediatric palliative care. *J Palliat Med* 11(9):1212–20.

Kimberly, M., Forte, A.J., Carroll, J.M., et al. 2005. Pediatric do not attempt resuscitation orders and public schools: A national assessment of policies and laws. *Am J Bioethics* 5(1):1–9.

Knapp, C., Madden, V., Marsten, J., et al. 2009. Innovative pediatric palliative care programs n four countries. *J Palliat Care* 25(2):132–36.

Lauer, M.E., Mulher, R.K., Wallskog, J.M., et al. 1983. A comparison study of parental adaptation following a child's death at home or in the hospital. *Pediatrics* 71: 107–12.

Lofstad, G.E., Reinfjell, T., Hestad, K., et al. 2009. Cognitive outcomes in children and adolescents treated for acute lymphoblastic leukemia with chemotherapy only. *Acta Pediatr* 98(1):180–86.

McSherry, M., Kehoe, K., Carroll, J.M., et al. 2007. Psychosocial and spiritual needs of children living with a life limiting illness. *Pediatr Clin North Am* 54:609–29.

Mercurio, M., Maxwell, M.A., Mears, B.J., et al. 2008. AAP Policy Statements on Bioethics: Summaries and commentaries: Part 2. *Pediatr Rev* 29:e15–22.

National Hospice and Palliative Care Organization, Children's Project on Palliative Care and Hospice Services (NHPCO ChiPPS). 2001. A Call for Change: Recommendations to improve the care of children living with life threatening conditions. www.nhpco.org/files/public/ChiPPSCallforChange.pdf (accessed April 19, 2010).

———. 2009. Standards of practice for pediatric palliative care and hospice. www .nhpco.org/i4a/pages/index.cfm?pageID=5874 (accessed April 19, 2010).

Pritchard, M., Burghen, E., Srivastava, D.K., et al. 2008. Cancer-related symptoms most concerning to parents during the last week and last day of their child's life. *Pediatrics* 121(5):1301–9.

Sirkia, K., Saarinen, U., Ahlgren, B., et al. 1997. Terminal care of the child with cancer at home. *Acta Paediatr* 86(10):1125–30.

Wolfe, J., Grier, H., Klar, N., et al. 2000. Symptoms and suffering at the end of life in children with cancer. *N Engl J Med* 342:326–33.

Youngblut, J., Brooten, D., Blais, K., et al. 2010. Grandparents' health and functioning after a grandchild's death. *J Pediatr Nurs* 25(5):352–59.

16

Palliative Care for the Child Who Has a Genetic Condition

Sara L. Perszyk, R.N., B.S.N., C.H.P.N., and Brian S. Carter, M.D.

In this chapter we discuss the following key points:

- Children who have diagnoses of genetic diseases have variable life spans, from hours to years.
- Children who have these conditions, as well as their families, will benefit from concurrent life-sustaining, supportive, and palliative care initiated from the point of diagnosis forward.

She is just part of what makes us a family. She is so much more than what we thought she could ever be, based on what we know about leukodystrophy....

Within the first 2 weeks after Katy was born, we knew things were not right. She did not startle at loud noises—ever. We called our pediatrician's office, and they told us not to worry because it was too early to jump to any conclusions. We attempted to startle her ourselves. I think we did this more out of a need to prove to ourselves that nothing was the matter. We decided that the problem had to be related to her hearing. We began trying to get her pediatrician to send her to an audiologist. We were told at this point, after several visits to the doctor, that she was a big baby and sometimes they developed more slowly and we shouldn't worry yet. We noticed that Katy did not move around as much as she did when she was born and she seemed to be sleeping an awful lot. Finally, at about 6 months, the pediatrician decided that Katy might have a hearing problem.

An audiologist tested Katy and said that there was no problem with her hearing. We went back to the pediatrician when Katy was 7 months old. When they measured her head, the circumference was off the growth chart.

They sent us to a neurologist at the children's clinic. An MRI was done and diagnosed Katy with leukodystrophy. Our lives were like a story out of *Reader's Digest*. It was like being in a dream. I was watching my life unfold, but it didn't seem real to me at this point. We cried a lot. We prayed a lot.

Coordinating regular checkups, sick patient visits, and therapies can be a logistical nightmare for a child with a rare condition. Emergency room visits are the worst. We try to avoid them at all costs because Katy has been subjected to unnecessary invasive testing in the ER when an attending refused to contact her primary physician at our request. We have since learned not to be so passive. Katy can spike a fever and in 3 hours it will be gone, leaving us wondering what is going on with her. On the other hand, a cold can develop into pneumonia overnight. We tend to overlook the obvious. When Katy was 3 years old, she was very ill. She kept spiking fevers and just could not seem to get better. She was admitted to the hospital because she was dehydrated and running a fever. On about the second day, they decided she had some sort of lung virus she had caught in the hospital. She was given breathing treatments several times a day. After about the fourth day, I knew she was not getting any better. I told Katy's pediatrician I thought I could take her home and give her breathing treatments myself. They sent me home with a nebulizer. I watched her at home and, as long as I gave her Tylenol and Motrin every 4 hours, she could sleep some, but she was not well. I called her geneticist and told him that Katy was not getting better and that she was going to end up in the ER again if we didn't do something. He told me to bring her in, so I did, and he looked in her ears and discovered a raging ear infection. What happened here is that everyone got so caught up in Katy's labored breathing (which is normal for her) that they forgot that she might just have a typical childhood illness that could be easily treated.

We did not think she would be able to respond much to the environment around her. We thought she would be homebound and unable to go on family outings. We have learned from her to take one day at a time. We have had way many more good days than bad days, and God has given us the grace and mercy necessary to make it through every single one of them. Some of our distant family members can only look at Katy and our family and pity her and pity us. They have no concept of what life with her is like. They think we just sit around and cry or stay depressed all the time. They cannot see how Katy could be anything but a burden. We feel sorry for them, because they have missed it.

We are not actively pursuing another pregnancy. In fact, we are using preventative measures to keep from becoming pregnant again. However, birth control is not foolproof, and if we become pregnant again, we would not abort that child even if we knew he or she had leukodystrophy. Children are a gift from God, and each life is important and valuable.

I cannot imagine my life without Katy. She has become such an important part of our family and has been the catalyst that has caused each of us to become a better person. We don't take many things for granted. We have become aggressive when it comes to choosing what is right for Katy. We have become more adaptable. We just look at the day and what we have to do and get creative in how we might accomplish what needs to be done. We have learned what is really important and have thus adjusted our priorities. Katy is our second born. She is lovely and fun. She gives pleasure to our family and brings much joy to us.

Katy's parents have survived earth-shattering news that their second-born daughter has Canavan leukodystrophy, a rare inherited disorder in which spongy degeneration of the central nervous system leads to progressive mental deterioration. She has increased muscle tone, poor head control, megalocephaly, and blindness. Her parents and sister have ridden the roller coaster of her degenerative illness with its inexorable decline in abilities. In spite of, or because of, her condition, her family is different and, in her parents' estimation, stronger and better. They clearly display many of the strategies Bluebond-Langner (1996) documented that parents adopt over the course of the illness:

- They have routinized treatment-related tasks, including gastrostomy feedings, nebulizer treatments, and trips to the doctor.
- They have redefined what is "normal" for their family.
- They have reassessed their priorities in life.
- They have reconceptualized the future. They unconditionally love their daughter and revel in the irreplaceable child she is.

Children with life-threatening genetic conditions, as well as their families, present distinctive challenges to the palliative care team. Frequently, these children have rare conditions that are unfamiliar to the family and health care providers. How do these families cope with caring for a child who has a rare condition? What approach should clinicians take when working with such a family? For many of these conditions, there is no cure; palliative care is the only option. Inherited conditions may lead to families dealing with overwhelming issues of guilt. Considerations of future childbearing may generate intense angst. How can the health care professional support the family in dealing with parental guilt for "passing down" an incurable genetic condition to present and perhaps future children? Parents and other family members deal with profound existential questions and may question why their God would allow an innocent baby to die before being born or why their God would permit a child to be born with a condition for which there is no cure.

The diagnosis of a life-threatening genetic condition may be made "out of the blue" with an amniocentesis, ultrasound, or birth of an affected baby. On the other hand, some children possess genetic conditions that will be diagnosed long after the parents first suspect that there is a problem, and some conditions will not be diagnosed until a second child is born with the same disorder. What methods are effective in assisting families to cope with the uncertainties of the child's condition, treatment, and future? Because palliative care is the only option for some children, parents may turn to unproven therapies, such as special vitamin mixtures. Given the rarity of many of these conditions, families may seek out information and support from the Internet. How can families' Internet searches be guided to provide good-quality results? Walking side by side with these families as they navigate the cataclysmic and often unknown journey of the child's illness requires knowledgeable, compassionate, and dedicated health care professionals.

Life-Threatening Genetic Conditions in Children

INCIDENCE

In 2005 there were 28,534 infant deaths in the United States. Almost 20 percent of these occurred in the face of congenital anomalies, making birth defects the leading cause of infant mortality (Martin et al., 2008). In a report of a 4-year period, genetic diseases and conditions contributed to 34 percent of all inpatient deaths at a university-affiliated children's hospital in the United States (Stevenson and Carey, 2004). In a report from Canada spanning 6 years (Siden et al., 2008), even among children managed by a palliative care team, in-hospital deaths were the norm for many children who had genetic diagnoses. The incidence of various genetic conditions affecting children ranges from common disorders, such as Down syndrome, neurofibromatosis, and fragile X syndrome, to a wide array of rare conditions, including nonketotic hyperglycinemia, spinal muscular atrophy type 1, and citrullinemia. Table 16.1 shows the incidence and mode of inheritance of selected life-threatening genetic conditions in children.

CHROMOSOMAL DISORDERS

The chromosomal anomaly conditions (aneuploidy, deletions, and duplications) are individually rare and each has many unique features, but collectively they constitute a sizable portion of the genetic disorders seen in infants and children. Multiple organ involvement is the rule, yet some individuals have few external abnormalities. Depending on the condition, up to one-half of the individuals born with chromosomal abnormalities do not have any obvious physical differences. The physiologic impact of a chromosomal disorder, however, can be significant: cardiac and brain anomalies often result in a shortened life span. Although some are exceedingly rare, the common thread of comparable problems seen in children leads to common support systems and groups. Feeding problems, failure to thrive, gastroesophageal reflux, seizures, and vision and hearing problems are all encountered. Yet the uniqueness of each child and family situation and values does not lend itself to making universal treatment decisions.

Chromosomal conditions often result in an assortment of static deficiencies. If surgical correction is feasible for a particular defect, such as a malformed heart or blocked intestine, the child may do physically or medically well for a period of time. But some reports question any net benefit of such specific interventions, as they ultimately do not reduce overall mortality (Goc et al., 2006). Irreversible cognitive and developmental disabilities are typically present in those infants who have chromosomal anomalies and go on to survive into childhood.

In recent years, the use of chromosomal microarray analysis has led to newly identified genetic conditions that, while able to be named, have less than fully known prognoses. In many instances, these tests are sought in the context of mental retardation or multiple congenital anomalies (Edelmann and Hirschhorn, 2009). Palliative care clinicians may find a measure of purpose in helping affected families as their children are managed by geneticists, neurologists, and developmental specialists through lengthy testing, supportive care, and management of symptoms.

INBORN ERRORS OF METABOLISM

Metabolic conditions are numerous and complex. A number of acute life-threatening conditions can complicate the daily routine of a child and be exacerbated when that child has surgery or encounters a stressor such as fever, vomiting, or diarrhea. Hypoglycemia, seizures, and lethargy are common sequelae of a deranged metabolic process.

A growing awareness of metabolic disorders has increased the case reports of these conditions. Hypoglycemia can occur in a fasting state as a result of inadequate release of stored sugars or fats. Sometimes the diagnosis is made at autopsy, after the first life-threatening event. The interventions for these groups of disorders can be both promising and time consuming. If the

Table 16.1 Incidence and mode of inheritance of life-threatening rare genetic conditions in children

Disease category	Genetic condition	Incidence	Mode of inheritance
Dysmorphic syndromes	Anencephaly	1:1,500	Autosomal and X-linked recessive
	Arthrogryposis multiplex congenita	1:100,000	Usually not hereditary
	Asphyxiating thoracic dystrophy	1:120,000	Autosomal recessive
	CHARGE association	1:25,000	Most often sporadic
	DiGeorge syndrome	1:10,000	Sporadic, familial
	Meckel syndrome	1:9,000 to 1:140,000	Autosomal recessive
	Osteogenesis imperfecta	1:20,000 to 1:50,000	Most common form autosomal dominant
	Potter syndrome	1:7,000	Sporadic
	Smith-Lemli-Opitz syndrome	170 cases recorded	Autosomal recessive
	Spondyloepiphyseal dysplasia congenita	1:100,000	Autosomal dominant
	Trisomy 13	1:12,000	Sporadic
	Trisomy 18	1:5,000 to 1:7,000	Sporadic
	Trisomy 21	1:800	Sporadic
	VACTERL association	Very rare	Sporadic

Inborn errors of metabolism	Adrenoleukodystrophy—childhood	1:100,000	X-linked
	Adrenoleukodystrophy—neonatal	1:100,000	Autosomal recessive
	Citrullinemia	Fewer than 1,000 diagnosed	Autosomal recessive
	Fabry disease	Fewer than 2,500 diagnosed	X-linked
	Glycogen storage diseases	1:150,000	Autosomal recessive
	Hunter syndrome—MPS II	1:100,000	X-linked
	Hurler syndrome—MPS I	1:100,000	Autosomal recessive
	Menkes disease	1:35,000 to 1:100,000	X-linked recessive
	Niemann-Pick disease	Rare	Autosomal recessive
	Nonketotic hyperglycinemia	1:250,000	Autosomal recessive
	Pompe disease	1:40,000	Autosomal recessive
	Sanfilippo syndrome—MPS III	1:50,000	Autosomal recessive
	Tay Sachs disease	1:50,000	Autosomal recessive
	Zellweger syndrome	1:100,000	Autosomal recessive
Neurological disorders	Batten disease	3:100,000	Autosomal recessive
	Duchenne muscular dystrophy	1:4,000	X-linked
	Krabbe leukodystrophy	1:40,000	Autosomal recessive
	Lissencephaly	Very rare	Autosomal recessive
	Metachromatic leukodystrophy	1:100,000	Autosomal recessive
	Spinal muscular atrophy—type 1	1:1,000,000	Autosomal recessive

metabolic disease cannot be adequately controlled, the likely consequence is the child's death. Even if the child is viewed as "stable," guilt may surface with each hospitalization or setback. Treatment and management of the disease may be feasible, but these disorders often prove unpredictable, following a roller coaster course that stresses most families.

DEGENERATIVE NEUROLOGICAL OR MUSCULAR CONDITIONS

A large group of rare disorders result in the degeneration of the brain. These can involve groups of enzymes, such as seen in the lysosomal or peroxisomal disorders, or the mitochondrial energy pathways. Early diagnosis may allow for the early intervention of both life-sustaining and supportive palliative care concomitantly, but this is not always possible (Grayer, 2005), as many genes remain to be fully understood. For some children, the only clear findings are the changes seen on serial brain imaging scans. A large number of conditions still require invasive diagnostic tests, such as nerve or muscle biopsy, for diagnosis. Support for these families is based on assisting them in recognizing that the changes taking place are not caused by parental neglect or lack of nutrition (e.g., secondary to recurrent vomiting); rather, the changes are rooted in the deterioration the child is experiencing as a result of the disease. The rate of progression of the child's condition affects the child's ability to "hold up" during illnesses and other stressors.

With medical interventions, the affected child's life span can be extended; however, the rate of disease progression is often not slowed. Recent examples of these difficulties include Hunter and Hurler syndromes and the matter of enzyme replacement therapy (Tokic et al., 2007; Wraith et al., 2008). Supportive, life-prolonging care can benefit the family, as it allows time for them to see the disease progression, have more time with the child, and gain support from friends and relatives. When a child experiences a rapid decline or sudden loss of life, the family does not have sufficient "prep" time and their grief is thus more complex. Table 16.2 lists symptoms, treatments, and life expectancy for selected life-threatening genetic conditions.

Neurodegenerative conditions come in a variety of forms. The process of losing skills and slowly changing focus from motor or nutritional concerns, to daily care, to supportive measures is gradual. Frequent visits are needed after the initial diagnosis and test results. The child and family need support and open, honest discussion. Common conditions are Batten disease, Duchenne muscular dystrophy, Krabbe leukodystrophy, lissencephaly, metachromatic leukodystrophy, and spinal muscular atrophy (SMA) type 1. Other less common disorders include Zellweger syndrome and nonketotic hyperglycinemia. The common pattern of decline with these disorders is progressive neurologic involvement. Some children have a period of normal or near-normal functioning. However, many have had minor problems along the way before the major problems are recognized. Different degrees of functional limitation and respiratory and feeding problems develop with time. Parents and family can recognize their child's habits, routines, likes, and dislikes. The personality of the child is often endearing, even if the child is not able to communicate verbally. Yet each decline may mark a juncture at which overall goals of care need to be reexamined and critical decisions made (Hardart and Truog, 2003; Roper and Quinlivan, 2010).

Patients' and Families' Needs

Who we are as human beings is more than just our DNA. Nonetheless, our genetic heritage is an essential part of who we are and who we will become. For children with life-threatening genetic conditions, their flawed paired bases of adenine, thymine, guanine, and cytosine propel them and their loved ones on a journey that can be filled with sadness, devastated dreams, and anguish for the perfect child who could have been. Then again, many of these families ultimately find love, joy, and delight in the special and unique human being who is their child.

Bluebond-Langner (1996) describes the "natural history of the illness" as the series of events from diagnosis to death that mark critical changes in the social and emotional life of the family, as well as in the clinical status of the child. The natural history of the illness closely parallels, but is not identical to, the clinical course. The needs of the family of a child with a life-threatening genetic condition fluctuate as the child and family move through this progression of events. Accordingly, the palliative care interventions essential to support this child and family vary with time.

> The impetus for living things to reproduce and create offspring who will survive them is so basic to life that it is one of the fundamental truths of our world, like gravity or the sun. Through it, continuity and a kind of immortality are achieved. The human impetus to reproduce and create offspring embraces both the biological and the symbolical. People both create life and give meaning to that life as part of existence and self-preservation. (Rubin and Malkinson, 2001)

Table 16.2 Presentation, treatment, and life expectancy of selected life-threatening genetic conditions

Genetic condition	Signs and symptoms	Treatment	Life expectancy
Anencephaly	Poor feeding, low muscle tone, head size often small, but may be large. Initial signs may be subtle, seizures or lack of social responsiveness are often a helpful tip-off. Some children have obvious spasticity.	Seizure medications, supportive care. In longer-lived individuals, therapies will benefit. Seizures, if not present initially, often develop by 3–4 months.	Minutes, days, a few weeks or months in 90%; a few live for many years.
Arthrogryposis multiplex congenita (more than 50 types)	Abnormal joint positions in the womb; fixed joints both distal and proximal; may involve the facial musculature. Amyoplasia type is often compatible with long-lived outcome and normal intelligence.	Casting and/or surgeries to correct malpositioning; supportive care; tube feedings; some may have seizures; some may have progression of symptoms.	If on ventilator at 30 days, would not expect long-term survival; some mild forms respond well to orthopedic therapies.
Asphyxiating thoracic dystrophy	Severe restriction of chest size; may initially not need respiratory support in 10%–20%; 5 subtypes, some with additional organ cysts in liver or kidney, clefting, etc. New types are being found.	Attempts to enlarge rib circumference have been moderately successful, but long-term complications and other organ involvement still make it a lethal condition for the most part.	Usually months; those who survive infancy have kidney failure later in life.
CHARGE association (this association can be variable with regard to the anomalies and specific combination present)	Coloboma (iris or retina or both); Heart defect (VSD TGV); Atresia of the choanal nasal passages (stenosis or partial blockage); Renal anomalies (dysplastic or missing); Genital hypoplasia; Ear anomaly (with or without deafness); small birth weight and facial asymmetry.	Surgical care to correct anomalies. Poor postnatal growth is common. Often chromosome abnormality is found and this changes outcome prediction.	Depends on the severity of the anomalies. Long-term survival is at least 75%.

DiGeorge syndrome	Classic features include heart anomaly, hypocalcemia, and immune deficit. Facial features may be subtle and easily overlooked. Many children have severe feeding problems, dysphagia, and GE reflux. Others may have a cleft palate.	Surgery to correct heart defects. Prophylactic antibiotics for possible immunodeficiency. Monitor and treat hypocalcemia, especially when under stress.	Severe cardiac defects; little immune function; shortened life span. Most children affected with mild to moderate severity. Survival to 2 years indicates probable long-term survival.
Potter syndrome	Any number of defects can lead to blockage of kidneys or little or no amniotic fluid (oligohydramnios). Long-standing oligohydramnios causes lung hypoplasia. Death occurs in the womb, or shortly after birth from respiratory failure.	Features of compression and deformation on the limbs, torso, and face are diagnostic and occur secondary to the lack of fluid around the baby.	There are no surgical interventions to correct lung hypoplasia. Supportive tube feedings can be attempted.
Trisomy 13*	Features include extra fingers and toes, but many babies are surprisingly large and healthy looking. Eye anomalies are common, along with clefting of the lip and heart defects. Clinical features are very helpful to make diagnosis, yet chromosome testing is often needed so others can also "see it."	Supportive measures may include oxygen per nasal cannula and a feeding tube to meet nutritional needs and sometimes surgery. They can assist family to care for child at home.	Many babies survive for a few days or weeks.
Trisomy 18*	These babies are small and have tight limbs. Poor feeding is common. Many babies look good, and most look like other family members.	These babies may live for several weeks. Most heart conditions are not immediately life threatening. Supportive care in the home is common.	Weeks to months. Respiratory and cardiac failure is commonly seen. Other babies develop poor growth patterns and get the "dwindles."

*Trisomies 13 and 18 are sometimes seen in live-born children. These conditions are lethal, yet at the start the children with these two trisomy conditions may be relatively fit babies who feed well and go home from the hospital. Time and again the prediction that the baby will die during childbirth does not come true. The parents often need to plan that the baby will do well for a while and then be prepared to keep the baby comfortable with support. These children can be more responsive to their caregivers than experts often predict.

DIAGNOSIS

When a fetus, baby, or child is diagnosed with a life-threatening condition, the parents' world, both present and future, is rocked to its core. Sensitive, intelligent, and accurate communication can make a difference in how the family initially copes with this trauma (Miguel-Verges et al., 2009; Skotko, Capone, and Kishnani, 2009). The parents will carry the memory of this conversation with them the rest of their lives; while they most likely will not recall all the details, they will remember the tone of the discussion and how caring or brusque the physician was. Results of the genetic workup, such as amniocentesis, uterine ultrasound, or DNA results, should not be given over the phone if it can be avoided. Both parents should be informed together, if at all possible. The physician should avoid the use of any medical jargon, especially because genetics can be confusing for lay people to understand. The clinician should provide sufficient details to the parents that they understand what is wrong with their child but are not overwhelmed. It is desirable for the physician and family to have a series of conversations over time, so that as the family moves out of shock and denial, they can begin to grasp the particulars of the condition and its treatment. The clinician should always present a plan for further workup, treatment, or follow-up with the initial discussion. This plan confers some sense of control to the family and furnishes a focal point for the family's actions in the near future. The fact that "something can be done" is reassuring to the family, especially when cure is not an option (Lipson, 2005).

Once the diagnosis is confirmed, the family may rush to the Internet for information and support, especially when a rare condition is diagnosed. Because the quality of the medical information available on the Internet is highly variable, the family may come away with erroneous information and perhaps false hope. On the other hand, the family may also receive tremendous support from other families who have children similarly affected. The parents may engage in an e-mail or instant message relationship with one or more families to compare their children's development and treatment. For example, the mother of an infant with SMA type 1 logs on to the Internet every night after her daughters go to bed to chat with other mothers of babies with SMA. Among all that she gleans from these conversations, she learns about the typical "do everything" treatment map for SMA. She now understands the gastrostomy–in-exsufflator–BiPAP–tracheostomy–ventilator progression well before her child requires any of these interventions and can begin to mull over the ramifications of this course of action for her child and her family. She and her husband have numerous discussions over time and are better prepared to make difficult decisions when their daughter's weight begins to "slip off" the weight chart and the clinician proposes a feeding gastrostomy. Because so many families turn to the Internet for information and support, it is prudent to discuss the use of the Internet early on in the course of the relationship to steer their searches toward good-quality websites.

DURING THE COURSE OF ILLNESS

Depending on the genetic condition, the child may experience a period of relative tranquility after diagnosis. The family may settle in to a routine of treatments, medications, therapies, and doctor's appointments. Some semblance of normal life is attained. Given that the child is doing relatively well, parents may begin to engage in what Bluebond-Langner (1996) labeled "redefinition of normal." This process involves expanding the realm of normal to encompass the ill child's condition and the family situation. The nebulizer treatments, night-time gastrostomy feedings, and physical therapy visits all become part of the family's everyday life.

As time goes on, the ramifications of their child's illness become more apparent. The reality of the nature and quality of the child's future existence and the impact this will have on the whole family system comes into clearer focus. This can be discouraging and depressing for the family. Some of the parents' initial hopes may be shattered. The family may require additional support from the interdisciplinary care team at this time. Palliative care professionals walk a fine line between acknowledging the "new" reality of the child's condition and at the same time preserving the family's hopes and dreams for their child. If the health care team errs too much on the side of reality, the family may turn away from them. It is common for parents to shun anyone who jeopardizes the foundation of their hopes. Among the parents' anxieties and fears for the future, they need to retain "threads of optimism" (Bluebond-Langner, 1996)—optimism for a newly found cure, for a miracle, for living longer than the doctor's prediction, and so on. Their hopes and threads of optimism help the parents get through each day (Feudtner, 2009). Palliative care clinicians can help in attending to such hopes, even—and perhaps especially—among an affected child's siblings, who may endure "guilt of normalcy."

COMPLICATIONS AND DETERIORATION

As the child's condition deteriorates, the family may begin a phase that many label "the roller coaster"—with exacerbation of the condition followed by recovery, each time not quite coming back to the previous baseline. For example, a child who has Menkes disease undergoes a series of episodes of aspiration pneumonia. With each episode, the child's overall condition is weakened, the child loses weight, and ultimately the child is unable to withstand the next pneumonia. At some point in this process, the family may reassess their priorities. It is common for one of the parents to be forced into full-time caregiving responsibilities.

There are no curative options for many genetic conditions. For this reason, a number of families with children with life-threatening genetic conditions will turn to unproven therapies, from oil mixtures to vitamin preparations. Purveyors may guarantee an outright cure or some substantial benefit, such as enhanced or normal intelligence for a child who has mental retardation. The family may be proffered this miracle cure from other families caring for a child with the same condition, or they might unearth these therapies on the Internet. Websites may show testimonials and before-and-after photographs illustrating how much healthier or smarter the treated child appears. If the family believes in the therapy, it may be best not to attempt to dissuade them from using it unless it has been proven to be harmful or is extraordinarily expensive. The relationship between the parents and the palliative care team can be adversely affected if the clinician pushes too hard on this issue.

Specific interventions at times of clinical or functional decline may be viewed as of short-term benefit, "buying time," or truly life extending. The points at which families address these interventions, their potential value, their relative risks, and the overall uncertainty of a child's prognosis with or without an intervention provide optimal circumstances for reevaluating the goals of care, the burdens accrued to the child by such care, and a more palliative than cure-oriented or life-extending paradigm of care. Palliative care clinicians may prove valuable to managing pediatricians, geneticists, and neurologists in facilitating these discussions. It is often the case that the child will die not directly from the genetic condition itself, but from circumstances in which, over time and in the context of an accrued burdens-versus-benefits analysis, the family may choose to intervene further or withhold further intervention. Honoring past decisions, yet acknowledging that circumstances may warrant new considerations, an interdisciplinary palliative care team can aid value assessments and directions for care.

DEATH AND BEREAVEMENT

When the child with a life-threatening genetic condition dies, a new and different work for the family begins. The experience they have had during the final chapter of the child's life can affect the family's abilities to cope with this devastating loss. The alternate extremes of sudden death (such as a still-birth) or a more lingering expected death (such as adrenoleukodystrophy or Canavan leukodystrophy) can overwhelm and erode the strengths and resilience of the child's parents. Given the magnitude of the entire experience, their ability to process the loss may be impaired. For parents of young children, this loss meets them at a point at which many are engaged in the responsibilities of raising a family, juggling work and family obligations, and trying to establish themselves as adults (Levinson, 1978; Gilbert and Smart, 1992). Many parents of young children are barely adults themselves. Any healthy coping mechanisms they possess may not be well established and their support systems may be nonexistent. These families will be best served by comprehensive long-term bereavement services provided by pediatric bereavement counselors.

The death of a baby in the perinatal period, through spontaneous miscarriage or abortion, or in the immediate neonatal period, through extreme prematurity, birth injury, or congenital or genetic conditions, presents additional challenges for the palliative care team. The demise of a fetus or infant during pregnancy or shortly thereafter is the loss of hopes, dreams, and expectations invested in the hoped-for child (Rubin and Malkinson, 2001). According to Riches and Dawson (2000), when a mother has chosen to have a fetus with a genetic condition aborted, her grief can be complicated by the social stigma of the nature of the loss, an inability to share her grief or experiences with others, the possibility of lack of support from the baby's father, and the ongoing ambivalence about the choice. The sense of isolation and loneliness felt by women who have undergone abortions may be seen by others as totally illegitimate, and the daydreams they may have over how their baby might have grown up had they lived are rarely shared by anyone (Riches and Dawson, 2000).

If the diagnosis was in doubt when the baby or child died, the family's grief may be complicated. While certainly not the norm, some families have waited up to 6 months for the entire autopsy results—including thorough genetic testing—to be concluded, and the results may come in when the family is reaching their grief nadir. Presenting these autopsy results to the family at this time can thus be a complex task, but an essential one for the physician involved. This information may aid the family in making sense of what transpired clinically with their child during his or her life and may facilitate the family's grief work. Some children will die without a firm diagnosis ever being made. This uncertainty can create appreciable hurdles for the family as they move through the grief process.

MISCARRIAGE OR STILLBIRTH

The family with a loss needs an understanding that the process of miscarriage or stillbirth data collection takes time. The wait for these results is interminable in the eyes of the mother and father. The parents cannot comprehend any good explanation for why this process takes so long. During this time, it is important for the couple to come in and meet with the doctor to review the details and discuss the workup in progress. The best approach is to make periodic phone contacts and follow up until all the studies are completed. It is desirable to give the control to the parents and allow them to call as often as they feel necessary for results or to review the details of the discussions and plans.

ISSUES CONCERNING CHILDBEARING

Issues concerning childbearing may have been discussed and dealt with during the course of the child's illness, particularly at the time of the initial diagnosis. These issues may resurface during the grief and bereavement phase as well. Many life-threatening genetic conditions are inherited in autosomal dominant, recessive, or X-linked patterns, and the parents are faced with a 25–50 percent chance of having another affected child. Some families may decide that this risk is too high, particularly if their religious tenets preclude prenatal testing if abortion may be the outcome for an affected fetus. However, prenatal testing and counseling with clinicians can also be used to psychologically prepare for the ill child or to provide adequate time to make a definitive diagnosis for rare disorders (Miguel-Verges et al., 2009). Prenatal testing is not an option for some genetic conditions, although the number of conditions that can be diagnosed in utero is increasing every year. Suggesting that the parents have a "substitute child" is inadvisable as a means of avoiding grief, as the possibility exists for confused boundaries between the deceased and the subsequent child (Rubin and Malkinson, 2001).

Parental guilt for bearing an imperfect child may result in the couple's having difficulties demonstrating affection to each other. Especially if the recurrence risk is understood to be high, the couple may do everything in their power to avoid an accidental pregnancy, including sterilization or even abstinence in extreme cases. Gentle inquiry about the health of the marital bond is appropriate.

DECISION MAKING

Differences in the distribution of the cause of death by age have important implications for the kind of end-of-life decisions that are made, and by whom.

A high percentage of infants and younger children die of birth-related, congenital, or genetic conditions. These children may never be healthy in the same sense as their cohorts in the general population. This situation raises complex quality-of-life issues. The parents are obliged to determine their child's best interests in the absence of information about the individual child's perceived life satisfaction (Sahler et al., 2000). Thus, quality-of-life concerns can be thorny for the family of a child with a life-threatening genetic condition. Because the child is often neurologically impaired and can't participate in consent or assent, and because there is often no curative treatment option for the child's condition, the burden is placed on the family to decide what to do.

Parents are often asked to make life or death decisions for their child at a time when they have just been confronted with the earth-shattering news of their child's diagnosis. They may be asked, for example, to make decisions about whether to intubate their child and start assisted ventilation, or place a tracheostomy tube; or perhaps to extubate him after a prolonged ventilator-dependent period; or to place a nasogastric or gastrostomy tube for feedings. The parents might have precious little practical information about the implications of such decisions and may have no concept of what that child's life (and subsequently what *their* life) will be like. They most likely have never met a child with the same condition that their child has. Given the rarity of many genetic conditions, the physician him- or herself may have limited or no experience in dealing with this condition, with the illness trajectory, and with palliative care. Thus, the family, which is most likely in a state of shock and disbelief, may be forced to make life or death decisions about their child, guided by a physician who knows little more than they do.

Often multiple subspecialists are involved in the care of the child who has a genetic condition. The child may be followed by pediatric specialists in genetics, neurology, pulmonology, cardiology, gastroenterology, surgery, otorhinolaryngology, orthopedics, nephrology, and others. Frequently, these specialists may offer widely varying predictions of prognosis, may propose treatment plans that conflict with each other, and may communicate poorly if at all with each other or the family, especially when dealing with rare conditions. Deciding what to do with all these opinions can be confusing and upsetting for parents. Conflicting information from caregivers constitutes a form of fragmented care (Hilden et al., 2000); parents report significant distress resulting from this seemingly avoidable but all-too-common occurrence. The American Academy of Pediatrics put forward a policy statement in 2005 to help clinicians address these concerns of care coordination for children who have special health care needs (AAP, 2005).

The geneticist or palliative care clinician can be helpful in unifying the various subspecialist opinions and discussing the input of the other doctors with the family. He or she should do so in conjunction with a primary care pediatrician or family physician, giving parents a forum to have questions answered about the various ideas and to consider the different "realities." The parents must balance the need to know with the need to care for their child. Not every test needs to be done, just for the sake of pinning down a particular diagnosis. Far too often the discussions are only focused on what test to do or lab to run. The family needs someone who will discuss the baby as a whole person, as a member of their family, and not just another case to "pick at until the diagnosis is found." Genetic testing is often vital to diagnose the condition with certainty and to quote accurate recurrence risks. However, the discussions should focus on the category of the disease and statements about the certainty of disease trajectory for that group of conditions. There may be several possible diagnoses that all have the same disease trajectory and outcome. If the outcomes are variable, this uncertainty should be pointed out. The framework of this discussion should be "how the patterns will reveal themselves" in the sense that the progression of illness to death is consistent, even if the exact cause is somewhat uncertain. Most families will at some point say they have learned enough to come to terms with the situation or to have sufficient understanding. They can then begin to move ahead with this knowledge and not keep coming back to the "what if" stage. (For example, parents might query whether exposure to a vapor from some chemicals or having an influenza vaccine last fall could have made their baby's cells change, leading to the demise or stillbirth of the baby.)

GUILT

Parental guilt is a prominent feature of families with a child diagnosed with a life-threatening condition. Most parents will question to varying degrees what they "did wrong" during the pregnancy. Almost every family will feel some degree of guilt, even if the condition is determined to be the result of a sporadic mutation. This can range from a transient sense of guilt experienced before the actual diagnosis is confirmed to incapacitating, lifelong guilt felt irrespective of any careful explanations of the inherited causality. Parental guilt for sick young children may be exacerbated by an unclear disease process. Until the diagnosis is known with certainty, some parents may feel this heightened sense of blame.

Careful, thorough explanations of genetics involved in the child's condition may ameliorate some parental guilt. Medical jargon should be avoided.

Simple words and sentences that both parents can understand are important, because the parents are in a state of shock and only the broad strokes of the discussion will be remembered. It is essential to engage in a series of conversations over time to reiterate the same information over and over again. Eventually the information will "sink in" and the parent's guilt will be assuaged to varying degrees.

Blame or guilt feelings are not always obvious. Sometimes the mother is a "Supermom" who seems to cope well and take every event in stride. The fact that the parent passed a genetic factor to the child, resulting in his or her suffering, is the factor that drives the parent (mother or father) to provide optimal care and to lessen the child's suffering as much as possible. Such parents may seek affirmation by asking about other families and how well the other children did by comparison. They need to know they succeeded in having a positive influence on their child's disease course.

The parent may strive to prove the doctor wrong. If the doctor prognosticated that the child wouldn't survive past 6 months, the parents may take pride in the fact that their child outlived this predicted life span. Various manifestations of parental guilt must be recognized. Families may insist on doing "everything" to prolong the life of their child, or the family might dress the child in nice outfits, or buy lavish toys for the affected child that they would not have considered buying otherwise. Some parents will spend an inordinate amount of time with the affected child, including performing complex daily procedures at home, attending numerous doctor visits, and going to therapy sessions while neglecting themselves, their marriage, and their other children. It is valuable to include a few questions about where the other children are and how they get to help out with their sibling as a part of each routine follow-up visit.

The reality of the child's disease becomes clearer as the suffering continues. Families begin asking more questions at their visits, possibly indicating a desire to discuss changing goals of care or indicating new worries in their ability to manage as the child's condition deteriorates. Asking the family when *they* want to return to the clinic gives them the control. It also acknowledges that they can change their mind and return sooner or later depending on the changes in the child. Palliative care professionals must work to empower parents as their child's true care managers.

Sometimes one parent experiences guilt more than the other. This can occur even if a condition is autosomal recessive and both parents have contributed equally genetically to the child's condition. This discrepancy in the parents' mind-set can create problems for the couple. One parent may not recognize the basis of his or her partner's feelings and may erroneously attribute their differences to a lack of caring. This intensifies the stress the couple is already experiencing.

Health Care Providers' Needs

PROFESSIONAL APPROACH TO THE CHILD WITH A LIFE-THREATENING GENETIC CONDITION

Developing an ongoing relationship with a family of a child who has a life-threatening genetic condition is a challenging undertaking. The physician and other professionals working with the family may not be knowledgeable about the child's particular condition, especially if it is rare. Families with rare conditions, first and foremost, would prefer a physician who is an expert on their child's condition, but in lieu of that ideal, they readily accept physicians who demonstrate a consistent, caring approach. Honesty about their lack of experience with this particular condition is desirable. The physician can suggest to the family that past experience with similar conditions can cross over and provide the knowledge base necessary to provide proper medical management. The physician can seek out expert medical opinions and inform the family that this is being done. This method of seeking out expert opinions does not undermine the parents' trust in the physician's care ("Why does our physician have to contact some other doctor to figure out what's wrong with our child? Doesn't he know?"), but rather will strengthen the trust the family has in the physician ("He cares enough about us to seek out others' opinions. He doesn't want to leave any stone unturned.").

The ideal psychological outcome for parents of a child who has a life-threatening genetic condition is to move from the initial grief for the loss of the perfect child they envisioned to acceptance for the imperfect, albeit unique, child they have created. For most parents this is a difficult and challenging journey requiring a tremendous amount of professional support. The fundamental approach to the child by the palliative care professional can make a substantial difference in helping the family reach acceptance. Many of these children have physical deformities and may "look funny" or unusual. It is inevitable that the child will be the object of numerous stares by strangers when the family is out in public. From the first encounter with the child and family, the physician and other palliative care professionals can demonstrate that despite the child's physical deformities and mental deficiencies, the child will not be treated any differently. The child should not be left in the parent's lap or on the exam table, but should be talked to, held, and touched. Normal or attractive features, any positive developmental gains, and any good behavior should be pointed out to the family. For example, a child born with massive hydrocephalus and an extensive bilateral cleft lip and palate may have beautiful, long fingers. Pointing this out to the parents can have tremendous meaning for them. In addition to identifying normal characteristics that the child possesses, the physician and other palliative care professionals can distinguish ways in which the child is distinctive and unique and maybe even better than the average child. For instance, some genetic conditions, such as Williams syndrome or Coffin-Lowry syndrome, are associated with pleasant, outgoing personalities.

The importance of the professional's approach to the child during the office visit cannot be overemphasized. In addition to the basic exam, it is beneficial, whenever possible, to take the time to examine the child out of his or her wheelchair and to remove any braces the child may be wearing. The exam should be done in part on the "impersonal" exam table, as well as on the parent's or professional's lap. A better assessment of muscle tone and functional ability can be done by touching and holding the child. There are structured steps of the neurological exam that can best be done on the exam table, but some parts should be done in the most comfortable way for the child. This includes sitting and holding the child on the examiner's lap, or getting down on the floor with a blanket and blocks to assess the child's abilities and skills.

Once a diagnosis is reached and the family realizes they have limited time with their child, a new set of medical concerns arises. The family's needs change from the immediate need to know the diagnosis and the reason for the condition to the care of the child in their home. The physician may find little to discuss once the diagnosis is made. The opposite is true for the family, because as they come to grips with the reality of the situation, they often need more time and attention from the professional team. The team's assessment ought to include not only the child's physical needs but also feeding issues, pain control, and infection control and prevention measures.

UNIQUE REACTIONS TO MEDICATIONS

Many genetic conditions limit the brain in its responses to medications and to painful stimuli. The use of major opioid medications for pain control must be cautiously approached and in some situations should be totally avoided in children who have these conditions. Children who have lysosomal disorders and "brain reduction" conditions, such as lissencephaly or holoprosencephaly, should not be prescribed morphine postoperatively. For example, when performing minor surgical procedures, such as gastrostomy placement, it is prudent to use non-opioid analgesics for such children, to ensure the recovery of respiratory drive postoperatively. Giving an opioid-naïve child with this condition a major opioid often results in apnea, necessitating respiratory support and an ICU stay. However, as the disease progresses, the child can and should be prescribed major opioids, while acknowledging the risk of apnea, as pain is often severe and is a predominant problem experienced by such children near the end of their lives.

The Use of Community Resources

Finding information about rare genetic conditions has become less complicated with the advent of the Internet. However, because information found on the Internet may be of questionable quality, health care professionals should steer parents toward long-standing websites sponsored by reputable organizations. Family goals of an Internet search include finding accurate information on their child's condition and seeking out other families with children who have the same or a similar condition.

Conclusion

Birth defects, including prematurity, account for the majority of childhood deaths. Feelings of guilt and blame are common in this setting, and it is critical for the survival of the family to receive clear and empathic explanations, in a staged manner, as well as affirmation that they did not intend for their child to be ill and did not cause his or her suffering. Means of accomplishing this goal include assisting parents to find community resources, accurate information on the Internet, and ongoing care to relieve the child's and family's distress. Parents may individually perceive differing amounts of guilt or blame, and counseling to assist them to accept each other's reactions may be helpful.

There are commonalities among these rare disorders. Patterns emerge that enable the astute clinician who is willing to reach out for consultative services to effectively assist families to remain in their communities, where they are most likely to receive support from family and friends. Families who receive care in tertiary centers are likely to receive conflicting information from a number of consultants. The geneticist or other qualified physician should serve as captain of the ship to streamline the information and assist families to think through their goals and treatment options. In this manner, the needs of families facing the deterioration and death of their child from a rare metabolic, degenerative, or developmental disease can be met, and the clinician will have the privilege of the amelioration and prevention of suffering of fellow humans.

References

American Academy of Pediatrics, Council on Children with Disabilities (AAP). 2005. Care coordination in the medical home: Integrating health and related systems of care for children with special health care needs. *Pediatrics* 116:1238–44.

Bluebond-Langner, M. 1996. *In the Shadow of Illness: Parents and Siblings of the Chronically Ill Child*. Princeton: Princeton University Press.

Edelmann, L., and Hirschhorn, K. 2009. Clinical utility of array CGH for the detection of chromosomal imbalances associated with mental retardation and multiple congenital anomalies. *Ann NY Acad Sci* 1151:157–66.

Feudtner, C. 2009. The breadth of hopes. *N Engl J Med* 361(24):2306–7.

Gilbert, K.R., and Smart, L.S. 1992. *Coping with Infant or Fetal Loss: The Couple's Healing Process*. New York: Brunner/Mazel.

Goc, B., Walencka, Z., Woch, A., et al. 2006. Trisomy 18 in neonates: Prenatal diagnosis, clinical features, therapeutic dilemmas and outcome. *J Appl Genet* 47(2): 165–70.

Grayer, J. 2005. Recognition of Zellweger syndrome in infancy. *Adv Neonat Care* 5(1):5–13.

Hardart, M.K.M., and Truog, R.D. 2003. Spinal muscular atrophy—type I. *Arch Dis Child* 88:848–50.

Hilden, J.M., Himelstein, B.P., Freyer, D.R., et al. 2000. Report to the National Cancer Policy Board: Pediatric Oncology End-of-Life Care.

Levinson, D.J., with Darrow, C.N., Klein, E.B., Levinson, M.H., and McKee, B. 1978. *Seasons of a Man's Life*. New York: Random House.

Lipson, M.H. 2005. Common neonatal syndromes. *Sem Fetal Neonat Med* 10:221–31.

Martin, J.A., Kung, H.S., Mathews, T.J., et al. 2008. Annual summary of vital statistics: 2006. *Pediatrics* 121:788–801.

Miguel-Verges, F., Woods, S.L., Aucott, S.W., et al. 2009. Prenatal consultation with a neonatologist for congenital anomalies: Parental perceptions. *Pediatrics* 124: e573–79.

Riches, G., and Dawson, P. 2000. *An Intimate Loneliness: Supporting Bereaved Parents and Siblings*. Buckingham: Open University Press.

Roper, H., and Quinlivan, R. 2010. Implementation of "the consensus statement for the standard of care in spinal muscular atrophy" when applied to infants with severe type 1 SMA in the UK. *Arch Dis Child* 95:845–49.

Rubin, S.S., and Malkinson, R. 2001. Parental response to child loss across the life cycle: Clinical and research perspectives. In *Handbook of Bereavement Research: Consequences, Coping and Care*, ed. M.S. Strobe, R.O. Hansson, W. Stroebe, and H. Schut. Washington, DC: American Psychological Association.

Sahler, O., Frager, G., Levetown, M., et al. 2000. Medical education about end-of-life care in the pediatric setting: Principles, challenges, and opportunities. *Pediatrics* 105:575–84.

Siden, H., Miller, M., Straatman, L., et al. 2008. A report on location of death in paediatric palliative care between home, hospice and hospital. *Palliat Med* 22: 831–34.

Skotko, B.G., Capone, G.T., and Kishnani, P.S., for the Down Syndrome Diagnosis Study Group. 2009. Postnatal diagnosis of Down syndrome: Synthesis of the evidence on how best to deliver the news. *Pediatrics* 124:e751–58.

Stevenson, D.A., and Carey, J.C. 2004. Contribution of malformations and genetic disorders to mortality in a children's hospital. *Am J Med Genetics* 126A:393–97.

Tokic, V., Barisic, I., Huzjak, N., et al. 2007. Enzyme replacement therapy in two patients with an advanced severe (Hurler) phenotype of mucopolysaccharidosis I. *Eur J Paediatr* 166:727–32.

Wraith, J.E., Scarpa, M., Beck, M., et al. 2008. Mucopolysaccharidosis type II (Hunter syndrome): A clinical review and recommendations for treatment in the era of enzyme replacement therapy. *Eur J Paediatr* 167:267–77.

17

Integrating Palliative Care with HIV Care and Treatment

Nancy Hutton, M.D., Cora K. Welsh, B.A., C.C.L.S., and Maureen E. Lyon, Ph.D., A.B.P.P.

James is a 19-year-old boy who is hospitalized for the third time in 4 months with fever, weight loss, abdominal pain, vomiting, and diarrhea. He was born with HIV and has lived through medical complications, family disruption, and emotional turmoil. He now has multi-drug-resistant HIV. He started taking a new combination of antiretroviral medications during his last hospital stay, but he has been unable to take them over the past week as a result of vomiting. His absolute CD4 count remains 7, indicating profound immunodeficiency. Blood cultures for *Mycobacterium avium* complex (MAC) are persistently positive, confirming systemic opportunistic infection.

Epidemiology

Pediatric and adolescent HIV and AIDS were first recognized less than 3 decades ago. In this period of time, the scientific understanding of and medical treatment for HIV infection have changed dramatically, altering the course of this life-threatening disease from relentlessly progressive and fatal to chronic and manageable with currently available treatment. Effective medical strategies reduce the risk of mother-to-child transmission of HIV from 20–35 percent to less than 2 percent. These advances have led to a new demographic of pediatric HIV in well-resourced countries. Now infants are rarely born infected with HIV. Many individuals born with HIV early in the epidemic have survived into adulthood with effective antiretroviral therapy. In the United States, death rates for HIV/AIDS have decreased significantly from 1994 to 2000 and have remained relatively stable through 2006 (Brady et al., 2010). The mean age at death in children infected with HIV-1 in the Pediatric AIDS Clinical Trials Group (PACTG) increased from 9 years in 1996 to 18 years in 2006. The majority of HIV-infected children can now be expected to live to adulthood. Despite these miraculous advances in treatment and prevention, HIV infection remains an incurable condition that threatens the survival and quality of life of children and adolescents throughout the world. The incidence of disease progression and death due to treatment failure is increasing again in older adolescents, often precipitated by poor adherence to complex treatment regimens and other psychosocial factors. James's story is typical of the final outcome of such difficulties. HIV care teams, families, and patients may become discouraged and hopeless when their best efforts do not achieve the goal of a long and healthy life for the HIV-positive individual.

The Role of Palliative Care in HIV/AIDS Care

Palliative care is a multidimensional model that offers specific benefits to those living with and affected by HIV/AIDS. Antiretroviral therapy (ART) is the most effective palliation for this disease. At its best, it stops HIV replication, reducing viremia to nondetectable levels with the goal of maintaining or regaining normal immune function and preventing other end organ damage. ART improves survival and quality of life but does not eradicate the underlying infection. There is still no "cure" for this disease (table 17.1).

Early on, the HIV community embraced the interdisciplinary, collaborative, and family-centered approach to care. Before the discovery of effective antiretroviral agents, all HIV care was supportive, aimed at reducing the morbidity and mortality of opportunistic infections while providing psychosocial support for patients and their loved ones. Specific HIV treatment was added to this care as it became available. In the United States, the Ryan White CARE Act authorized federal funding to all states and many cities to prioritize and deliver a wide array of health and support services, including hospice care, to uninsured and underinsured people living with HIV/AIDS. The President's Emergency Plan for AIDS Relief (PEPFAR), a U.S. government program that provides funding for HIV care and treatment to countries that have constrained resources, specifically designates palliative care as a key service. Experience has confirmed that antiretroviral medications must be provided in concert with supportive services to achieve the intended goals of improving survival and quality of life. ART alone is insufficient, regardless of the patient population or setting.

Table 17.1 Integration of palliative care with the care and treatment of HIV

National Consensus Project (2009) domains for high-quality palliative care	HIV care and treatment examples of palliative care
Structure and processes of care	Interdisciplinary clinical teams Coordination of multispecialty care Continuity over time and across venues
Physical aspects of care	Management of medication side effects Antiretroviral therapy to control HIV Antibiotics and vaccines to prevent infections Pain and symptom prevention and management
Psychological and psychiatric aspects of care	Emotional support at diagnosis and throughout the course of disease progression Coping with repeated medical procedures Multiple loss—grief
Social aspects of care	Family meetings HIV disclosure to child patient HIV disclosure to friends and intimate partners Financial, disability, and housing issues Grandparenting and parenting Legacy concerns
Spiritual, religious, and existential aspects of care	Influence of religious beliefs and practice on health care decisions Concerns that HIV is punishment for past behavior Issues of meaning, affirmation of importance
Cultural aspects of care	Understanding cultural health beliefs Input from community advisory board Cultural competency for staff related to ethnicity, socioeconomic status, sexuality and gender, age Allay suspicion and mistrust of health care institutions
Care of the imminently dying patient	Ryan White funds hospice care for uninsured patients
Ethical and legal aspects of care	Respect beliefs, values, goals in care planning Guardianship for orphans Advance directive and health care proxy for young adults (>18 years) or involving adolescents under the age of 18 in decision making about their own end-of-life care as recommended by the IOM and AAP Capacity to make decisions

Source: Domains referenced in National Consensus Project for Quality Palliative Care, 2009, www.national consensusproject.org.

HIV Is Different from Other Life-Threatening Conditions

The stigma surrounding HIV/AIDS arises from moralistic attitudes about the sexual and drug-using behaviors that expose people to infection, its infectious mode of transmission, and its incurable and potentially lethal outcomes. The introduction of antiretroviral treatment into communities eases the difficulty of living with this illness by offering hope and the opportunity to actively control the infection and its impact on one's health and life. However, stigma persists and too often interferes with the implementation of successful public health and medical interventions to control the spread and progression of this disease. Attitudes among all stakeholders can undermine the benefits of existing prevention and treatment options. These include the following:

- *Personal:* "I am contaminated." "It doesn't really matter. I'm going to die anyway." "It's not fair. I didn't do anything to deserve this."
- *Family:* "It's your own fault." "I am ashamed of my daughter's behavior." "Every time I give her the medicine, I remember that this is all my fault."
- *Community:* "Only bad people get HIV." "Your child can't play with my kids." "You look like you have AIDS."

Adherence and Viral Resistance

HIV infection is uniquely unforgiving of the normal human pattern of partial adherence to medical recommendations. Early adherence research found that people on average take 75 percent of prescribed doses of a 10-day course of antibiotics. It would appear that many people who have chronic conditions, such as asthma, hypertension, and diabetes, maintain reasonable control, despite missing some doses of medication. If they miss enough doses to precipitate a medical crisis, the reinstitution of the previous regimen brings the condition back under control. There is still another chance to succeed.

Antiretroviral therapy must be given with 90–100 percent accuracy to be effective and to prevent the accumulation of drug-resistant viral mutations. When doses are missed, the viral load increases immediately and natural mutants are selected based on the presence of subtherapeutic drug levels. The first indication of a problem comes at a routine medical visit, when the viral load test spikes, revealing the suboptimal adherence. Viral resistance may have developed, prompting a change to a more complex medication regimen that will be more difficult to adhere to completely. A cycle of less-than-perfect adherence, leading to greater resistance, leading to disease progression and the potential for life-threatening complications occurs in the social context of assigning guilt to the young patient for failure to adhere completely.

When James was 14 years old, his HIV doctor suggested that he start the new combination treatment, taking "one pill once a day" to simplify his medication regimen as he entered high school. He initially took the medicine routinely at bedtime. Now 15, he stays up late talking with friends and has begun skipping the bedtime dose if it is past midnight, figuring it is now the "next day." At his next routine clinic visit, his viral load is up from nondetectable to 6,000 copies/mL. Resistance testing reveals high resistance to the major drug class in his pill, so he must change to a regimen consisting of three pills twice daily. He will never be able to use the single pill regimen again. He feels frustrated and guilty. His grandmother says, "But I trusted you! You are old enough to know better. You're going to die if you don't take your medicine!"

HIV in Families

HIV wreaks havoc in families. It is transmitted between sexual partners and from mothers to their children. It infects multiple members of the same generation who inject drugs. It sickens and kills the young adults who would normally bear the responsibility for financial support and child rearing. As a result, families experience the grief of multiple losses and on multiple levels, interfering with the essential fabric of their lives (Neugebauer et al., 1992; Nord, 1996). The losses often go beyond the death of a parent or sibling. Children may be aware of the health needs of elderly caregivers and fear that they too might die. Elders, themselves often disabled and rarely with sufficient financial resources even for themselves, are burdened with the care and support of orphans, while coping with their own guilt, shame, and anger about the behavior of their adult children. Aging and sick elders must attempt to meet their own care needs while caring for sick children and youth. Families often experience social isolation due to secrecy about the diagnosis.

James's mother died when he was 4 years old. He went to live with his maternal grandmother, who only then discovered that her daughter had hidden the fact that she and James were HIV positive. She felt angry that her daughter had not trusted her, ashamed that her daughter must have been using drugs, and guilty that she should have found a way to protect both her daughter and her grandson from this disease.

Unique Needs of Adolescents Born with HIV

James's HIV doctor has always prescribed the recommended available antiretroviral therapy for him. Initially this was a single medication, given four times daily. Over time, treatment guidelines recommended giving two and then three medications at a time. New, highly active drug classes provided dramatic control of the HIV virus. Although dose frequency improved to once or twice daily, the pill burden (number and size) became significant. James, like many patients, had trouble swallowing large pills. Newly available blood tests showed that James's viral load was not well controlled and that he had developed multiple drug resistance mutations. As James's doctor struggled to find a new combination of medicines that might successfully suppress his drug-resistant HIV infection, she recognized that the early, less-potent treatments she offered contributed to the current clinical situation.

With access to highly active antiretroviral therapy (HAART), infants born with HIV can be treated promptly and successfully, allowing them to remain healthy and to survive well into adulthood. However, there exists a unique cohort of young people who have survived with lifelong HIV who were born before public health efforts to prevent mother-to-child transmission and before the availability of fully suppressive HAART. The current health status of these young people varies from healthy to severely ill and dying. They are different from age-matched peers who acquired HIV through "adult" risk behaviors in numerous ways (table 17.2).

Physical Distress Related to HIV

HIV infection is a multisystem disorder; its complications and treatment commonly cause physical distress (O'Neill, Selwyn, and Schietinger, 2003). The hallmark of HIV/AIDS is immunodeficiency and opportunistic infection. Infections are best managed by prompt diagnosis and specific anti-infective treatment while managing the associated physical pain and other symptoms. Physical pain often involves the oropharynx and gastrointestinal system, interfering with normal caloric intake. Nutritional supplementation provides energy until a normal diet can be resumed. The need to endure

Table 17.2 Characteristics of adolescents and young adults who have perinatally-acquired HIV

Lifelong HIV infection

Lifelong medication

Grew up with expectation of limited life expectancy

Experience of profound immune suppression and medical complications

Antiretroviral drug resistance very common

Visible sequelae of chronic and early HIV infection: short stature, delayed puberty

Learning problems, multiple school absences due to illness

Frequently orphaned, abandoned by family, living in foster care

"Innocent victims"

---

procedures is common for these patients, but, with forethought and preparation, procedural pain can be minimized (table 17.3).

Medical Management of HIV Symptoms

Many antiretroviral medications, specifically protease inhibitors (PIs) and non-nucleoside reverse transcriptase inhibitors (NNRTIs), are inhibitors, inducers, and substrates of the cytochrome P450 (CYP450) enzyme system in the liver. Each drug has a unique profile of interactions with other antiretrovirals and with other medications metabolized via the CYP450 enzyme subsystem (Pham and Flexner, 2008). Certain palliative care drugs fall into this category and must be used with caution or avoided if the patient remains on antiretroviral therapy (table 17.4).

> James received intravenous fluids for dehydration, acetaminophen for fever, prochlorperazine for nausea and vomiting, and morphine for pain and diarrhea. He is feeling a bit better and can now take small amounts of nutritional supplements by mouth, but he is afraid to take any other medicines for fear of vomiting again. The inpatient care team urges him to restart his HAART regimen in addition to the three antibiotics treating the disseminated MAC infection. His grandmother is not present; she is in another hospital after becoming short of breath as a result of congestive heart failure. James begins to feel anxious and agitated; he refuses to take any other medicines and does not allow the team to perform daily physical exams. The team is concerned that he is depressed and is not making good decisions.

Table 17.3 Examples of symptom distress with HIV infection

Clinical condition	Experience of symptoms	Disease-directed therapy	Symptom-directed therapy
Procedures	Fear Pain	• Child-life preparation	• Distraction • Topical anesthetics • Sedation for invasive procedures
Medication side effects	Nausea Vomiting Diarrhea Headache Neuropathic limb pain Dysphoria	• Consider alternate medications • Review total medication regimen	• Antiemetics • Antidiarrheals • Anticipatory counseling
Candida esophagitis	Chest pain Dysphagia Wasting and malnutrition	• Fluconazole or alternate	• Analgesics • Nutritional supplements
Cryptococcal meningitis	Headache Stiff neck Fever	• Fluconazole or alternate	• Analgesics • Antipyretics
CNS toxoplasmosis	Altered mental status	• Cotrimoxazole or alternate	• Personal care and supervision
Pneumocystis pneumonia	Shortness of breath Cough	• Cotrimoxazole or alternate	• Oxygen • Opioids

Condition	Symptoms	Treatment	Supportive care
Disseminated Mycobacterium avium complex	Fever Chills, sweats Abdominal pain Diarrhea Wasting	• Double or triple drug therapy: azithromycin, ethambutal, fluoroquinolone • HAART	• Antipyretics • Analgesics • Nutritional supplements
Cryptosporidiosis	Diarrhea Dehydration Wasting and malnutrition	• HAART	• Antidiarrheals • Nutritional supplements
Bacterial pneumonia	Chest pain Shortness of breath Fatigue Fever	• Antibacterials	• Analgesics • Antipyretics • Oxygen
Renal failure	Fatigue Edema Altered mental status	• Renal dialysis • Renal medications	• Salt and fluid restriction
Peripheral neuropathy	Pain in feet	• Stop offending agents (d4T, ddI, ddC)	• Adjuvant analgesics (tricyclics, antiepileptic agents)
Stroke	Headache Focal weakness Disability	• Antithrombotics if indicated	• Analgesics • Physical therapy
Dementia	Memory loss Delirium Altered mental status Coma	• HAART	• Personal care and supervision • Antipsychotics
IRIS (Immune reconstitution inflammatory syndrome)	Fever Pain Lymphadenitis	• Anti-inflammatory agents	• Antipyretics • Analgesics

Table 17.4 Palliative care medications and HIV

- Recommended medications—minimal interactions
  - Acetaminophen
  - NSAIDs
  - Morphine, hydromorphone
  - Prochlorperazine
  - Metoclopramide
  - Ondansetron, granisetron, dolasetron
  - Levetiracetam
  - Topiramate
  - Valproic acid
  - Lorazepam
  - Olanzepine
  - Sertraline
  - Citalopram, escitalopram
- Contraindicated
  - Midazolam
  - Fentanyl
  - Phenobarbital
  - Phenytoin
- Caution—check specific interactions
  - Dexamethasone
  - Methadone
  - Amitriptyline
  - Antacids
  - Famotidine, ranitidine
  - Omeprazole, lansoprazole, esomeprazole, pantoprazole

Emotional Distress

Anxiety, fear, and depression are common among people who have HIV; however, these distressing emotions can be managed. Nonpharmacologic techniques are first-line interventions to prevent and relieve emotional distress. Medication use should be encouraged when nonpharmacologic techniques are insufficient to restore a better quality of life. All patients benefit when health care professionals do the following:

- Provide a calm and listening presence.
- Answer questions honestly and in understandable language; answer only the question asked, then reassess to see if that response fulfilled the need for information.

- Offer relaxation exercises and guided imagery.
- Recognize and validate practical and psychosocial concerns with appropriate interventions. In the case of James, talk with him about his concern for his grandmother and help him get information about her health status.
- Enable and encourage discussion of fears (including fear of death), previous losses, grief.

If distress continues or worsens despite the interventions listed above, further evaluation is warranted. For distress that manifests as anxiety, a trial of medication can be offered; lorazepam is an anxiolytic that can be safely coadministered with HAART. For distress that manifests as depression, formal inventories, such as the Beck Depression scale or other scales designed for pediatric patients, can help elicit pertinent symptoms. It is important to remember that the vegetative "symptoms" of depression occur commonly in advanced stages of illness as a result of the medical condition itself; the distinguishing feature of depression is a feeling of hopelessness and helplessness on the part of the patient. Asking about prior personal and family history of mental health concerns and illnesses and talking with others (family, staff) who have known the patient over time to assess for new or changing symptoms complete the assessment. There are antidepressants that can be safely coadministered with HAART; drug-drug interactions should always be checked before initiating one of these agents.

In reviewing James's past mental health history, the team learns that he was hospitalized at age 15 for depression and passive suicidal ideation. He was refusing his HIV medicines and was feeling hopeless that he could ever control his HIV. Medical evaluation at the same time revealed that although his HIV had developed resistance to one class of medicines, it was still controllable with conventional combination therapy. He was treated with antidepressant medication with improved mood and renewed ability to take his HIV medicines. In contrast, evaluation during the current admission reveals that he is appropriately concerned about his deteriorating health and the health of his grandmother. He recognizes that his HIV has become difficult to control and is considering limiting the number of medications he takes to those that help him feel better. He declines medicine for anxiety or depression, preferring to meet daily with the child-life specialist to make a scrapbook of memories.

In 2009, Dr. Lori Wiener and her colleague at the National Cancer Institute published a board game, *Shop Talk*, to use with patients living with cancer or HIV. The object of the game is to have a fun time "shopping" while talking about the child's/adolescent's life, interests, illness, and feelings; the game can be "played" with one or more people at a time. The therapist can use the player's response as a point of departure for further discussion or exploration.

Shop Talk is designed for children age 7 to 16. Because critical information can be revealed through the course of play—suicidal feelings, for example, or nonadherence to medication regimens—the game should be used only with the supervision of a trained therapist so that opportunities for intervention aren't missed.

Shop Talk players visit 10 different "shops" around the board, selecting one of six "gifts" from each store to place in an individual shopping bag when they choose to answer the question. The shops are named according to different themes: The Ball's in Your Court sports store, for example, allows players to explore how they would respond to various social scenarios during treatment.

The beauty of the game lies in its flexibility. Questions can be simple, such as, "What is the nicest thing you have ever done?" or they can be deeper, such as, "If you had a mock will, what would be the hardest things to give away?" In this way, a therapist can tailor the game to the needs of the players, delving deeper with each round or altering the questions to address an individual's concerns or needs.

After hearing the question, the player is asked if he would like to buy the gift. If he's not comfortable answering, he can say, "No thanks, just looking." Questions can also be addressed to the entire group of players, allowing someone who isn't comfortable talking about his or her own problem to learn through the experience of others.

Although couched in amusement, *Shop Talk* clearly enters into emotionally charged territory. It is important for children and adolescents to talk about the thoughts that keep them awake at night, rather than struggling alone and in silence. Many of these patients are concerned about sharing information that will upset their parents, but their parents are often having these same thoughts. This game provides a safe opportunity to find coping strategies together, so that they can focus their energy on healing, rather than avoidance. Getting concerns out in the open also prevents the health care team from engaging in the ethically troublesome and energy-consuming collusion of silence.

Shop Talk is available in two versions: one for HIV patients and one for their siblings. All questions in both versions of the game are written in Spanish and in English. It can be played in a small-group setting or one-on-one with a patient. Developed with the help of patients, including those who have HIV and cancer, this game is available free of charge. Therapists who are interested in obtaining a copy of the game should contact Lori Wiener at wienerl@mail.nih.gov.

Social Distress

Many parents of children and teens who have HIV infection are faced with an array of social, educational, financial, and medical difficulties. Some parents struggle with past or present chemical dependence; they may be socially isolated within their family and community; they may be stressed about their child's well-being and their own. Parents are at high risk to be overwhelmed by guilt, particularly mothers who passed HIV on to their children. Many mothers say that the tasks of helping their children take medicine every day and keeping frequent medical appointments are inescapable reminders of the responsibility they hold in passing on the illness to their children. This guilt can be a strong barrier to good care, at the end of life and before. Professional caregivers working with individuals infected or affected by HIV must be willing to reach out when they are missing multiple medical appointments, to hear this anguish in the context of adherence discussions, and to help parents sort through the effects of these feelings so they do not jeopardize their child's care. This can prevent medical providers from being in situations in which they struggle with whether or not to report medical neglect, especially at the end of life.

When a child is orphaned, a grandparent often becomes the child's dedicated and stable caregiver. Grandparents as parents offer a unique set of strengths and challenges. Their memories of their own children growing up provide the orphaned child with an important opportunity for connectedness with their now-deceased parents. Grandparents have raised a family already and can bring wisdom and insight that a first-time parent may not have. The challenge arises when grandparents cannot let go of the "way things were when they were young," which can result in communication difficulties. Talking about sex and sexuality is one area with which grandparents seem to particularly struggle. Grandparents, being older, are prone to have their own health problems. A child who has already lost a parent may worry about being abandoned again; grandparents' medical appointments and hospital stays can exacerbate these concerns. Some grandparents are too exhausted to think about the process of raising children again. While they may feel a sense of responsibility to care for their orphaned grandchildren, they may begrudge the related financial, social, emotional, and physical burden.

Although attitudes toward people who are HIV positive have improved over the past 25 years with advances in HIV treatment and prevention, myths and misunderstanding continue to circulate within affected communities. All individuals have the right and responsibility to share their personal health information judiciously, but people living with HIV continue to feel a heightened need to limit the circle of others who know their HIV status. For this reason, many HIV-infected children and teens have family members (even those living in the same home) who do not know the young person's diagnosis. When someone in the family is dying with undisclosed HIV disease, other individuals are likely to ask why the individual is so ill. This can be a difficult question to answer honestly, without disclosing the patient's HIV status. Often, children in the same household are told not to ask questions, which can be detrimental to their coping with the situation. It is important to help parents and caregivers have responses on hand that both protect privacy and validate the child's questions. Saying things like "That is a great question. I wonder what makes you ask it?" is sometimes enough to satisfy a young child. A caregiver can also provide part of the information. A simple explanation that their brother's or sister's body has a sickness that is stronger than the medicine can be a good way to respond to young children. Older children may require a more complex explanation, and the caregiver may benefit from discussing potential answers (and even role-playing the conversation) with a member of the treatment team.

Disclosing an HIV/AIDS Diagnosis to the Patient

Clinicians have many things to consider when disclosing a child's HIV status to him or her. Age, developmental level, and family feelings and readiness are important. The American Academy of Pediatrics (AAP COPA, 1999) recommends that children be told diagnosis and prognosis commensurate with their developmental level. In a statement specific to HIV, they suggest that an ongoing approach to disclosure that eventually includes the name of the illness is recommended. Disclosure does not happen in a moment, nor should it be talked about once and never revisited (Gerson et al., 2001). Ideal disclosures are gradual and part of a process over many weeks, months, or years; children are given information as they seek it and as their caregivers feel they are able to handle it. Disclosure should be on the minds of all those in the interdisciplinary team when meeting a new HIV-affected family (table 17.5).

Table 17.5 Recommendations for disclosure of HIV diagnosis to children

Stage 1: Information gathering and trust building
- Meet medical team; review patient and family history, including disclosure status; affirm partnership with the family in care of the child.

Stage 2: Education
- Educate parents and guardians about HIV and its treatment and prevention.
- Anticipate the need and prepare adults to respond to child and family questions about medicine, clinic appointments, blood tests, etc.
- Never lie. The simplest answer is often best. Telling a 4-year-old that she takes medicine because it keeps her healthy usually adequately addresses her concerns.

Stage 3: Determining when the time is right for disclosure
- Once children reach school age, it is important to plan specifically for disclosure of the HIV diagnosis.
- Explore family fears about disclosure. Emphasize the benefits and address worries. Explore the child's understanding of privacy (Has she started closing the door when dressing or using the bathroom? Does he understand that some family conversations are private and not to be repeated outside the home?). This approach is usually effective in achieving agreement to disclose the diagnosis to the child.

Stage 4: Actual disclosure
- Disclosure may take several visits, depending on the child's interest, attention, and cognitive level of understanding.
- First, assess the patient's understanding of basic health concepts (germs and infection can cause illness, body immune system helps fight off infection, blood contains cells that fight infection, medicines help the body fight infection).
- Discuss why it is important to take medicine (virus in your body tries to hurt your immune system, medicines keep it from causing damage to immune system, this keeps your body healthy).
- Name the illness (this virus is called HIV—have you ever heard of it?) and respond to any questions or misconceptions.
- Share with the patient that he or she is being told this medical information because he or she is now old enough to understand and participate more fully in the care. Add that part of the more grown-up responsibility includes maintaining privacy. Make a distinction between talking about personal medical information with one's parent or health care provider and discussing it with friends at school ("your body isn't anyone else's business").
- Assess understanding commensurate with developmental stage.

Stage 5: Monitor after disclosure at subsequent visits
- Reassess understanding of medical information especially as patient matures in cognitive ability.
- Assess personal and family coping with the disclosed information.
- Plan for future disclosures to friends and intimate partners over time.

Table 17.6 Children's awareness of disease progression and death

Children often overhear or understand more than adults around them realize

Children are aware of their own bodily changes

Children are familiar with treatment protocols and generally recognize when unexpected tests/procedures are performed

Children are sensitive to changes in the mood and behavior of those around them

---

Talking with children who are very sick and may be dying is difficult for the adults who care for them. Adults worry that children will lose hope and become emotionally distraught if given candid information about their health status. However, children and teens usually know how sick they are and how upset the adults around them are about this. They may not raise questions or worries out of concern that they will cause further distress for their loved ones. Yet it is at precisely these times that trusted adults need to find ways to allow and promote conversation with the child or adolescent about their illness and the possibility of death (table 17.6).

Health Care Decisions

A majority of children and teens who have perinatal HIV are cared for by adults other than their biological parents. Whether these arrangements are short or long term, children need clearly defined guardians to make decisions in their best interest. This takes on critical importance as children and adolescents approach the end of life (Wissow, Hutton, and Kass, 2001; table 17.7).

Older children and adolescents develop the capacity for mature decision making over time and with experience. Assess the patient's decision-making capacity by asking the following:

- Does the patient understand the medical information currently being presented?
- Does he or she recognize the risks and benefits, short and long term, of the choice at hand?
- Can he or she make and communicate his or her choice?
- Is his or her choice based on more than momentary preferences?

Step back and assess the medical situation. What is medically possible? Are treatments likely to help? In what way? What are the benefits and bur-

Table 17.7 Including children in health care decisions

Infant/toddler (birth through 3 years)	• Unable to participate in theoretical decisions • Able to make choices about concrete *a* or *b* decisions • Able to express preferences through physical gestures, words, crying, facial expression
Preschool, early school age (4 through 7 years)	• Unable to reason abstractly, not able to participate in most theoretical decisions • Can make choices about things they see, feel, taste, experience, hear • Able to express preference through physical gestures, words, facial expression, some written communication
Middle to late school age (8 through 12 years)	• Able to make some abstract decisions, but may frequently change their minds as they try to understand • Can make choices about what they can sense and make limited decisions about what they can imagine • Able to express preferences through physical gestures, words, facial expression, written communication • Sometimes appreciate the permanence of death
Adolescent (13 through 21 years)	• Able to think and decide about abstract and concrete concepts • Can make choices about what they sense and imagine • Able to express preferences through physical gestures, words, facial expression, written communication • Usually understand the permanence of death

dens of available treatment options? Critical decision-making points relevant to James's case include the following:

• How treatable is the underlying HIV infection at this point? Updated resistance testing should be performed if not recently obtained; multi-class resistance can be impossible to treat. In this setting, it is reasonable to discontinue antiretroviral medicines or to continue them with the intent of maintaining partial control of HIV to prolong life or in the hope that new medicines may become available in the future. The burden of the side effects associated with these medications should be considered when making this decision.

- How treatable is the disseminated MAC? Although combinations of antibiotics can decrease MAC bacteremia, eradication of this infection requires a year of treatment in combination with HAART, provided that the CD4 count can be raised out of the severely deficient range. Patients with multiply resistant HIV are unlikely to achieve this goal.

- How important is it to him to take medicine to try to treat these infections? How burdensome is taking all these medicines? Patients vary in the meaning they associate with HAART. Some need to fight the HIV as long as possible. Others decide that the burden and side effects outweigh the benefits. A treatment plan can be developed that supports the patient's values and goals of care.

Family-Centered Advance Care Planning

Tools are now available for health care providers and families to assist children and adolescents living with HIV in making decisions about end-of-life care. In 2009, Maureen Lyon and colleagues at Children's National Medical Center (Lyon et al., 2009a, 2009b) published the results of their FACE study, helping HIV-positive adolescents talk with their families about wishes for their own end-of-life care with the assistance of a trained facilitator.

The three sessions are scheduled at 1-week intervals. Session 1 is the independent completion of the Lyon Family Centered Advance Care Planning Survey by the adolescent and legal guardian or chosen proxy. This survey, for example, asks adolescents whether they want to be involved in decision making about their own end-of-life care and, if so, when in the course of illness they would like to have these conversations. The family/proxy version checks for the family's/proxy's understanding of what he or she thinks the adolescent wants.

Session 2 is the Respecting Choices Interview, developed by Linda Briggs and colleagues at Gunderson Medical Lutheran Foundation. Using Leventhal's theory of self-regulation model and the patient's representation of illness, the trained/certified interviewer brings the patient and family together to explore the following subjects: (1) the adolescent's understanding of his or her illness, possible complications, and the patient's associated values and beliefs; (2) what has sustained the patient and family during difficult times;

and (3) family members' experiences with death and dying. As each section of the interview with the patient is completed, the interviewer checks in with the proxy/family to deepen this exploration. This process provides an opportunity to clarify the family's values and experiences with death and dying. The interview then shifts to the Statement of Treatment Preferences, giving three scenarios of increasing illness severity that could happen in the future, asking the adolescent what his preference would be (e.g., to continue all treatments, to discontinue disease-directed treatments and continue symptom management, or don't know). The family is then encouraged to discuss these options, weighing the benefits and burdens of each choice. Standardized training and certification in the *Respecting Choices Interview* is available by contacting Linda Briggs at labriggs@gundluth.org.

Session 3 is the completion of the *Five Wishes* document, which helps a person express how he or she prefers to be treated in the event of serious illness accompanied by the inability to speak for him- or herself. *Five Wishes* is legally valid for adults in most states in the United States. It can also be useful as a tool to help adolescents participate in shared decision making, discussing their preferences for their own end-of-life care with their family. *Five Wishes* is developmentally appropriate with respect to age and cognitive capacity for adolescents living with a life-threatening illness and is available on the Internet for a minimal cost; there is a video that accompanies it, explaining how to complete the form.

The three-session FACE intervention was effective in increasing congruence in treatment preferences between HIV-positive adolescents and their families, decreasing decisional conflict compared with control families. FACE families were confident that they knew what their adolescents wanted. For information about the FACE protocol, contact Maureen E. Lyon at mlyon @cnmc.org.

End of Life

How do we know when the end of life is near? Classically, all medicines have failed to achieve their purpose, complications are not reversible, and disease progression leads to organ failures and ultimately death. A variation of this scenario in HIV infection is the patient with "terminal" nonadherence, whether due to neurocognitive or behavioral disorders, complete breakdown of social and family support, depression, or inability to come to terms with living with HIV or with taking medicine—often despite heroic efforts to help the patient get through this high-risk period. When this patient says,

"I want to live, I don't want to die," but behaves in ways that interfere with successful treatment, the involved health care professionals must grapple with the limits of what they can do for the patient. Issues of competence and capacity for decision making may be raised and the need for referral to child or adult protective services considered.

Sometimes everyone agrees that the end is near, yet the patient continues to survive or even enjoy a somewhat improved quality of life for a time. This may lead to disbelief when later counseled that death is near ("You told me that last year, and you were wrong!"). Counseling to hope for stabilization or improvement while preparing for the possibility of death allows the maintenance of trust with the patient, no matter what the outcome.

Even antiretroviral regimens that are failing to help the patient achieve the standard goals of a nondetectable viral load and improved CD4 count may have survival benefit, allowing the patient to await new drugs with different resistance profiles. The patients for whom this strategy works are those for whom the availability of a new regimen coincides with the patient's achieving the age and maturity to successfully adhere to the treatment plan and thus achieve viral suppression. Unfortunately, some patients have such severe multiclass resistance that there is no hope for viral suppression or immunologic recovery; they might experience some slowing of disease progression, but eventually the medication burden and increasing toxicity lead to the recommendation to discontinue ART. It remains reasonable to continue antibiotic prophylaxis if not too burdensome to the patient. Even that minimal treatment may offer survival benefit that allows time for a new primary therapy option to become available.

Legacy

When an infected teen is nearing the end of life, his or her thoughts may turn toward his or her legacy. Some challenges arise in legacy building with an HIV-infected child or teen and the family. First, the dying child may be orphaned, either owing to parental death or because he or she has been permanently separated from the parents by child protective services. Second, many HIV-affected families deal with housing instability, financial hardships, and sometimes addiction issues or other serious health concerns. In light of these many challenges, some traditional legacy-building activities may not be practical. Where possible, it may be helpful for the outpatient clinic to keep physical possession of legacy items until the family is in a more stable situation (table 17.8).

Table 17.8 Legacy-building activities

• Scrapbooks / memory books	• Parties
• Workbooks	• Cards/letters/poems
• Hand molds	• Scholarships/programs for others
• Photographs	• Wishes
• Plates	• Rituals
• Gardens	• Music—*Songs of Love*
• Journals	• Objects
• Wills	◦ Some items they loved/made
• Movies / home video	◦ Toys or characters that remind us
• Arts/crafts	

Maintaining Rapport until the End

HIV disproportionately affects racial and ethnic minority groups that continue to experience disparities in health. Professionals must remain cognizant of the powerful influence of suspicion and trust in the patient-family-provider relationship. Families may already believe that they do not receive the best care as a result of their illness, race, economic status, or educational level. In this context, raising the option of limiting medical interventions at the end of life may sound like the health care team "giving up" on the child. The interdisciplinary team must have conversations with the family about their hopes, needs, and goals and be empathetic and candid about what can and cannot happen. Meeting families "where they are," maintaining open body language, and asking open-ended questions that invite further conversation ("tell me more about that," "help me understand," "what else?") are all steps to continuing a trusting relationship with HIV-affected families.

Impact on Health Care Professionals

Sometimes health care providers have difficulty coping with or feel a sense of responsibility or failure after the death of a patient. Helping each other while helping patients and families is a vital part of ensuring that good care remains available. Some suggestions for mutual support are found in table 17.9.

Table 17.9 Peer support for health care professionals

Helpful things to do or say

- Provide genuine reassurances (e.g., "You worked really hard," "You helped him as best you could," "You are very dedicated").
- Remind that all reasonable medical interventions were offered.
- Recall the variety of interventions offered (e.g., "We tried helping her with adherence," "We spent a lot of time figuring out what the deeper issues were," "You spent hours with the family every time you saw the patient").
- Acknowledge that the grief is real, that it hurts, and that it is to be expected among loving and dedicated providers—the kind you would like to have if you were ill.
- Tell your colleagues and yourself it is okay to grieve and feel sad about this patient's death.
- Be gentle with one another; realize that different people grieve differently. Some may want to share, whereas others may want to be alone in their grief.
- Provide opportunities to remember the patient, formally or in conversation.

Things to avoid doing or saying

- Judgments about the care provided are particularly difficult to hear at this time.
- Questions about staff member's professionalism.
- Suggestions about what could have been done differently to achieve a different outcome (e.g., "If she were my patient, I would have . . .").
- Statements that disenfranchise or devalue grief or feelings of regret (e.g., "It was just a patient" or "You will get over it").
- Statements that suggest that either the staff person or the patient did not work hard enough (e.g., "It is his own fault that he died. He knew what would happen if he stopped taking medicine.").

Conclusion

Palliative care is a critical aspect of support and good care throughout the continuum of HIV illness. Its elements include the following:

- Comfort, support, and counseling at time of diagnosis
- Coping and minimizing distress of procedures, visits
- Psychosocial support for living with HIV
- Symptom prevention and treatment at time of ART initiation
- Symptom treatment with disease complications and progression
- Open, honest, compassionate, clear communication about disease, condition, future
- Support in health decisions
- Nonabandonment

- Care in the last hours/days
- Bereavement support for loved ones and for staff

References

American Academy of Pediatrics, Committee on Pediatric AIDS (AAP COPA). 1999. Disclosure of illness status to children and adolescents with HIV Infection. *Pediatrics* 103(1):164–66.

Brady, M.T., Oleske, J.M., Williams, P.L., et al.; Pediatric AIDS Clinical Trials Group 219/219C Team. 2010. Declines in mortality rates and changes in causes of death in HIV-1 infected children during the HAART era. *J Acquir Immune Defic Syndr* 53(1):86–94.

Gerson, A.C., Joyner, M., Fosarelli, P., et al. 2001. Disclosure of HIV diagnosis to children: When, where, why, and how. *J Pediatr Health Care* 15(4):161–67.

Lyon, M.E., Garvie, P.A., Briggs, L., et al. 2009a. Development, feasibility and acceptability of the Family-Centered (FACE) advance care planning intervention for adolescents with HIV. *J Palliat Med* 12(4):363–72.

Lyon, M.E., Garvie, P.A., McCarter, R., et al. 2009b. Who will speak for me? Improving end-of-life decision-making for adolescents with HIV and their families. *Pediatrics* 123(2):e1–8.

National Consensus Project for Quality Palliative Care. 2009. *Clinical Practice Guidelines for Quality Palliative Care*, 2nd ed. www.nationalconsensusproject.org.

Neugebauer, R., Rabkin, J., Williams, J., et al. 1992. Bereavement reactions among homosexual men experiencing multiple losses in the AIDS epidemic. *Am J Psychiat* 149(10):1374–79.

Nord, D. 1996. The impact of multiple AIDS-related loss on families of origin and families of choice. *Am J Family Therapy* 24(2):129–44.

O'Neill, J.F., Selwyn, P.A., and Schietinger, H. 2003. *A Clinical Guide to Supportive and Palliative Care for HIV/AIDS*. Health Resources and Services Administration.

Pham, P.A., and Flexner, C.W. 2008. *Antiretroviral Drug Interactions, 2008–2009*. Baltimore: Johns Hopkins University School of Medicine, Division of Infectious Disease.

Wissow, L.S., Hutton, N., and Kass, N. 2001. Preliminary study of a values-history advance directive interview in a pediatric HIV clinic. *J Clin Ethics* 12(2):161–72.

18

Integrating Palliative Care with Pediatric Hematology/Oncology

Sarah E. Friebert, M.D., Brian Greffe, M.D., and Janice Wheeler, Ed.D.

Pediatric hematology/oncology is a gratifying field, largely because so many children who have cancer are cured and because health care providers enjoy long-term relationships with children and their families. Both of these facts can make integrating palliative care into pediatric hematology/oncology care particularly challenging, especially when the child is likely to survive.

- What essential elements of palliative care should be part of every hematology/oncology practitioner's skill set?
- What added value can a palliative care team bring to an interdisciplinary hematology/oncology team?
- How can the disciplines of pediatric hematology/oncology and pediatric palliative care best complement each other's strengths to provide seamless, comprehensive care to families?

This chapter explores these and other elements of palliative care unique to the pediatric hematology/oncology patient and family. While the primary focus of the chapter will be on oncology, children who have severe hematologic conditions (such as sickle cell disease) and their families are another population who benefit from palliative care, and issues surrounding their care will be interwoven throughout the text.

Vanessa was a mature 12-year-old when she was diagnosed with stage IV Ewing sarcoma. Because of her disease stage and the known burdens associated with her journey, Vanessa's oncology team consulted the hospital's pediatric palliative care team at the time of diagnosis, to help with decision making, establishing goals of care, and anticipatory guidance related to symptom management and quality of life. During Vanessa's long treatment with chemotherapy and radiation, she always participated in consultations and decisions about her care. The palliative care team provided recommendations to the oncology team to minimize the side effects of Vanessa's treatment, while preserving her primary relationship with her oncology team. The teams also worked together to provide psychosocial, spiritual, and emotional support to Vanessa's family, especially her sister.

After a year, Vanessa was declared "disease free"; unfortunately, 7 months later, sharp back pains led to further testing, and the evaluation revealed recurrence. Understanding that curative options for recurrent Ewing sarcoma were limited, Vanessa decided she was not willing to undergo "just any old treatment." Of the available options, Vanessa chose gene therapy treatment at the National Cancer Institute. She was rejected as a candidate because her life expectancy was felt to be too short. The family was devastated. Their palliative care team then engaged the services of a pediatric hospice to provide additional support.

The home-based team quickly established a good relationship with Vanessa and her family. Vanessa saw herself as a normal teenager with a limited life span. She dated, entertained friends, pursued her talent in art, and traveled whenever she could. Vanessa received additional radiation treatments for pain and blood transfusions to combat fatigue and promote her overall quality of life. Members of the oncology team, including her primary oncologist, made personal visits to Vanessa as death grew nearer. The palliative care team also made visits, providing additional "eyes and ears" in the home to maximize Vanessa's symptom control. A close circle of friends and family supported Vanessa on her journey. Throughout the 7-month hospice experience, Vanessa's pain was well controlled; she died peacefully at home with her parents and sister present. The palliative care and hospice teams continue to offer bereavement support to the family.

Vanessa's mother reflects, "We are changed forever, but we have not lost hope. We are going to be okay." Now an ardent advocate for the widespread availability of high-quality pediatric palliative care, her mother realizes, "We were at the far end of the bell curve. We had an excellent oncology team, a pediatric palliative care team, a pediatric-specific hospice program, a supportive community, and a strong family unit. That should be the goal for the care of every child with a life-threatening illness, no matter what the outcome is."

Vanessa and her family had good control of symptoms and a continuous relationship with their child's oncology team throughout the illness. They had access to systematized information that facilitated shared, informed decision making as Vanessa's condition and prognosis changed. The family realized the importance of involving Vanessa directly in important decision making and ensured that she had the opportunity to participate. They had the help of a hospice team with pediatric experience. In addition, Vanessa's family had community support and help with siblings.

All of the services provided to Vanessa's family are recognized as crucial for good palliative care for children (AAP COB/COHC, 2000). The challenges for providers include finding answers to the following questions:

- How can the core components of good palliative care be integrated and systematized throughout the continuum of the pediatric hematology/ oncology experience?
- How do we provide continuity of care, good symptom control, help with siblings, and, most importantly, assistance for parents making difficult decisions for and with their child in a way that minimizes suffering for all?
- How do we do so while still respecting the frequent desire to proceed with disease-directed treatment, including phase I or other experimental therapies?
- How do we ensure that children and families are truly informed with respect to alternatives, that their emotions are appropriately addressed, and that their final choices are honored? (Vickers and Carlisle, 2000)

More than 12,000 children and adolescents younger than 20 years are diagnosed with cancer each year in the United States. Despite the good news that at least 80 percent of these children will be cured, childhood cancer remains the leading cause of disease-related mortality among children 1–14 years of age. Approximately 2,100 children and adolescents will, in fact, die each year from cancer (Gurney and Bondy, 2006). Given the life-threatening nature of pediatric cancer, integration of pediatric palliative care into the treatment plan for these patients and their families would seem ideal. Prognosis aside, however, many diagnoses encountered in pediatric hematology/ oncology involve high-intensity treatment protocols, including bone marrow transplantation, with the potential to cause multidimensional suffering for children and their families. Children who have severe sickle cell disease represent another cohort of patients for whom palliative care can offer benefit: years of chronic pain, psychosocial issues, and possible bone marrow transplantation are all amenable to palliative care services (McClain and Kain, 2007; Benjamin, 2008).

Pediatric palliative care has evolved into an organized, accredited subspecialty over the past decade, and there is strong evidence that more tertiary pediatric care institutions are now offering palliative care to patients diagnosed with cancer and sickle cell disease and their families. Unfortunately, the percentage of institutions where such care is available is well below the ideal number of 100 percent. In a survey of Children's Oncology Group member institutional practices and resources surrounding palliative and end-of-life care, only 58 percent of institutions acknowledged that they offered such care to their oncology patients and families (Johnston et al., 2008). This represents a significant improvement over a previous survey done by the American Society of Clinical Oncology in 1998 that indicated that only 36 percent of pediatric oncology centers offered some type of palliative care (Hilden et al., 2001); nevertheless, many pediatric oncology patients and their families are still not offered this state-of-the-art care. Further, even in institutions where palliative care is offered, service provision appears only to be scratching the surface. Respondents to the 2008 survey (187 of 232, 81% response rate) reported a median of 45 newly diagnosed patients and 8 deaths in a 12-month study period in 2005. However, even where palliative care was available, only a median of 3 newly diagnosed and 0 relapsed patients per institution used the service (Johnston et al., 2008).

The availability of pediatric palliative and end-of-life care to the pediatric oncology population outside of the United States is also variable, yet intriguing. A 2001 survey of Canadian pediatric oncology centers demonstrated that 88 percent of these institutions offered palliative care (Johnston et al., 2008). A more recent report described an integrative model of care offered at a medical center in Israel (Golan et al., 2008). The goal of this model is to introduce palliative care to every child with cancer at the time of diagnosis. Although patients with a poor or terminal prognosis were given priority for admission to this inpatient palliative care unit, almost 50 percent of good-prognosis patients during the study period benefited from services as well. Surprisingly, the percentage of deaths at home among this population decreased after the opening of the unit, indicating a high level of familiarity and comfort with the inpatient palliative care unit. Results from this study and the work of others show that parents and families are able to maintain dual goals of cure-directed and palliative care concurrently and can benefit from palliative care when services are offered in a balanced manner (i.e., not after all cure-directed therapy has been abandoned; Bluebond-Langner et al., 2007).

As discussed elsewhere in this text, the American Academy of Pediatrics (AAP COB/COHC, 2000) has emphasized the importance of offering the components of palliative care from the time of diagnosis of a life-threatening illness, even if the medical outcome is cure. Nowhere is this position more germane than in pediatric oncology. Statistics aside, oncologists' ability to prognosticate accurately with regard to an individual patient's likely trajectory is widely variable (Wusthoff, McMillan, and Ablin, 2005). Yoking access to palliative care to prognosis disenfranchises a significant number of families who could benefit from the multiple services offered by a specialized pediatric palliative care team. Ideally, therefore, palliative care should be offered to every child who has a new cancer diagnosis and his or her family. At present, this would represent a new paradigm in how many pediatric oncology patients receive palliative care. In truth, however, any cancer-directed intervention is potentially palliative, depending on the goals of treatment; while the focus may fluctuate from cure-directed to palliative, both are possible and should coexist (Wolfe, Friebert, and Hilden, 2002; Friebert and Wiener, 2009).

The Relationship between Hematology/Oncology and Palliative Care

Barriers to early integration of palliative care in the course of a child's life-threatening condition are numerous and are explored fully elsewhere in this text. Briefly, they include technologic advances in medicine leading to treatments that may be inappropriately burdensome; the complex ethical, legal, and health care policy issues affecting children; inability of community-based hospice providers to offer palliative care due to lack of training or restrictive regulatory guidelines; fragmented medical care affecting children who have complex medical conditions such as cancer; and difficulty in assessing and managing pain and other symptoms in children, particularly at the end of life (Himelstein et al., 2004). Furthermore and unfortunately, the use of the word *palliative* has become synonymous with the word *hospice*, making the introduction of palliative care into the overall care plan for a child difficult. Parents, other family members, and some health care providers may view palliative care as representing an acknowledgment of death as the final outcome—in other words, "giving up."

Early integration of palliative care into the care of children who have hematologic or oncologic diagnoses is a worthwhile goal but presents some unique challenges. As with cystic fibrosis and HIV/AIDS, pediatric hematology/

oncology care is usually provided by comprehensive management teams who develop long-term relationships with patients and families. If palliative care teams are viewed as "other," it may be difficult to reconcile the presence of another team, another group of people whose job descriptions may, in fact, overlap many of those on the primary team. Further, palliative care consultation is not infrequently met with skepticism about its added value— "I already do that" is a commonly encountered barrier throughout the field of palliative medicine. Pediatric oncologists have historically been considered the "experts" in managing symptoms (particularly nausea, vomiting, and pain) and in caring for dying children. Thus, discerning the differences between good palliative care principles applied by all clinicians and expert-level pediatric palliative care brought by a highly skilled team is of particular importance in this environment.

Additionally, children who have cancer or sickle cell disease often have an understanding and acceptance of illness and its ramifications beyond their chronological age. While this maturity may not extend beyond the illness, their capacity for health care decision making is often sophisticated. This reality creates additional layers of complexity in communication for oncology and palliative care teams but offers increased opportunity for empowerment and self-efficacy for these children and their families during illness and especially at the end of life, if that occurs.

Another barrier that is particularly relevant is the fact that oncology care is often painful and burdensome, but the proven benefit usually makes it worthwhile. In fact, treatment with intent to cure has been, is, and should be the norm for children who have newly diagnosed malignancies in most cases, especially for young children for whom the potential of long years of life and productivity lost outweighs the potential for even significant discomfort—or in common oncology parlance, "makes the fight worthwhile." Our current excellent outcomes are a direct result of "pushing the limits" over the decades in which multidisciplinary, clinical trial-based oncology care has become the standard. However, this "fight" stance creates a difficult hurdle to overcome when the posture of care needs to change to one of maximizing comfort and quality of life with acceptance of alternate outcomes.

Historically, models of comprehensive palliative care have largely derived from the Medicare hospice model, meant to structure care in the last phase of life for the majority of adult cancer patients. But payment structures and reimbursement have not matched well with the population of children and families who would benefit from palliative care provided concurrently with curative therapy. In particular, hospices have often been reluctant to enroll children who continue to receive any type of life-extending, invasive, or expensive therapy, including total parenteral nutrition, palliative chemotherapy or radiation, or transfusion support. While these elements add up to an untenably expensive plan of care under the hospice benefit, in fact they represent the usual course for most pediatric hematology/oncology patients and often contribute to an improved quality of life. Again, then, tying enrollment in hospice and palliative care to abandonment of usual, cure-directed therapy creates a difficult-to-surmount barrier.

All of these factors have slowed the acceptance of interdisciplinary interdigitation between pediatric hematology/oncology and palliative care teams. However, the currently available models of care are far more flexible and integrative than the models of the past. The risks of not including palliative care early in the trajectory for children who have oncology diagnoses more clearly outweigh the risks of waiting until "the family is ready" or the curative therapy is done. Recognition of the opportunity to minimize suffering, even in the face of cure-oriented treatments, can increase earlier implementation of palliative care and put the team in place to carry on with the family if the child's cancer does not respond to treatment. For children who have sickle cell disease, compassionate care focused on prevention and relief of suffering to preserve dignity, meaning, value, and quality of life—all core components of pediatric palliative care—is appropriate from birth until the end of life (Benjamin, 2008). So how should this be accomplished?

Advantages and Strategies for Early Integration

Despite the apparent rationality of early integration of palliative care, few data exist at present regarding the effectiveness of such a model. In fact, the majority of the current literature speaks to the introduction of palliative care in the terminal phase of cancer. Although such care plays a major role in reducing pain and suffering during this difficult time, patients and families have in some sense missed out on the benefits of palliative care earlier in the trajectory of the child's illness. These benefits include closer monitoring of symptoms and quality of life; improved emotional and psychological adjustment for parents and other family members, allowing them to better cope with the loss of the child over time; and better preparedness on the part of the parents regarding what to expect in the end-of-life care period (Mack and Wolfe, 2006). In particular, parents are more likely to rely on relational aspects rather than biomedical indicators to rate the quality of their child's care, even if the child dies. Palliative care teams can contribute a great deal to informed, ongoing, and sensitive communication with families; thus, integration of the services early on will likely improve family perception of quality of care (Mack et al., 2005).

To avoid abrupt transitions in care approaches or personnel, palliative care should be viewed as always being part of the care paradigm (Malin, 2004). In this way, the transition to exclusively comfort and supportive care goals can occur gradually, intuitively, and effectively (Wolfe and Sourkes, 2006). One clear advantage to this approach is that it removes the pressure on families to "accept" a referral to palliative care, which they may equate with giving up hope for a cure. "The family isn't ready" is a frequent caregiver-derived reason for postponement; whether accurate or not, such delays also result in missed opportunities for collaboration. Research shows that families become aware of the likely terminal outcome of their child's condition a full 3 months after clinicians do (Wolfe et al., 2000b). Therefore, relying on family initiation or acceptance of palliative care team involvement again creates unnecessary delay. Further, and perhaps most salient, in no other medical subspecialty is consultation dependent on family request or acceptance. For example, families are not asked if a neurology or infectious disease consultation is desired; certain clinical scenarios necessitate consultation with these and other subspecialists as circumstances and best practices dictate. Palliative care consultation should not be an exception.

Another potential benefit is that the child and his or her parents will view palliative or comfort care as an integral part of good cancer treatment, rather than as an indicator that all hope for cure has been extinguished. While standard-risk acute lymphoblastic leukemia may carry an 85 percent cure rate at the present time, patients and families are living with a life-threatening illness for several years, even when cure is obtained. Introducing the palliative care team at the time of diagnosis could be of tremendous emotional benefit. "Even with outstanding outcomes research, it must be remembered that each family and patient handles adversity differently. It is our task to attend to these diverse signals, whether they are personal, psychosocial, cultural, or spiritual, and to modify our approach accordingly. The ultimate outcome is the comfort and well-being of our patients and their families" (Harris, 2004).

The barrier to early integration may not, as mentioned above, only be one of philosophy. In our present health care system, resources play a major role and the reality of their scarcity often forces palliative care teams to focus primarily on the child who is terminally ill. In pediatric hematology/oncology, however, there are clearly other populations who should be offered palliative care services before the terminal phase.

Nadine was a 4-year-old girl who presented to the emergency department (ED) with a short history of drooling, ataxia, and dysarthria. Physical exam revealed right fifth, sixth, and seventh nerve palsies, dysarthria, ataxia, and increased tone on the left side, with 4/5 strength in the left lower extremity. CT scan of the head revealed a large hypodense posterior fossa mass posterior to the basilar artery and anterior to the fourth ventricle, most consistent with a brainstem tumor. MRI of the head confirmed the diagnosis.

Nadine was started on dexamethasone and subsequently referred to a radiation oncologist. She received 6,000 cGy to the brainstem over several weeks, with significant improvement in her symptoms. Nine months after her diagnosis, Nadine's symptoms returned and an MRI revealed progressive disease. Her neuro-oncologist referred Nadine to the oncology division's Experimental Therapeutics Program (ETP), which offered her family a phase I study; the family agreed to participate.

As part of her referral to the ETP, Nadine and her family were also introduced to the palliative care team, which has become standard for all oncology patients offered experimental therapy at her treating institution. The physician and nurse practitioner from the inpatient palliative care team discussed the palliative care program in detail with Nadine's parents. They were particularly open to receiving as much emotional support as possible for the immediate family, including Nadine's siblings. The day after her discharge from the hospital, members of the outpatient palliative care team (chaplain, nurse, and social worker) met with Nadine and her family. Over the next 3 months, the outpatient team worked closely to support them as Nadine's physical condition began to deteriorate from her disease process. Memory-making activities and funeral arrangements were completed. During the terminal phase of her illness, the palliative care nurse, whom the family had met earlier, became closely involved with Nadine's medical comfort care. She died peacefully at home with her family close by.

Several approaches may facilitate the integration of palliative care earlier in the course of a child's illness. First, palliative care providers along with pediatric oncology care providers need to determine what diagnoses should trigger involvement of the palliative care team. Second, it is crucial to educate families and the oncology staff that palliative care can be undertaken alongside curative therapy. Patients and families must be made aware of what palliative care has to offer with respect to decision making and identification of goals of care, pain and symptom management, psychosocial support, and spiritual support. Initially the role of the palliative care team can be "supportive," helping patients and families identify their goals and values and then make informed choices regarding offered therapies in the context of those values, while simultaneously helping them identify quality-of-life priorities. The palliative care team may then assume a larger role in the care of the patient and family, depending on how the child's disease responds to therapy.

Third, institutional support of the palliative care team is crucial to ensuring its success. It takes time to structure and implement a successful palliative care program. In a cure-oriented setting, this will certainly involve consensus building at multiple institutional levels. A recent report from St. Jude Children's Research Hospital discusses a low-key "zig-zag" strategy, which involved taking an indirect approach to pediatric palliative care before making a formal request to create a new program (Harper et al., 2007). The authors describe doing preliminary institutional feasibility studies, followed by creation of a task force comprising clinical team leaders interested in palliative care. Focus groups, the creation of a vision statement and strategic plan, and institutional research efforts followed. All of these components lay the groundwork for the introduction of a program that ideally will facilitate successful early referral for appropriate palliative care.

Fourth, integration requires that pediatric oncologists acknowledge the benefits that subspecialty-level pediatric palliative care can contribute to the care of patients and families. By the same token, palliative care professionals must work collaboratively with oncology teams to enhance a culture of mutual collaboration, respect, and acknowledgment of expertise. An analogy can be drawn with the intersection of oncology and infectious disease. Pediatric oncology clinicians are highly skilled in the care of children who have complex infectious disease issues, and a solid general understanding of infectious disease is part of oncology training. However, subspecialty-level infectious disease consultation is also crucial in the ongoing care of children who have cancer or blood disorders and represents best practice. As mentioned, pediatric hematology/oncology teams have been providing components of palliative care all along. Over time, as the field develops, pediatric palliative care teams need to clearly demonstrate the value added of subspecialty-level pediatric palliative care, such that integration of the two services will also represent best practice.

As palliative care providers strive to integrate services as early as possible, it is important to recognize that this approach can certainly lessen the suffering of pediatric oncology patients, particularly in the terminal phase of disease. Wolfe et al. (2000a) conclude that earlier recognition of prognosis,

Table 18.1 Benefits of integrating palliative care early

Prevents disruptive transition to new care team at the worst possible time for the family

Decreases feelings of abandonment for families and for care teams

Minimizes fragmentation of care and lack of coordination among providers

Improves symptom management

Provides umbrella of support through entire illness experience

Allows patient and family self-determination about treatment options

Empowers parents / decision makers to maintain dual goals of care concurrently

Provides additional support for the oncology team (time, resources, self-care, prevention of caregiver suffering)

Improves relational aspects of care

Source: Friebert, 2008, p. 514. © Jones & Bartlett Learning, Sudbury, MA. www.jblearning.com. Adapted and reprinted with permission.

followed by earlier introduction of palliative care, was associated with improved quality of home care, earlier institution of do-not-resuscitate (DNR) orders, less use of cancer-directed therapy during the last month of life, and a higher likelihood that the goal of cancer-directed therapy identified by both physician and parent was to lessen suffering. A follow-up study in a later cohort—presumably reflecting more available and pervasive palliative care services and practices—demonstrates that changing patterns of care have resulted in earlier and more frequent hospice discussions, earlier documentation of DNR orders, and fewer deaths in the hospital or intensive care unit (Wolfe et al., 2008; tables 18.1 and 18.2).

At the very least, palliative care should play an early and major role in treating those patients whose prognosis is poor or who have progressive and/or recurrent disease. Where to set the bar for determination of a "poor prognosis" is not well defined at present; one might argue that a less than 30 percent chance of disease-free survival would be a good starting point for oncology programs that have not yet integrated palliative care into the repertoire of services provided. Table 18.3 lists examples of palliative care integration by illness progression along the hematology or oncology trajectory.

Ethical Issues

Lindsey will be 14 years old soon. She wants to have control about what's happening to her. I don't want to just say, "Let's go ahead and try it," without

Table 18.2 Strategies to accomplish early integration of palliative care and oncology teams

1. Consider palliative care as an adjunct medical specialty that comes as part of a package with oncology services, not as an optional service
2. Prioritize symptom management and find a symptom or reason to introduce the team to the family early on (e.g., pain control, spiritual distress, dyspnea, anxiety, pruritus)
3. Remove idea of prognosis altogether: the difficulty of the journey merits involvement of additional support people (this approach avoids having to decide who is appropriate and who is not)
4. If access to full palliative care team is limited, educate care team members to practice palliative care principles
5. Structure the collaboration such that families do not have to have a whole other team if only certain services are needed
6. Think about list of diagnoses or conditions appropriate for palliative care at or soon after diagnosis:
   a. Acknowledge likelihood of cure
   b. Acknowledge burdensome treatment course
   c. Perform honest appraisal of "doing to" vs. "doing for"
7. Evaluate various time points on illness trajectory to think of incorporating palliative care:
   a. Overwhelmed at diagnosis
   b. Phase I enrollment
   c. Relapse/recurrence
   d. Serious complications (multiorgan failure with sepsis, spinal cord compression)
   e. Intensive care unit admissions/transfers

Source: Friebert, 2008, p. 515. © Jones & Bartlett Learning, Sudbury, MA. www.jblearning.com. Adapted and reprinted with permission.

Table 18.3 Examples of the integration of palliative care

At diagnosis of any malignancy for which the journey will be burdensome or support resources are limited

At diagnosis for poor-prognosis malignancies

At diagnosis for a malignancy for which the patient and family choose not to pursue curative therapy

Early in treatment for comprehensive symptom management, including chronic pain associated with sickle cell disease

At consideration of stem cell transplant for relapse or recurrence of cancer or as curative therapy for sickle cell disease

At the time of on-therapy progression or development of metastatic disease

At entry onto Phase I/II clinical trial

At the onset of serious complications of treatment +/− PICU admissions/transfers

Source: Adapted from Friebert, 2008; Friebert and Wiener, 2009.

helping her fully understand what she is getting herself into ... she's not an adult, but she isn't a child anymore.

ADOLESCENTS WHOSE TREATMENT-RELATED
WISHES ARE DIFFERENT FROM THEIR PARENTS'

Decision making for adolescents who have cancer can be particularly challenging because of ethical and legal considerations raised in this age group (discussed in depth in other sections of this text). As exemplified in the case of Vanessa, decision making at this stage of illness relates to the adolescent's physical condition, school, family, social relationships, intellectual capacity, as well as the emerging personal independence that normally seeks expression during these years. The most fundamental decision facing teenagers with advanced cancer is whether or not to discontinue efforts to treat the underlying disease. In approaching this decision, most adolescents are in a position to draw on their considerable medical experience, accumulated since the initial diagnosis. Rarely, a teenager may be faced with a decision not to begin antineoplastic therapy at all, in the light of a particularly dismal prognosis. More commonly, patients with advanced or recurrent disease will have experienced a medical course characterized by gradual debilitation resulting from prolonged attempts at cure.

Because they are more mature than much younger patients, at each relapse, *informed* adolescents will be aware of both their diminishing potential for cure and the benefits and burdens of continued disease-directed treatment. How they weigh these considerations and to what extent their opinions hold sway in determining goals of care largely reflect their own developmental maturity, preexisting family dynamics, and the biases of the involved clinical personnel. Nevertheless, most adolescents with advanced cancer are able to participate in complex decision making. In the setting of terminal illness, in particular, consensus supports the presumption of decision-making capacity for chronically ill, intellectually intact patients in the adolescent age range of approximately 10–20 years, unless there is evidence to the contrary. Families and health care personnel can support an adolescent's decision-making role, irrespective of the patient's exact legal status, by engaging the adolescent in a relationship-based framework (Hinds et al., 2005).

How to best support the minor's autonomy varies according to particular circumstances. Older adolescents who clearly possess functional competence should be given full decisional authority. In these cases, the decision to continue or discontinue antineoplastic treatment is communicated to the legally responsible adult who then executes the decision through "modified substituted judgment" (the application of a minor's expressed preferences in a decision made on his or her behalf) (Freyer, 2004). It should be noted that the purpose is to apply the *minor's stated wishes*, not those of a responsible adult seeking decisional control. Advance directives also have been advocated for older adolescents (Weir and Peters, 1997). In practice, however, intrafamily conflicts over decisions are rarely resolved in such a straightforward manner and may obligate the treating oncologist, through fidelity to the child patient, to attempt to negotiate on behalf of the child's wishes, if the adolescent is determined to possess decisional capacity.

As discussed previously, inclusion of children in phase I and phase II studies raises important issues. Exaggerated hope for clinical benefit without full acknowledgment of the risk for burden or toxicity may lead to undue pressure for the adolescent to enroll in such a study. On the other hand, in the face of bleak odds, a highly motivated or altruistic adolescent may wish to continue treatment in the context of a phase I or II study but be discouraged from doing so by parents with faltering hopes for cure and alternative goals for the remaining time. In every case, it is critical that the adolescent's true desires be carefully distinguished from a natural tendency to please authority figures such as parents, physicians, or other adults.

It is also essential that the clinician provide the adolescent and family with a forum that promotes the acquisition of accurate information and decisional integrity. One successful means for this is the "final stage conference" first described by Nitschke et al. (1977). The final stage conference is a communication approach employed at the time of cancer relapse, with the goal of communicating essential information concerning the disease, treatment options, and possible course, including palliative care options. The child, even if very young, is routinely included in the conference (with parental permission). Nitschke et al. reported numerous benefits of this approach, including optimal involvement of the child, improved intrafamily communication, and increased trust in the medical team. At every stage of the process, involvement of the palliative care team with the adolescent and his or her family can facilitate informed decision making, empowering both the adolescent to make individual choices and the family to honor the patient's wishes.

IS THERE "TRUE" INFORMED CONSENT FOR PEDIATRIC CANCER PATIENTS?

For pediatric ethics, informed consent is more properly understood as a combination of informed parental permission and (when appropriate) the assent of the child.

—*Kodish (2003, p. 90)*

The ethical dilemma in cases involving children is that permission and assent are intertwined, somewhat a tangled web in pediatric cancer research. Parents can give informed consent for themselves only. Unless legally determined to be an adult for that purpose, minors can provide informed *assent*, not consent. Another problem in the consent process is the errant focus on the completion of forms, rather than ensuring an understanding of the goals and likely outcomes of the proposed clinical trial. Despite modern efforts to the contrary, these forms are often voluminous, intimidating, legal in tone, and fraught with unfamiliar terminology. Moreover, there is ethical concern that parents and children may not understand that they are involved in research rather than clinical care, treatment arms that include placebos, and/or the actual possibility of direct benefit.

> When Ewing sarcoma recurred, Troy (age 15) asked, "Is there anything else I can do?" In consultation with Troy and his family, the oncologist suggested "gene therapy."

By labeling gene transfer research in this way, children like Troy and their families are at risk for confusing research with standard clinical care (Lysaught, 1998). The process of obtaining consent and permission should encourage dialogue, discussion, and time for questions. Phase I trials may offer a glimmer of hope for parents faced with the death of their child while minimizing, reducing, or sacrificing the child's quality of life. There is also the risk that consent to research provides emotional and psychological benefits to the parents, but not to the child (Oberman and Frader, 2003; Goldberg and Frader, 2009).

PHASE I/II CLINICAL TRIALS

Many tertiary pediatric oncology centers offer experimental therapies as part of phase I/phase II studies for patients with advanced or recurrent cancer. While these therapies may offer both hope and control of symptoms such as pain, patients and families need to be made aware of the true goals of such trials. Given the prognosis of children considered for phase I/II trials, the team should simultaneously be discussing with the family palliative goals of care and concurrent involvement of palliative care and hospice professionals (AAP COB/COHC, 2000). Ideally, the institutional pediatric palliative care team should be considered part of the experimental trials team (as was the case for Nadine and her family), so that goals of care, symptom control, psychosocial and spiritual concerns, quality-of-life management, and advance care planning are discussed before and during enrollment into such studies.

Phase I and II clinical trials for pediatric oncology patients offer continued cancer-directed therapy but only a small chance of life-prolonging benefit to the specific patient. To make the best decision, the child and parents need detailed and clear information regarding these therapies, including realistic short- and longer-term individual benefits; known and potential burdens (side effects, procedures, time at clinic or in the hospital); alternative options and their associated burdens and benefits; and how participation may contribute to the care of future patients.

A recent study of parental perceptions of their children's participation in phase I trials indicated that 62 percent of parents felt that study participation was not a "decision," as the alternative of "no treatment" was simply not an option for them. Their expectations about study enrollment included receiving treatment to prolong the child's life, buying time for a potential new therapy, having more time with their child, hoping for a cure or a miracle, and helping other children (Deatrick, Angst, and Moore, 2002).

The clinician should state clearly to patients and families that the scientific goal of phase I research is to determine the toxicity and maximum tolerated dose of an investigational agent. The chance of tumor response (some degree of shrinkage) in phase I trials is low (4%-6% historically, 2.5% in a meta-analysis; Roberts et al., 2004), and remission or cure is even less common (Decoster, Stein, and Holdener, 1990; Daugherty et al., 1995; Shah et al., 1998). Not uncommonly, physicians tend to communicate and/or families tend to hear more positive potential benefit from experimental chemotherapy than is justified (Daugherty et al., 1995). Further, pediatric oncologists have historically deferred discussion of palliative goals of care to the time when "there is no viable therapy to offer," if the topic is ever mentioned at all (Hilden et al., 2001). Although these biases are not intentional, they may invalidate the informed consent process, raising further ethical questions (Emanuel and Patterson, 1998).

Thus, in obtaining informed consent and assisting families and children to define the goals of care, the clinician should impart all of the information noted in table 18.4 to the family and patient who has advanced cancer.

Pediatric oncology teams well trained in communication will approach clinical trial discussions from a balanced, ethical, goal-directed perspective. In this scenario, what are the benefits of linking palliative care consultation with enrollment in a phase I clinical trial? Palliative care teams can partner with oncology teams to ensure that families have more realistic expectations

Table 18.4 Information that should be imparted to the patient with advanced cancer and the family

All available treatment goals and options, including those that are "palliative"

Diagnosis and prognosis, including the likelihood of death

Likely effects of the disease on the patient

Likely effects of various treatment options on the patient, including possible hospitalization, clinic visits, discomfort, fatigue, isolation, and invasive procedures

Any relevant physical or emotional problems likely to impact the child and family

Uses and interactions of medications

Availability of pharmacologic and nonpharmacologic interventions to ease suffering

The availability of hospital, community-based, and national professional and nonprofessional resources to aid the family, including palliative care, symptom control, hospice, support groups, and practical assistance

Predictable changes in the child's functional status and their anticipated time course

Impact, as predictable, on the child's quality of life

Impact on the family, including marital stress, sibling concerns, financial and practical concerns, and spiritual and grief-related issues

What death will look and be like with and without artificial interventions

Impact on school, peers, and community

of the trials; that control in end-of-life decision making is maintained; that a supportive, nonjudgmental climate exists in which goals of care and advance care planning can be discussed; and that pain and symptom management issues arising from the toxicity of the protocol and/or from progression of the tumor are expertly addressed. Providing palliative care concurrently with enrollment in a clinical trial affords children and parents the opportunity to share experiences, fears, and concerns about the clinical course, which will enhance the trusting relationship with all health care providers.

NONDISCLOSURE: "DON'T TELL MY CHILD SHE HAS CANCER!"

One of the most difficult clinical situations for families and health care providers alike is conflict surrounding how much and when a child who has cancer should be told about the diagnosis, treatment, and prognosis. This issue is perhaps best addressed through prevention: consistent, age-appropriate inclusion of the child in discussions and decisions about his/her treatment from the start. Full exploration of disclosure is covered in other sections of this text. For the pediatric oncology population in particular, the

Table 18.5 A stepwise approach to nondisclosure

Prevention: engage in open dialogue from the start of the relationship

Remain calm and respond empathically throughout

Understand disclosure as a process, not a "tell-all" moment in time

Determine cultural/religious context for information sharing and hierarchy for decision making

Try to understand family's viewpoint: what are you afraid will happen?

Determine what child already knows, has questions about

Brainstorm possible solutions together with the family

Assure family information disclosure will occur in stepwise fashion

Engage interdisciplinary team in information gathering and sharing

Negotiate a solution: reiterate honesty and fidelity to child as primary patient but respect family-centered approach

Create mechanism for involved caregivers to discuss issues/concerns, or opt out of direct care

If impasse: "outside advisor" (extended family, ethics consultant, family religious leader)

Source: Zieber and Friebert, 2008; Chaitin and Rosielle, 2009.

work of Kreicbergs et al. (2004) indicates that disclosure should generally be encouraged and facilitated by providers. In this study, no parent whose child had died regretted being honest with the child about his or her diagnosis. In contrast, parents who did not disclose regretted their decision at least 25 percent of the time; further, parents indicated that it should be the oncology provider's responsibility to help guide disclosure conversations. There are circumstances, however, in which disclosure should not be forced, such as in families for whom cultural or religious traditions handle information sharing differently. Table 18.5 shows a helpful stepwise approach to address nondisclosure.

The Management of Symptoms Specific to Oncology Diagnoses

Emerging work from multiple investigators demonstrates that there are many under-recognized and undertreated symptoms associated with significant suffering for children who have cancer (Collins et al., 2000; Wolfe et al., 2000b, 2008; Ullrich and Mayer, 2007). Although pain management should be part of good basic oncology care, pain is often undertreated. Other physical symptoms such as nausea, dyspnea, anorexia, constipation, diarrhea, and mucositis may be difficult to manage. Infection and bleeding are two of the major risks for the terminally ill child with cancer, each with its unique symptomatic presentation. Finally, more subjective and difficult-to-measure symptoms such as fatigue, spiritual distress, anxiety, and depression may be ignored. To provide good-quality symptom management, clinicians must recognize the importance of considering the distress associated with cancer-related symptoms, not just the presence of the symptom itself (Collins et al., 2000), and must also be aware of a recognition gap, with parents reporting presence of symptoms and related distress much more frequently than physicians (Wolfe et al., 2000a).

Untreated symptoms cause suffering and isolation, unnecessary fear, and interference with relationships, not only for the child but also for caregivers, health care providers, and the extended community. With good proactive symptom control, many children are able to truly live with their diagnoses, not in spite of them. While pain and symptom management related to pediatric palliative care is discussed in another section of this text, this section briefly explores the control of symptoms as it relates to the pediatric oncology patient. Interested readers are referred to several outstanding and more comprehensive resources for more in-depth exploration of pain management in children (WHO, 1998; Drake and Hain, 2006; Friedrichsdorf and Kang 2007; see also chap. 10).

CONTROL OF PAIN AND OTHER SYMPTOMS

Control of pain and the recognition and treatment of side effects associated with the medications used to achieve good pain control are imperative in providing state-of-the-art pediatric palliative care throughout the trajectory of the illness. While terminally ill children and their families experience psychosocial and spiritual pain at the end of the child's life, there is clear evidence that untreated or undertreated physical pain is also present much of the time. Wolfe et al. (2000a) reported that 89 percent of pediatric oncology patients had at least one symptom during the last month of life. The most common symptoms included pain, fatigue, and dyspnea. Similar retrospective parental recall data from Germany demonstrated that the most common symptoms experienced by children with cancer at the end of life were (in descending order) fatigue, pain, loss of appetite, and dyspnea; symptoms that caused the most distress, in contrast, were dyspnea and anxiety (Hechler et al., 2008).

Further, symptom distress remains undertreated. The German study demonstrated that while pain, constipation, and nausea were successfully managed, fatigue, loss of appetite, dyspnea, and anxiety were not. A more recent cohort study reveals that parents of children with cancer who died continue to report prevalent pain, dyspnea, fatigue, and anxiety during the last month of life, but note decreased suffering in their children related to those symptoms compared to previous studies (except fatigue; Wolfe et al., 2008). The impact of poor symptom control cannot be overstated. In addition to causing more complicated bereavement for families whose children die, children with poorly controlled pain are more likely to have difficulty with nutritional status, sleep, and tolerance of disease-directed therapy. Effective symptom management in the pediatric oncology population is therefore of paramount importance.

ASSESSMENT AND MANAGEMENT OF PAIN

Pain has been defined as "an unpleasant sensory and emotional experience associated with actual or potential tissue damage, or described in terms of such damage" (International Association for the Study of Pain, 1979). It is modulated by physiologic, environmental, developmental, behavioral, familial, and cultural factors. While the majority of pain occurs as a result of therapy rather than disease in children who have cancer, the opposite is true when the child becomes terminally ill. It is estimated that more than 80 percent of children who have advanced stages of cancer will experience pain, regardless of the underlying diagnosis (Wolfe and Sourkes, 2006).

There are several barriers to achieving effective pain management in children who have cancer at the end of life. Barriers not unique to the oncology population include deficits in knowledge and experience among health care providers, unwarranted fears of inducing addiction on the part of parents and providers, and fear of hastening death as a result of respiratory depression, excessive sedation, or both. For pediatric oncology patients in particular, pain may not be adequately reported owing to fears about its meaning— disease progression, more trips to the hospital/clinic—which can complicate effective treatment. Further, families and providers may not want to add medications or side effects to an already complex regimen.

Barriers notwithstanding, an approach to the treatment of pain in the child who has advanced cancer should include several practical principles. Careful and complete assessment must be performed initially and frequently throughout treatment (Hunt, 2006). Patients should be administered pain medication based on the World Health Organization Analgesic Pain Ladder (WHO, 1998), which recommends a stepwise approach to pain management, tailored to the patient's level of pain and modified by the patient's response. Pain medications need to be administered on a "round-the-clock" basis rather than PRN so the child does not need to ask for pain medications as a result of breakthrough. Invasive procedures and intermittent pain exacerbations—such as incident (movement- or treatment-related) pain—should be addressed by additional appropriate pain medication dosing. The easiest route for administration of pain medications should be used. Fortunately, many children who have advanced cancer will already have central venous access that can be used if the oral route is no longer effective or an option. Pain should be approached logically, selecting an appropriate opioid or adjuvant therapy to target the mechanism of pain most likely responsible for the patient's symptoms.

In addition to general principles of pain treatment, pediatric oncology patients benefit from several unique considerations related to the management of pain and symptoms. Of particular importance in oncology is the treatment-related avoidance of nonsteroidal anti-inflammatory medications. If a child is still receiving antineoplastic therapy, this section of the WHO ladder will need to be modified and options may be more limited, depending on treatment goals. Also, rectal medications are rarely used and are usually contraindicated in pediatric oncology patients. Both of these issues may necessitate additional education for pediatric hospice and/or palliative care providers more familiar with nononcologic diagnoses. In addition, many families have had previous experience with opioid and nonopioid medications as a result of treatment-related pain; these patients are often not opioid naïve and may already know what will work best for them.

It is imperative that all children who have advanced cancer and are started on opioids also be given a bowel regimen to avoid constipation, which occurs in virtually 100 percent of patients. Constipation may be a more troubling symptom in children who have cancer because of the location of the tumor and/or previous treatment (especially surgery). Nausea is also a common side effect, and an antiemetic should be made available on an as-needed basis. Obviously, children who have cancer and their families usually have a long history with antiemetics and can often guide therapeutic choices based on past successes and failures. Additional opioid-induced side effects include myoclonus, pruritis, and hallucinations, which can be treated symptomatically or by changing the opioid. Again, palliative care and/or hospice providers may need education to guide therapeutic choices for these patients based on previous experience and personal choice; in particular, use of more "expensive" antinausea medications may be troubling for hospice providers used to prescribing drugs based on restricted formulary choices, whereas these drugs may be preferred by families and oncologists.

An important point to remember about pharmacologic management is that medications should be reevaluated periodically as to their continued effectiveness. Many times medications are added for symptoms and continued without reconsideration, resulting in children and families juggling multiple medications every day. This can increase the risk of side effects, medication interactions, and serious drug errors.

Medications are the cornerstone of effective pain management in this population. However, interventional pain management treatments such as radioisotopes and bisphosphonates, short-course radiation therapy, surgical procedures, and nerve blocks are also important components of symptom management. In fact, many of these techniques were developed specifically for oncologic problems and are therefore likely to be effective. When chosen carefully, these modalities can replace or augment medications to decrease dose-limiting side effects. Examples of indications include the following:

- Short-course radiation therapy or debulking surgery for spinal cord compression
- Short-course radiation therapy or surgical removal of a protruding, fungating tumor
- Nerve block for neuropathic pain secondary to a pelvic tumor unresponsive to high doses of medications
- Insertion of a pigtail catheter chest tube to drain reaccumulating malignant pleural fluid, palliating severe dyspnea
- Pamidronate disodium infusion for extreme tumor-related or metabolic bone pain

Limitations of these and other therapies do exist, such as the ability to perform surgery or interventional blocks in a patient who has severe thrombocytopenia or the willingness of the family to travel to and from radiation therapy. After careful consideration of burdens and benefits, each patient's goal-directed plan of care needs to guide appropriate therapeutic choices.

As well, nonmedical/pharmacologic or integrative therapies such as imagery, expressive therapy, massage, biofeedback, hypnosis, acupuncture, pet therapy, and play therapy should be incorporated into the overall pain management plan. Occupational and physical therapy can also be of tremendous benefit in regard to positioning and adaptive devices to maximize comfort.

Monte was an 18-year-old young man who initially presented to the ED with urinary incontinence, left leg pain, and weakness. He reported that he had been walking with a limp for a year. His exam was remarkable for decreased strength and sensation in the left lower extremity as well as ataxia. An MRI revealed a large enhancing left pelvic mass pressing against the anterior sacrum and displacing the bladder superiorly. There was no invasion of the spinal canal. A biopsy of the lesion revealed osteogenic sarcoma. He had no evidence of pulmonary or bone metastases. He agreed to start chemotherapy with cisplatin, doxorubicin, and methotrexate. Pain and neurologic symptoms were controlled with oral methadone and gabapentin.

Monte completed 10 weeks of standard chemotherapy but was lost to follow-up for 3 months after he was told that local control would consist of amputation of his left leg, with probable loss of bowel and bladder function. Six months after the initial diagnosis, he returned to the oncology clinic reporting back pain, left leg pain, and constipation. A CT scan revealed a slight increase in the size of the pelvic mass. Monte declined additional chemotherapy, but he did agree to consultation with a radiation oncologist and decided to proceed with palliative radiation therapy. Pain control consisted of extended-release morphine, intermediate-release morphine for breakthrough pain, and gabapentin.

Eight months after his initial diagnosis, Monte was referred to the institutional palliative care program as an outpatient. Although his pain was initially controlled with oral analgesics, the pain related to disease progression now necessitated IV hydromorphone for better pain control. The palliative care team began to work with Monte and his family to prepare them for his eventual death. Monte's pain remained well controlled and he was able to spend significant quality time with his family. He discussed his spiritual concerns with the palliative care program's chaplain and reconnected with his local church. Additional symptom management included placement of a Foley catheter to assist with urinary retention, treatment for a decubitus ulcer, and two courses of antibiotics to treat urinary tract infections. He was also begun on a midazolam drip for agitation.

Nine months after his enrollment into the palliative care program and 17 months after his initial diagnosis, Monte began to experience myoclonic jerks while on continuous infusion hydromorphone. His opioid was changed to fentanyl with improvement of symptoms, and he was also started on promethazine for nausea and vomiting. He was offered an admission to the inpatient oncology unit but was determined to stay at home. His palliative home care team (nurse, chaplain, and social worker) helped Monte achieve his goals of graduating from high school and becoming an honorary fireman. He died comfortably at home 2 months later.

PALLIATIVE CHEMOTHERAPY AND RADIATION

Pediatric oncologists have many chemotherapy agents available to them that can be used in an "off-label" manner to help control symptoms. Oral agents include etoposide, 6-mercaptopurine, hydroxyurea, topotecan, cytarabine, and steroids. Some of the newer agents that can also be given orally are temozolomide, idarubicin, capecitabine, imatinib, and irinotecan (Ashley et al., 1996; Demario and Ratain, 1998; Royce, Hoff, and Pazdur, 2000). Most of these agents are relatively well tolerated. Radiotherapy may play a role in controlling painful bone metastases seen in advanced neuroblastoma or bone malignancies. Radiotherapy should also be considered in those patients with spinal cord compression secondary to recurrent tumor. Radioisotopes such as Samarium and 131-MIBG (Serafini, 2000; Matthay et al., 2009) may be useful in treating bone metastases and neuroblastoma. Importantly, a recent study reveals that bereaved parents report that their child experienced at least some suffering resulting from cancer-directed therapy; in retrospect, they would not recommend such therapy to other families, especially when there is no realistic chance for cure. At the very least, physicians should help parents develop realistic expectations about the possibility that suffering may occur and should tailor recommendations to family-directed goals (Mack et al., 2008).

PALLIATION OF BONE MARROW
FAILURE IN THE HOME SETTING

Bone marrow failure manifests itself as progressive fatigue, bleeding, and risk of infection due to infiltration of the marrow by disease (leukemia, lymphoma, neuroblastoma) or secondary to the myelotoxic effects of chemotherapy or radiation therapy.

Supportive care with respect to blood products should be discussed with the patient and family, and a plan should be agreed on regarding how often platelet and red cell transfusions should take place. In many instances, families will want to continue platelet transfusions to avoid excessive bleeding or hemorrhage at home; although the actual incidence of this complication is rare, if and when it does occur, it can be highly upsetting to the patient and/or family. Patients may be able to receive blood products in the home, obviating the need to come to the clinic, depending on the specific experience and policies of an involved home care or hospice agency. At a minimum, families should be instructed to keep dark towels on hand to minimize distress in the event that bleeding occurs.

For those patients who are comfortable and want to continue to interact with friends and family, periodic red cell transfusions are appropriate to help overcome fatigue. Occasional patients may, however, experience increased pain as a result of transfusion due to increased oxygen delivery, and this potential side effect should be discussed with families. It is worth remembering and discussing as well that progressive anemia is not a painful way to die, so discontinuation of routine red cell transfusions may offer a peaceful end, depending on the patient's and family's goals of care.

Potentially life-threatening infections do occur at end of life as a result of marrow failure. Institution of antibiotics—whether oral or IV, and whether empiric or based on evaluation—needs to be discussed with the patient and family as part of advance care planning.

FATIGUE

As reported in several series (Wolfe et al., 2000a; Jalmsell et al., 2006; Hechler et al., 2008), parents of children dying of cancer noted that fatigue was the most common and disturbing symptom during the terminal phase of their child's illness. The etiology of fatigue at the end of life is multifactorial; it includes side effect of medications (e.g., chemotherapy and opioids), anemia, endocrine dysfunction, increased work of breathing, impaired sleep, muscle abnormalities, and a variety of psychological factors, including depression. Symptoms may include weakness, weight loss, insomnia, impaired cognition, irritability or other emotional manifestations, and lack of participation in daily activities (Ullrich and Mayer, 2007).

The care team should first and foremost directly assess fatigue, either through the routine use of fatigue scales (Hockenberry et al., 2003) or in routine review of systems evaluation. If fatigue is concerning to the patient and/or family, therapy should be based on the etiology and can include red cell transfusions, sleep hygiene, psychosocial strategies, or exercise. The use of stimulants such as methylphenidate, or other pharmacologic agents such as corticosteroids or megestrol acetate, has been reported anecdotally; an evidence base is currently lacking to support their routine use or recommendation (Ullrich and Mayer, 2007).

NEUROLOGICAL SYMPTOMS

Patients who have recurrent CNS neoplasms, as well as those with metastatic disease to the brain, may be at risk for recurrent seizures. Seizures may also be the result of metabolic disturbances or a side effect of chemotherapy or radiation therapy. Prophylactic anticonvulsant therapy should be considered for those at high risk, and maintenance anticonvulsants may be indicated for patients with documented seizures. It may be prudent for families to have rectal diazepam on hand at home in the event of intractable seizures. Midazolam IV as a continuous infusion is also effective in controlling intractable seizures.

Increased intracranial pressure may occur as a result of primary, recurrent, or metastatic CNS disease. Symptoms include headache, photophobia, irritability, lethargy, nausea and vomiting, or transient neurological deficits. The cornerstone of medical therapy is the combination of steroids (usually dexamethasone) and acetazolamide. Analgesics, antiemetics, and benzodiazepines introduced early, when symptoms present, may be beneficial in controlling distressing symptoms. There may also be a role for radiotherapy, chemotherapy, or occasionally surgery. Again, goals of care need to drive the choice of intervention; neurosurgical intervention may be appropriate for a cystic lesion that can be decompressed with relatively little morbidity, and placement of a shunt may be indicated if the child has the potential to live with a good quality of life for a significant amount of time. The course of action should consistently result from informed, bidirectional decision making with the family, rather than a standard or knee-jerk response to a scan result.

Insomnia may occur as a result of undertreated symptoms such as pain, pruritis, anxiety, depression, or dyspnea. In the event that nonpharmacologic approaches fail, it is reasonable to consider an antidepressant or hypnotic to help facilitate sleep.

Additional Special Considerations

PREVIOUS EXPERIENCE WITH THE
MANAGEMENT OF PAIN AND SYMPTOMS

A review of a patient's previous experience with opioids, antiemetics, seizure medication, etc., and their effectiveness may be helpful in charting an end-of-life medication plan. A discussion with the parents and patient, if appropriate, about relevant choices may also be helpful.

ROUTINE MRIS/SCANS

Typically, when patients enter into a pediatric hospice program, routine imaging is no longer indicated. Except in the event of a potentially reversible medical situation allowing the patient to return to a good quality of life where imaging may be required or for family peace of mind, scans should not be performed.

RECTAL MEDICATIONS

To avoid a potential blood-borne infection, patients undergoing palliative chemotherapy should not use rectal medications. During the terminal phase of illness, rectal medications can be useful, particularly if the patient is unable to swallow or does not have a central line. Rectal diazepam may be of particular use in patients who are having seizures at the end of life or who have brain tumors/metastases that may cause seizures.

NSAIDS

Typically NSAIDs are not given to pediatric oncology patients pursuing disease-directed chemotherapy, as they can result in platelet dysfunction, which could lead to bleeding complications in a thrombocytopenic patient. At end of life, however, these types of analgesics may be useful adjuncts to treat fever and/or pain and should be offered if the patient is able to take them.

EXPENSIVE NONFORMULARY MEDICATIONS

When children transition to hospice care, many may be receiving expensive, nonformulary medications. Pediatric oncology professionals should discuss the role of each of these medications and whether the medication is benefiting the child as he or she moves into the terminal phase of illness. The goal should be to use the lowest number of medications that allow for good quality of life.

TOTAL PARENTERAL NUTRITION AND INTRAVENOUS FLUIDS

Total parenteral nutrition (TPN) plays a limited role in hospice medicine, except in scenarios where a reasonable time and quality of life are still expected. Families, however, may have a difficult time discontinuing intravenous (IV) nutrition, as they worry that their child might "starve to death." In these situations, the pediatric oncology provider should explain that during the terminal phase of illness patients become less hungry and many will refuse food. In patients who are fluid sensitive, TPN and IV fluids may in fact increase discomfort and hasten death owing to worsening of pulmonary edema or CHF. Patients who are in renal failure should have minimal if any IV fluids at the end of life.

INTRAVENOUS ANTIBIOTICS

A discussion about the use of antibiotics, either empirically for fever or for documented infection, is a critical part of any end-of-life care plan. Their use should be discouraged in patients who are in the terminal phase of their illness; with appropriate symptom control, sepsis is a comfortable mechanism of death. However, localized infections, mucositis, and abscesses can be painful, and the child may benefit from the use of antibiotics in these circumstances. Expensive antifungal agents generally also do not play a role in hospice care. For families who are uncomfortable with doing "nothing" for fever or infection, a broad-spectrum oral antibiotic may be a reasonable compromise.

As Death Becomes Imminent

Families need to be prepared for the changes that will occur in their child near the time of death. Changes that might be seen include

- altered mental status or state of awareness;
- respiratory changes such as agonal, Cheyne-Stokes, or rattling patterns of breathing;
- changes in skin color or temperature, including mottling;
- relatively rapid changes in body habitus, especially if the child is no longer eating or drinking;
- seizures;
- preterminal bowel and bladder evacuation;
- bleeding (rare).

Education of families regarding what may occur around the time of death will help minimize fear and anxiety. Information written specifically for parents and other nonmedical caregivers may prove to be helpful. While treatment of pain and symptoms should continue until the time of death, it is also crucial to recognize the psychosocial and spiritual issues that are present at the end of life for patients and families. In particular, parents report that staff presence helps ameliorate difficult moments of death and affects bereavement outcomes even years later (Kreicbergs et al., 2005).

The Role of the Oncology Team during Aftercare, Dying, and the Bereavement Process

Despite health care professionals' fears of causing pain by making contact after a child has died, many families wish to continue relationships with their child's primary hematology/oncology team. In fact, acute withdrawal of a long-term relationship can aggravate the family's sense of loss. Attending the funeral or at least sending a written condolence letter is recommended, as is offering families the opportunity to participate in a follow-up conference to discuss the child's disease path or autopsy results, if one was performed (Meert et al., 2008). Further, families greatly benefit from structured bereavement opportunities, such as remembrance services, organized by professionals who knew their child, and including other families whose journeys have been similar (James and Johnson, 1997).

Individual hematology/oncology practitioners need to acknowledge the cumulative grief and burden of caring for children who die, and come to terms with their own feelings. To be fully present to families before, during, and after a child's death, involved professionals must carefully attend to boundary issues and personal feelings of regret and/or failure. Families greatly appreciate bereavement home visits by team members and any opportunities to keep the child's name and memory alive.

It may be comforting for hematology/oncology teams to realize that palliative care and hospice programs provide in-depth ongoing services to families in their care. Many offer individual, group, and community-based programming that is usually not time limited. Further, involved professionals can help assess families (and clinicians) for signs and symptoms of prolonged, complicated, or disenfranchised grief and facilitate appropriate interventions and referrals (Friebert and Wiener, 2009).

Conclusion

Pediatric hematology/oncology is an extremely rewarding field, offering clinicians long-term relationships with patients and their families. Palliative care represents a set of principles and practices that are completely complementary to the goals of pediatric hematology/oncology care. Well-integrated palliative care and hematology/oncology teams bring to children and families the best that holistic, family-centered, longitudinal, interdisciplinary care has to offer. The journey of a life-threatening illness is difficult for any child and family, whether the outcome is cure or death. By recognizing the expertise each discipline delivers, together with the added synergy of the combination of approaches, unified pediatric palliative care and hematology/oncology teams can do much to alleviate the physical, psychosocial, emotional, spiritual, and practical suffering accompanying the journey, dramatically improving the quality of life for children affected by cancer, their families, and health care providers.

References

American Academy of Pediatrics, Committee on Bioethics and Committee on Hospital Care (AAP COB/COHC). 2000. Palliative care for children. *Pediatrics* 106(2): 351–57.

Ashley, D.M., Meier, T., Kerby, F.M., et al. 1996. Response of recurrent medulloblastoma to low-dose oral etoposide. *J Clin Oncol* 14:1922–27.

Benjamin, L. 2008. Pain management in sickle cell disease: Palliative care begins at birth? *Hematology Am Soc Hematol Educ Program* 2008:466–74.

Bluebond-Langner, M., Belasco, J.B., Goldman, A., et al. 2007. Understanding parents' approaches to care and treatment of children with cancer when standard therapy has failed. *J Clin Oncol* 25(17):2414–19.

Chaitin, E., and Rosielle, D.A. 2009. Responding to requests for non-disclosure of medical information. *Fast Facts and Concepts* Sept; 219. www.eperc.mcw.edu/fastfact/ ff_219.htm (accessed April 30, 2010).

Collins, J.J., Byrnes, M.E., Dunkel, I.J., et al. 2000. The measurement of symptoms in children with cancer. *J Pain Symptom Manage* 19:363–77.

Daugherty, C., Ratain, M.J., Grochowski, E., et al. 1995. Perceptions of cancer patients and their physicians involved in phase I trials. *J Clin Oncol* 13(5):1062–72.

Deatrick, J.A., Angst, D.B., and Moore, C. 2002. Parents' views of their children's participation in phase I oncology clinical trials. *J Pediatr Oncol Nurs* 19:114–121.

Decoster, G., Stein, G., and Holdener, E.E. 1990. Responses and toxic deaths in phase I clinical trials. *Ann Oncol* (3):175–81.

Demario, M.D., and Ratain, M.J. 1998. Oral chemotherapy: Rationale and future directions. *J Clin Oncol* 16:2557–67.

Drake, R., and Hain, R. 2006. Pain-pharmacologic management. In *Oxford Textbook of Palliative Care for Children*, ed. A. Goldman, R. Hain, and S. Liben, pp. 304–31. New York: Oxford University Press.

Emanuel, E.J., and Patterson, W.B. 1998. Ethics of randomized clinical trials. *J Clin Oncol* 16(1):365–71.

Freyer, D. 2004. Care of the dying adolescent: Special considerations. *Pediatrics* 113(2): 381–88.

Friebert, S. 2008. Palliative care. In *Cancer in Children and Adolescents*, ed. W.L. Carroll and J.L. Finlay, pp. 513–22. Sudbury, MA: Jones and Bartlett Publishers.

Friebert, S., and Wiener, L.S. 2009. Integrating palliative care into the pediatric oncology setting. In *Quick Reference for Pediatric Oncology Clinicians: The Psychiatric and Psychological Dimensions of Pediatric Cancer Symptom Management*, ed. A.E. Kazak, M.J. Kupst, M. Pao, et al., pp. 260–67. Charlottesville, VA: American Psychosocial Oncology Society.

Friedrichsdorf, S.J., and Kang, T.I. 2007. The management of pain in children with life-limiting illnesses. *Pediatr Clin N Amer* 54:645–72.

Golan, H., Bielorai, B., Grebler, D., et al. 2008. Integration of a palliative and terminal care center into a comprehensive pediatric oncology department. *Pediatr Blood Cancer* 50:949–55.

Goldberg, A., and Frader, J. 2009. Holding on and letting go: Ethical issues regarding the care of children with cancer. In *Ethical Issues in Cancer Patient Care*, 2nd ed., ed. P. Angelos, p. 177. New York: Springer.

Gurney, J.G., and Bondy, M.L. 2006. Epidemiology of childhood cancer. In *Principles and Practice of Pediatric Oncology*, 5th ed., ed. D. Poplack and P. Pizzo, pp. 1–13. Philadelphia: Lippincott Williams and Wilkins.

Harper, J., Hinds, P., Baker, J., et al. 2007. Creating a palliative and end-of-life program in a cure-oriented pediatric setting: The zig-zag method. *J Pediatr Oncol Nurs* 24(5):246–54.

Harris, M.B. 2004. Palliative care in children with cancer: Which child and when? *J Nat Cancer Instit Monographs* 32:144–49.

Hechler, T., Blankenburg, M., Friedrichsdorf, S.J., et al. 2008. Parents' perspective on symptoms, quality of life, characteristics of death and end-of-life decisions for children dying from cancer. *Klin Padiatr* 220:166–74.

Hilden, J.M., Emanuel, E.J., Fairclough, D.L., et al. 2001. Attitudes and practices among pediatric oncologists regarding end-of-life care: Results of the 1998 American Society of Clinical Oncology Survey. *J Clin Oncol* 19(1):205–12.

Himelstein, B., Hilden, J., Morstad-Boldt, A., et al. 2004. Pediatric palliative care. *N Engl J Med* 350:1752–62.

Hinds, P.S., Drew, D., Oakes, L.L., et al. 2005. End-of-life care preferences of pediatric patients with cancer. *J Clin Oncol* 23(36):9146–54.

Hockenberry, M.J., Hinds, P.S., Barrera, P., et al. 2003. Three instruments to assess fatigue in children with cancer: The child, parent and staff perspectives. *J Pain Symptom Manage* 25(4):319–28.

Hunt, A. 2006. Pain assessment. In *Oxford Textbook of Palliative Care for Children*, ed. A. Goldman, R. Hain, and S. Liben, pp. 281–303. New York: Oxford University Press.

International Association for the Study of Pain, Subcommittee on Taxonomy. 1979. Pain terms: A list of definitions and notes on usage. *Pain* 6:249–52.

Jalmsell, L., Kreicbergs, U., Onelov, E., et al. 2006. Symptoms affecting children with malignancies during the last month of life: A nationwide follow-up. *Pediatrics* 117(4):1314–20.

James, L., and Johnson, B. 1997. The needs of parents of pediatric oncology patients during the palliative care phase. *J Pediatr Oncol Nurs* 14(2):83–95.

Johnston, D., Hagel, K., Friedman, D., et al. 2008. Availability and use of palliative care and end-of-life services for pediatric oncology patients. *J Clin Oncol* 26(28): 4646–50.

Kodish, E. 2003. Informed consent for pediatric research: Is it really possible? *J Pediatr* 142(2):89–90.

Kreicbergs, U., Valdimarsdóttir, U., Onelöv, E., et al. 2004. Talking about death with children who have severe malignant disease. *N Engl J Med* 351(12):1175–86.

———. 2005. Care-related distress: A nationwide study of parents who lost their child to cancer. *J Clin Oncol* 23(36):9162–71.

Lysaught, M.T. 1998. Commentary: Reconstruing genetic research as research. *J Law Med Ethics* 26(1):48–54.

Mack, J., and Wolfe, J. 2006. Early integration of pediatric palliative care: For some children, palliative care starts at diagnosis. *Curr Opin Pediatr* 18:10–14.

Mack, J.W., Hilden, W.M., Watterson, J., et al. 2005. Parent and physician perspectives on quality of care at the end of life in children with cancer. *J Clin Oncol* 23(36):1–7.

Mack, J.W., Joffe, S., Hilden, J.M., et al. 2008. Parents' views of cancer-directed therapy for children with no realistic chance for cure. *J Clin Oncol* 26(29):4759–64.

Malin, J.L. 2004. Bridging the divide: Integrating cancer-directed therapy and palliative care. *J Clin Oncol* 22(17):3438–40.

Matthay, K., Quach, A., Huberty, J., et al. 2009. Iodine-131—metaiodobenzylguanidine double infusion with autologous stem-cell rescue for neuroblastoma: A new approach to neuroblastoma therapy phase I study. *J Clin Oncol* 27(7):1020–32.

McClain, B.C., and Kain, Z.N. 2007. Pediatric palliative care: A novel approach to children with sickle cell disease. *Pediatrics* 119(3):612–14.

Meert, K.L., Eggly, S., Pollack, M., et al., for the National Institute of Child Health and Human Development Collaborative Pediatric Critical Care Research Network. 2008. Parents' perspectives on physician-parent communication near the time of a child's death in the pediatric intensive care unit. *Pediatr Crit Care Med* 9(1):2–7.

Nitschke, R., Wunder, S., Sexauer, C.L., et al. 1977. The final-stage conference: The patient's decision on research drugs in pediatric oncology. *J Pediatr Psychol* 2(2): 58–64.

Oberman, M., and Frader, J. 2003. Dying children and medical research: Access to clinical trials as benefit and burden. *Am J Law Med* 29:301–17.

Roberts, T.G., Goulart, B.H., Squiteieri, L., et al. 2004. Trends in the risks and benefits to patients with cancer participating in phase I clinical trials. *JAMA* 292(17): 2130–40.

Royce, M.E., Hoff, P.M., and Pazdur, R. 2000. Novel oral chemotherapy agents. *Curr Oncol Rep* 2:31–37.

Serafini, A.N. 2000. Smaanirum Sm-153 lexidronam for the palliation of bone pain associated with metastases. *Cancer* 88:2934–39.

Shah, S., Weitman, S., Langevin, A.M., et al. 1998. Phase I therapy trials in children with cancer. *J Pediatr Hematol Oncol* 20(5):431–38.

Ullrich, C.K., and Mayer, O.H. 2007. Assessment and management of fatigue and dyspnea in pediatric palliative care. *Pediatr Clin N Amer* 54:735–56.

Vickers, J., and Carlisle, C. 2000. Choices and control: Parental experiences in pediatric terminal home care. *J Pediatr Oncol Nurs* 17:12–21.

Weir, R.F., and Peters, C. 1997. Affirming the decisions adolescents make about life and death. *Hastings Cent Report* 27(6):29–40.

Wolfe, J., Friebert, S., and Hilden, J. 2002. Caring for children with advanced cancer: Integrating palliative care. *Pediatr Clin N Amer* 49:1043–62.

Wolfe, J., Grier, H., Klar, N., et al. 2000a. Symptoms and suffering at the end of life in children with cancer. *N Engl J Med* 342:326–33.

Wolfe, J., Hammel, J.F., Edward, K.E., et al. 2008. Easing of suffering in children with cancer at the end of life: Is care changing? *J Clin Oncol* 26(10):1717–23.

Wolfe, J., Klar, N., Grier, H., et al. 2000b. Understanding of prognosis among patients of children who died of cancer: Impact of treatment goals and integration of palliative care. *JAMA* 284:2469–75.

Wolfe, J., and Sourkes, B. 2006. Palliative care for the child with advanced cancer. In

Principles and Practice of Pediatric Oncology, 5th ed., ed. D. Poplack and P. Pizzo, pp. 1531–55. Philadelphia: Lippincott Williams and Wilkins.

World Health Organization (WHO). 1998. Guidelines for analgesic drug therapy. *Cancer Pain Relief and Palliative Care in Children*, pp. 24–28. Geneva: WHO/IASP.

Wusthoff, C.J., McMillan, A., and Ablin, A.R. 2005. Differences in pediatric oncologists' estimates of curability and treatment recommendations for patients with advanced cancer. *Pediatr Blood Cancer* 44:174–81.

Zieber, S., and Friebert, S. 2008. Pediatric cancer care: Special issues in ethical decision making. In *Ethical Issues in Cancer Patient Care*, 2nd ed., ed. P. Angelos, pp. 93–116. New York: Springer.

INDEX

anxiety, 266, 279, 295, 425; and benzodiazepines, 408; and communication
with children, 210, 211, 212; and
hematology/oncology, 506, 507; and
HIV/AIDS, 474, 475; medication for,
256, 404; and PICU environment,
392, 398
anxiolytics, 376
appetite, 258–59
arthrogryposis multiplex congenita, 446,
450
arts / art therapy, 208, 212–13, 266–69,
270, 334, 420, 427
asphyxiating thoracic dystrophy, 446, 450
assent, by children, 77. *See also* informed
assent; informed consent
Association of Medical School Pediatric
Department Chairpersons
(AMSPDC), 95, 96
Association of Pediatric Hematology
Oncology Nurses (APHON), 90
autonomy, 27, 29, 31, 41, 42, 43, 44,
46–47
autopsy, 185–86, 279, 369, 407, 410, 455
azithromycin, 473

Baby Doe regulations, 353
barbiturates, 404
Batten disease, 447, 448
Beck Depression scale, 475
benzodiazepines, 155, 256, 257, 258, 261,
376, 379, 404, 408, 513
bereavement, 21, 28, 121, 275–304, 417;
acknowledgment and processing of,
332–33; and child's decision making,
157; common themes in, 276–87; and
communication, 286, 302; community resources for, 300; and connection to medical team, 291; and
contact with child's body after sudden
death, 293; and continuity of care,
301–2; counseling for, 300–302; and
expression of feelings, 278–79; and
families, 11, 276, 285–87, 333, 515–16;
and follow-up support, 301–2, 335;
and genetic diseases, 456; and
hematology/oncology care, 515–16;
and home care, 424, 438; and ICU

environment, 392, 393, 397; and
nursing education, 86, 87, 89; and
open communication with child, 190;
packets for, 298; and parents, 276,
290; and perinatal death, 293–302;
and PICU, 410; plan of care for,
285–87; and prenatal period, 357; and
religious support, 194; resources for,
299–300, 302, 308; satisfaction with
support in, 301; and school groups,
433; and siblings, 290; and sudden
death, 291–93; support for, 58, 96;
support groups for, 279, 284, 300,
301–4; and uncertain prognosis,
287–91; and unknown factors, 160;
updates for, 335. *See also* grief
birth defects, 354, 355–56, 435, 462
bisphosphonates, 509
blood pressure medications, 405
bone marrow failure, 511–12
bone marrow transplant, 490–91
brain, 256, 257, 264, 461
brain death, 49–50, 62
bronchodilators, 261
buprenorphine, 253, 255
butyrophenone, 404

California Department of Health Care
Services, 130
cancer, 10–11, 12, 13, 88, 255, 263, 476,
477. *See also* hematology/oncology
Candida esophagitis, 472
Candlelighters Childhood Cancer
Foundation, 434, 438
capecitabine, 511
cardiac anomaly, 355
cardiac pacing, 434
cardiopulmonary resuscitation (CPR),
367, 405, 434
cardioversion, 434
caregivers. *See* health care professionals;
nurses; parent(s); physicians;
suffering, caregiver
care teams, early involvement of, 59, 68,
75, 79, 80, 82, 145, 195, 207–8
care/treatment: burdens of, 38, 60, 67,
140, 400, 492, 499; child-centered,
27; continuity of, 34, 78–79, 89, 96,

death (*cont.*)

planning for, 153, 156; and post-mortem evaluation, 160–61; and pregnancy, 293; pregnancy after, 299, 302; preparation for, 275, 293, 368, 407, 427, 515; probability of, 4, 5; rate of infant, 8, 10; and reference to child by name, 302, 303; responsibility for, 39; and return to school, 428; risk of, 4; rituals for, 298–99, 437; signs of, 261–62, 407, 515; sudden, 88, 291–93; support for, 152, 155; in tertiary hospitals, 74; time frame for, 4; and tissue and organ donation, 161, 369; understanding of, 28, 234–35, 368; unexpected, 293. *See also* bereavement; dying; end-of-life care; grief; hospice

decision making, 46–47; and acute and unexpected terminal conditions, 148–49; and adolescents, 144–45, 500–501; after live birth, 349–50; after treatment trial, 350–52; and Baby Doe regulations, 353; and care goals, 151–52; child's participation in, 44, 95, 139, 144–45, 149–50, 157–59, 163, 186–90, 208, 209, 211, 480–82, 490, 493, 500–501, 504–5; and chronic conditions, 149–50; collaborative, 98, 141, 350; and communication, 148–49; and debriefing, 160; and delivery room, 348–49; and diagnostic certainty, 146; documentation of, 160; evolution of, 139, 143; fact-based vs. value-based, 350; by families, 63, 95, 139, 141, 149–50, 163, 208, 348–50, 367–69, 408, 500–501; and genetic diseases, 456–58; and graduate medical education, 103; and hematology/oncology, 490, 493, 497, 500–501, 504; and HIV/AIDS, 480–82; and location of death, 156; and nurses, 365; and parents, 32–33, 46–47, 49–51, 157, 161–63, 277, 303, 349–51, 360, 399, 456–58; and perinatal period, 347–54; and primary care physician, 194; as process, 139; and prognostic certainty, 145–46; and psychosocial

needs, 203, 207; reflection on, 159–60; and respect, 331–32; and siblings, 219; and site of care, 156; and sudden death, 292; suffering and distress accompanying, 317, 318; and technology, 153–55; and time element, 63; and trust, 146–47; as value laden, 349

depression, 249, 256–57, 279, 295, 325, 425, 475, 506, 512

developmental stages, of children, 121, 187, 266–67, 427

dexamethasone, 263, 474, 513

diagnosis: certainty in, 146; of fetal anomaly, 364; and genetic diseases, 369, 444, 452–53, 455, 458, 461; and hematology/oncology, 490, 492, 495, 499, 504, 505; and HIV/AIDS, 467, 478–80; and hospice, 121; initiation of palliative care at, 204–5, 207–8, 417, 492, 495, 496; of metabolic conditions, 369; and prenatal period, 347–48, 357; stress of new, 204–6; uncertain, 205, 314, 357

diamorphine, 251, 253, 254, 255

diarrhea, 17, 260–61, 506

diazepam, 256, 258, 264, 427

DiGeorge syndrome, 446, 451

digoxin, 377

dihydrocodeine, 253

diphenhydramine, 258

dolasetron, 474

do-not-resuscitate (DNR) orders, 20, 37, 79, 369, 405, 409; and hematology/oncology, 498; and home care, 421, 434–36; inexperience discussing, 106

doulas, 377, 380

dry lips/mouth, 377

Duchenne muscular dystrophy, 447, 448

dwarfism, 347, 355

dying: exploring feelings related to, 267–68; high risk for, 390; interpretation of, 28; meaning and purpose in, 206; as normal process, 58; and nutrition and hydration needs, 376–77; prolongation of, 353. *See also* death

dysmorphic syndromes, 446

dysphoria, 472

HIV/AIDS (*cont.*)
distress, 477–78; and stigma, 468;
and symptoms, 467, 471–73; and
treatment adherence, 468–69; and
viral resistance, 468–69
Hodgkin disease, 262
holoprosencephaly, 347, 461
home, 64, 103, 208, 276; and continuity
and coordination of care, 78; death
at, 15, 17, 156, 190, 367, 431, 436–38,
491; transition to, 367, 420–24; visits
to, 105
home care, 66, 414–39; and bereavement, 424, 438; and care plan, 432;
and child's needs, 427–30; clinical
challenges of, 424–27; and end-of-life
care, 436–38; family responsibilities
in, 423–25; goals of, 424; and grief,
424; and hematology/oncology, 498;
information for PICU staff about,
399; and integrated models of care,
417; and medication, 424–27; and
needs assessment, 421–23; and neonatal period, 358, 359, 376–78; and
nursing, 57, 65; and out-of-hospital
DNR orders, 421, 434–36; and pain
management and symptom control,
425; and palliative care teams, 432;
pilot programs in, 416; problems
with, 414–15; safety of environment
for, 422; and stress on family, 432;
and treatment plan, 422; and trust,
426
home care teams, 78, 420, 421, 423, 432
hope, 32, 206–7, 208, 326, 349; and
family, 183–84, 453; and hematology/
oncology, 495; and HIV/AIDS, 480;
meaning of, 36–37; and spirituality,
236–37
hospice, 57, 61, 63, 118, 132, 156, 335, 415;
access to, 48, 56, 415; for adults, 66;
and bereavement, 276, 300, 301,
424; community-based, 194, 208;
and continuity of care, 79, 89; and
curative care rules, 121; and curative
treatment services, 130; and death vs.
life enhancement, 208–9; and doulas,
377, 380; eligibility criteria for, 92;

and finances, 65; and Florida health
care system, 72; and graduate medical education, 100, 102, 103; and
hematology/oncology, 490, 493–94,
504, 508, 514; and HIV/AIDS, 466,
467; and home care in neonatal
period, 359; and hope, 208; and
hospitals, 208, 209; and integrated
models of care, 417; lack of training
of, 492; and Medicaid, 416; and
neonatal period, 376; open access to,
6; and palliative care team, 194;
payment of, 69; and preparation for
death, 275, 437; referral to, 208, 303;
sibling support by, 217. *See also* death
Hospice of the Florida Suncoast, 377,
380
hospice teams, 215, 216, 433
hospitals, 120, 216, 222; access to, 56;
adequate staff for, 77–78; and
bereavement, 298–99; and care
continuity and coordination, 78–79,
89; community, 367; death in, 14, 16,
18; duration of terminal care in,
18–20; education specific to, 93;
facilities of, 81; and graduate medical
education, 103; inpatient palliative
care programs of, 208; interface
between home and, 60; and medication, 402; parents' continued contact
with staff of, 424; and partnerships
with community hospice programs,
208, 209; transition to home from,
420–24; and visitation protocols, 216
Hunter syndrome, 447
Hurler syndrome, 447
hydration, 51–52, 352–53, 367, 368,
376–77, 514
hydrocephalus, 359
hydromorphone, 251, 253, 255, 403,
474
hydroxyurea, 511
hyoscine, 262
hyoscyamine, 262
hypnotic agents, 404
hypoglycemia, 445
hypoxic-ischemic encephalopathy,
356

medications (*cont.*)
depression, 256–57; for disordered sleep, 257–58; and DNR orders, 434; and dosing and safety issues for newborns, 371; and end-of-life plan, 513; enteral, 403; family record keeping of, 424–25; and fatigue, 512; for feeding problems, 258–59; for gastrointestinal complaints, 259–60; and genetic diseases, 461–62; and gradual discontinuation of treatment, 407; and hastening of death, 368, 373, 408; and hematology/oncology, 504, 506–11; and hemodynamic instability, 402, 403, 404; for hemorrhage, 264–65; and HIV/AIDS, 466, 467, 468, 469, 470, 471–73, 474, 475, 477, 479, 482, 484; and home care, 423, 424–27; and infusions vs. intermittent dosing, 403; for intractable seizures, 264; intravenous forms of, 403; and medical history, 402–3; need to adjust comfort, 405; and neonates, 377, 378–79; periodic reevaluation of, 509; and PICU, 402–4; for raised intra-cranial pressure, 263; rectal, 514; refusal of, 475; for respiratory symptoms, 261–62; side effects of, 47, 403, 434, 506, 508, 509; for skin problems, 262; for spinal cord compression, 263; for superior vena cava obstruction, 263–64; and symptom management with life-support discontinuation, 408; titrating dose of, 244, 253–54, 368, 373, 408, 426. *See also* analgesia; *specific medications*
meditation, 334, 427
megestrol acetate, 259, 512
melatonin, 258
memories/memorials, 285, 286, 298, 302; creation of, 401; and NICU, 364; of neonates, 380; rituals for, 334, 335; services for, 286
Menkes disease, 447, 454
mental health care, 299, 300
meperidine (pethidine), 255
6-mercaptopurine, 511

metabolism, inborn errors of, 355, 356, 445, 447, 448
metachromatic leukodystrophy, 447, 449, 461–62
metastatic CNS disease, 513
methadone, 255, 373, 379, 403, 474
methylnaltrexone, 254
methylphenidate, 512
metoclopramide, 258, 379, 474
midazolam, 256, 258, 264, 265, 376, 379, 474
midazolam IV, 513
minority groups, 64, 66, 68, 81
miscarriage, 294, 455, 456
moral distress, 313, 318, 319–20, 331, 365. *See also* ethics/morality
morphine, 244, 251, 252, 253, 254, 261, 353, 377, 379, 403; effectiveness of, 373; and EMS providers, 434; and genetic diseases, 461; and HIV/AIDS, 471, 474; and home care, 426–27
mothers, 279–81, 295–96, 359, 364, 465, 469, 470, 477
Mount Ida College, 108
mouth/lips, 261, 265, 353
mucolytics, 261
mucosal bleeding, 261
mucositis, 506
muscle relaxants, 252, 376
Mycobacterium avium complex (MAC), 471, 473, 482
myoclonus, 508

naloxone, 254, 262, 379
nasogastric tubes, 259, 260
National Association of Children's Hospitals and Related Institutions (NACHRI), 95, 96
National Center for Complementary and Alternative Medicine (NCCAM), 246
National Consensus Project, 417
National Hospice and Palliative Care Organization (NHPCO), 65, 107–8, 122, 417; Children's Advisory Council, 415; Standards of Care, 419
National Institutes of Health, 246
nausea, 17, 259, 260, 377, 506, 507, 508

opioids (*cont.*)
of, 254; and neonatal period, 373, 376, 378, 379; and oncology, 508; pain responsiveness to, 249, 250; and pruritus, 262; relative potencies of major and minor, 253; titrating dose of, 244, 253–54, 408; weaning from, 402
osteogenesis imperfecta, 446
out-of-hospital (OOH) DNR orders, 434–36
outpatient clinics, 103, 421
oxycodone, 251, 255
oxygen, 377

pain, 17, 27, 247–67, 312; assessment of, 250–51, 255, 370–76, 403, 492; avoidance of, 32; baby's response to, 247–48; and best practices, 91; and board certification requirements, 106, 107; and bone pain, 509; breakthrough, 244, 252, 253, 254; and cancer, 248; children's experience of, 247–48; and Children's Pain Checklist, 403; child's management of, 187; classifications of, 250; diagnosis of, 247–50, 255; discussion of, 140; and ethics, 42–43; experience of, 247–48; failure to relieve, 31; and genetic diseases, 461–62; and graduate medical education, 102; and hematology/oncology, 497, 505–11; and HIV/AIDS, 467, 470–71, 472, 473; holistic approach to, 246; and home care, 425; inexperience with, 105; and medical education, 108; and medical history, 402–3; medications for, 49, 251–55; musculoskeletal, 244, 252; neuropathic, 244, 249, 252, 255, 257, 509; in newborns, 370–76; nonpharmacologic interventions for, 371; and nonverbal or preverbal children, 249–50; and nursing education, 86, 87; and pain ladder, 251, 252; parental perceptions of, 406; perception of, 250; in perinatal period, 370–76; physicians' knowledge of, 92; physiologic, metabolic, and behavioral

changes from, 370; PICU management of, 402–3; poorly coordinated management of, 80; and premature babies, 370; and premature infants, 371; procedure-related, 371, 373; and quality of life, 58; reduction of, 95; and responsiveness to opioids, 249, 250; scales for, 371, 403; soft tissue, 249; and spiritual advocacy, 241; as subjective phenomenon, 248; titration to relief of, 42–43, 373, 426; total, 244–45; treatment-related, 508; undermedication of, 313; undertreatment of, 506; and withdrawal of non-oral nutrition and hydration, 52. *See also* analgesia; suffering
pamidronate disodium infusion, 509
panic spiral, 256
pantoprazole, 474
paraldehyde, 264
paralytic agents, 367, 403, 408
parent(s), 79; abandonment of family by, 277; and ability to say goodbye to child, 276; acceptance by, 36–37, 278; and advance care planning, 142, 193–94; advocacy by, 40, 41, 123; affirmation of, 173; anticipatory guidance for, 359; assessment of needs of, 124–25, 127–28; and assurance of continued good care, 41; autonomy of, 46–47; and bereavement, 290–91, 301–2, 424; blame by, 277; brief interactions at bedside with, 34; care by, 221; care plan development with, 432; children's relationship with, 187; and child's attitude, 256; and child's best interests, 67; and choosing to give up, 67; of chronically ill children, 174; communication with, 33–35, 79; and communication with children, 187–90; and connection with children after death, 237; and connection with children before death, 285, 288; and connection with medical staff, 287, 424; control of medications by, 425; counseling of, 36, 39, 424; and daily rounds, 400; and death of other children, 277; and denial of poor

prognosis, 35–36; and developing prognosis, 32–33; and disagreements over effectiveness of care, 37–41; discussion of autopsy with, 369; and discussion of death with children, 213, 286, 289; discussion of tissue and organ donation with, 369; division of labor by, 221; emotional support for, 32, 34–35, 279; and end-of-life care, 436–37; entrenched positions of, 40–41; and experience of conditions, 173; as expert on illness, 173; expression of feelings by, 278–79; family meetings with, 34; and feeding, 258, 259; financial stress on, 215; and future childbearing, 443–44; and genetic diseases, 452–53, 454–55, 458–60; grief of, 214, 279–84, 295–96; guilt of, 39, 214–15, 277, 295, 322, 458–60; and hematology/oncology, 494, 495, 503–4, 505; and HIV/AIDS, 469, 477, 479, 480; and hydration, 352, 353; and informed consent, 502; as integral members of care team, 360; and limitation of life support, 405; and marriage, 215–16, 279; and meaning of hope, 36–37; and media, 129; and neonatal home care, 359–60; and neonatal treatment trial, 350–51; network for sharing experiences of, 287; and NICU, 360, 362–64; and nutrition, 52, 352, 353; and opportunity to see and hold newborns, 364; and panic spiral, 256; as partners, 173–77, 363, 423, 424; and perinatal period, 346–47, 349–51, 356, 357–58, 359; perspective of, 79–80, 173–74, 175–77; and phase I and phase II studies, 501; physical contact with, 182; post-death conference with, 279; and prenatal tests, 356; and preparation for death, 293, 368, 427, 436–37; preparation for discontinuation of interventions, 406–7; preparation for grief, 205–6; as protected by children, 32, 210, 235, 289; protector role of, 293; psychosocial needs of, 214–16, 221–23; and quality of life, 149, 406;

resources for, 125; respect for, 32, 41; and respite care, 286; restoration of daily functioning of, 276; review of medical events by, 277; right to accurate information, 32; role as, 295; and satisfaction with care, 20–21; and siblings, 215, 216, 217, 218, 277, 431; spirituality and religious faith of, 150; stress of new diagnosis on, 205; and sudden death, 291–93; suffering of, 17–18; suitable rooms and furniture for, 81; supervision of outpatient caregivers by, 222–23; support for, 286, 432; support groups for, 215; and trust, 79, 80, 178; and uncertainty, 314; understanding and priorities of, 179; understanding of perinatal options, 351, 357; and value judgments, 38, 39; volunteering by, 81. *See also* decision making; families

Partners in Care: Together for Kids (PIC:TFK), 72

Partners in Pediatric Palliative Care, 89

pastoral care, 150, 364, 420. *See also* chaplains

Patient Protection and Affordable Care Act (PPACA), 130, 132

pediatricians, primary care, 80, 421, 458

pediatric intensive care unit (PICU), 60, 387–410; and advance care planning, 404–6; and bereavement, 410; care after discharge from, 409; case identification in, 394; collaborative and educational approaches with staff of, 388–89; communication with families about, 398–402; deaths in, 76; enhancing awareness of palliative care principles in, 392–98; environment of, 403, 406–7; and family meetings after death, 409–10; and forgoing unbeneficial or burdensome treatments, 404–9; pain management in, 402–3; value of palliative care in, 389–97

pediatric oncologists, 493, 497, 503

Perinatal Grief Scale, 297

perinatal loss doula service, 377, 380